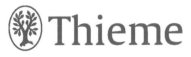

# Neurovascular Anatomy in Interventional Neuroradiology

## A Case-Based Approach

**Timo Krings, MD, PhD, FRCPC**
Professor of Radiology and Surgery
Director, Neuroradiology Program
University of Toronto, Toronto Western Hospital
Toronto, Ontario, Canada

**Sasikhan Geibprasert, MD**
Staff Neurointerventionalist and Lecturer
Department of Radiology
Ramathibodi Hospital, Mahidol University
Bangkok, Thailand

**Juan Pablo Cruz, MD**
Staff Neuroradiologist and Assistant Professor
Department of Radiology
Hospital Clínico de la Pontifica Universidad Católica de Chile
Santiago, Chile

**Karel G. terBrugge, MD, FRCPC**
The David Braley and Nancy Gordon Chair in Interventional Neuroradiology
Professor of Radiology and Surgery
Head, Division of Neuroradiology
University of Toronto, Toronto Western Hospital
Toronto, Ontario, Canada

Thieme
New York • Stuttgart • Delhi • Rio de Janeiro

Thieme Medical Publishers, Inc.
333 Seventh Avenue
New York, New York 10001

Executive Editor: William Lamsback
Managing Editor: J. Owen Zurhellen IV
Director, Editorial Services: Mary Jo Casey
International Production Director: Andreas Schabert
Vice President, Editorial and E-Product Development: Vera Spillner
International Marketing Director: Fiona Henderson
International Sales Director: Louisa Turrell
Director of Sales, North America: Mike Roseman
Senior Vice President and Chief Operating Officer: Sarah Vanderbilt
President: Brian D. Scanlan
Printer: King Printing Co., Inc

**Library of Congress Cataloging-in-Publication Data**

Krings, Timo, author.
 Neurovascular anatomy in interventional neuroradiology: a case-based approach / Timo Krings, Sasikhan Geibprasert, Juan Pablo Cruz, Karel G. terBrugge.
    p. ; cm.
 Includes bibliographical references.
  ISBN 978-1-60406-839-9 (paperback) – ISBN 978-1-60406-840-5 (e-book)
  I. Geibprasert, Sasikhan, author. II. Cruz, Juan Pablo, author. III. Brugge, K. G. ter (Karel G. ter), author. IV. Title.
  [DNLM: 1. Cerebrovascular Disorders–radiotherapy–Case Reports. 2. Central Nervous System–blood supply–Case Reports. 3. Radiology, Interventional–methods–Case Reports. WL 355]
  RC386.6.R3
  616.8'10757–dc23
                    2014026030

Copyright © 2015 by Thieme Medical Publishers, Inc.

Thieme Publishers New York
333 Seventh Avenue, New York, NY 10001 USA
+1 800 782 3488, customerservice@thieme.com

Thieme Publishers Stuttgart
Rüdigerstrasse 14, 70469 Stuttgart, Germany
+49 [0]711 8931 421, customerservice@thieme.de

Thieme Publishers Delhi
A-12, Second Floor, Sector-2, Noida-201301
Uttar Pradesh, India
+91 120 45 566 00, customerservice@thieme.in

Thieme Publishers Rio de Janeiro, Thieme Publicações Ltda.
Argentina Building 16th floor, Ala A, 228 Praia do Botafogo
Rio de Janeiro 22250-040 Brazil
+55 21 3736-3631

Printed in the United States of America          5 4 3

ISBN 978-1-60406-839-9

Also available as an e-book:
eISBN 978-1-60406-840-5

**Important note:** Medicine is an ever-changing science undergoing continual development. Research and clinical experience are continually expanding our knowledge, in particular our knowledge of proper treatment and drug therapy. Insofar as this book mentions any dosage or application, readers may rest assured that the authors, editors, and publishers have made every effort to ensure that such references are in accordance with **the state of knowledge at the time of production of the book.**

Nevertheless, this does not involve, imply, or express any guarantee or responsibility on the part of the publishers in respect to any dosage instructions and forms of applications stated in the book. **Every user is requested to examine carefully** the manufacturers' leaflets accompanying each drug and to check, if necessary in consultation with a physician or specialist, whether the dosage schedules mentioned therein or the contraindications stated by the manufacturers differ from the statements made in the present book. Such examination is particularly important with drugs that are either rarely used or have been newly released on the market. Every dosage schedule or every form of application used is entirely at the user's own risk and responsibility. The authors and publishers request every user to report to the publishers any discrepancies or inaccuracies noticed. If errors in this work are found after publication, errata will be posted at www.thieme.com on the product description page.

Some of the product names, patents, and registered designs referred to in this book are in fact registered trademarks or proprietary names even though specific reference to this fact is not always made in the text. Therefore, the appearance of a name without designation as proprietary is not to be construed as a representation by the publisher that it is in the public domain.

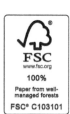

This book, including all parts thereof, is legally protected by copyright. Any use, exploitation, or commercialization outside the narrow limits set by copyright legislation without the publisher's consent is illegal and liable to prosecution. This applies in particular to photostat reproduction, copying, mimeographing or duplication of any kind, translating, preparation of microfilms, and electronic data processing and storage.

*To our students*

# Contents

# Foreword

We have witnessed a dramatic evolution in the management of various cerebrovascular diseases in the last 20 years, triggered by better understanding of the pathophysiology of each disease and by development of new innovative technologies. From the beginning of our specialty, termed interventional neuroradiology in early 1970s, there have been many ingenious moments that have elevated the endovascular management of cerebrovascular diseases. For instance, the introduction of detachable balloons by Serbinenko in 1974 made traumatic carotid–cavernous fistulas treatable via the endovascular route, the development of variable-stiffness microcatheters in 1986 enabled us to reach far distal in the cerebral circulation, and the invention of detachable coils in 1991 changed the management strategy for intracranial aneurysms.

When the detachable coil system was introduced, many clinicians, especially those in the neurosurgery community, were skeptical of this technique and its initial results and claimed that "it is only for surgically difficult or untreatable aneurysms, as its efficacy is not as good as surgical clipping." Diligent efforts in clinical and basic research, however, proved endovascular treatment of aneurysms is safer than and as efficient as surgical clipping. Furthermore, continuous refinement of tools made it easier to reach targets and succeed with results comparable to, and even better than, surgery. Even those who were skeptical of endovascular treatment of aneurysms until recently became convinced of its efficacy and are now themselves actively involved in this specialty.

As technology advances and more new interventionalists are trained around the world, the tenet of interventional neuroradiology—knowledge of the vascular anatomy—became diluted or ignored. It is easy to recognize aneurysms or vascular malformations readily on advanced imaging tools, such as computed tomography angiography, magnetic resonance imaging and angiograms, and three-dimensional angiography. Many teaching programs focus their training more on techniques of how to use tools and a number of cases trainees participated, and less on teaching fundamental basics and vascular anatomy, either because of a lack of interest or insufficient knowledge. Many young interventionists do not get enough exposure to the basic vascular anatomy, and therefore cannot build a sound foundation for the future advancement of their careers.

I still have a vivid memory of what Professor Alejandro Berenstein said to me when I started training as a fellow in interventional neuroradiology at New York University Medical Center in 1982. He was explaining to me his relationship with the late Professor Pierre Lasjaunias. Professor Berenstein was the one who knew how to drive a car, but did not know the roads. However, Pierre had a map of the roads. Together, they were able to accelerate their understanding and treatment of cerebrovascular diseases and contributed a great deal to make interventional neuroradiology an essential part of neuroscience.

Pierre wrote in the preface of the second edition of *Surgical Neuroangiography* the following: "Anatomy is a language, and mastering this language is essential for physicians involved in the management of patients with vascular diseases of the central nervous system." He was the one who taught us all about functional anatomy. He changed the way vascular anatomy was interpreted and illustrated all variations on the basis of embryology.

I am delighted Timo, Sasikhan, Juan-Pablo, and Karel put together case-based illustrations of the functional anatomy of the intracranial as well as extracranial circulations. I hope many young interventionalists will study each case with enthusiasm. I am sure this book will help build a sound foundation in understanding of the functional anatomy.

*In Sup Choi, MD, FACR*
*Professor of Radiology*
*Tufts University School of Medicine*
*Boston, Massachusetts*
*Director of Interventional Neuroradiology*
*Lahey Hospital and Medical Center*
*Burlington, Massachusetts*

# Preface

The importance of neurovascular anatomy when managing patients, using endovascular techniques, was emphasized by neuroanatomists such as Pierre Lasjaunias some three decades ago. Over the years, many neurointerventional therapists have remained unaware of the pertinent details of neurovascular anatomy and its relevance for safe therapy. This often resulted in "unexpected" neurological complications after embolization and, eventually, the perceived need to perform various testing procedures to avoid complications at the time of embolization. Not only were these testing procedures unnecessary if available knowledge of the regional anatomy had been applied, but these testing procedures were also often false-negative because of the fact that increased flow associated with arteriovenous shunts would simply sump the testing material away from the territory to be assessed.

The tools that have become available during the last two decades are more and more sophisticated, making it technically possible to reach very distal positions in the head and neck arterial vasculature. It is thus not surprising that once such positions were reached, embolization with liquid material resulted in an anatomical cure of the target lesion but could also result in neurological complications because the distal arterial supply to the region, including collaterals, was completely eliminated. This has significant practical implications; for instance, transarterial embolization of lesions in the cavernous sinus region may result in disruption of the arterial supply to the cranial nerves in this region. This, in turn, may correctly sway the neurointerventional therapist to not use the arterial approach but, rather, use the safer transvenous route.

The recognition of the presence of arterial variations is relevant in many clinical circumstances:

- Variations in the arterial vascular anatomy may be responsible for "unexpected" neurological symptoms not in the classic distribution of the parent vessel; therefore, protocols to examine the regional vascular anatomy are of practical importance for understanding clinical symptoms and guiding therapy.
- Variations in the arterial anatomy indirectly indicate a lack of full maturation of the vessels, and therefore, a vulnerability to vessel wall disorders such as aneurysm formation.
- Variations in the vascular anatomy, such as the presence or lack of collateral leptomeningeal anastomoses, will have a profound effect on the outcome of patients presenting with acute cerebral ischemia, so evaluation of such collateral flow is critically important.

Understanding the role of the heritage of the human neurovasculature is relevant because it will explain that although the vessel represents a continuum of the lumen, each vessel wall segment phylogenetically will have a different background, and therefore, a different vulnerability to develop in a given segment certain types of diseases and not others. It also represents the impetus to asses (image) the vessel wall to understand better the various causes of luminal changes.

The venous vascular anatomy has been difficult to understand because of its high degree of variability. Venous pathology has therefore been more difficult to recognize, and delayed diagnosis has been frequent. With improved awareness and appropriate early noninvasive imaging, our ability to recognize venous vascular disease has significantly improved.

As our understanding of the venous vascular anatomy and function has progressed, it has become clear that many symptoms a patient may present with were related to venous hyperpressure phenomena such as in dural arteriovenous shunts with leptomeningeal cortical venous reflux interfering with the normal drainage of venous blood in the region. Depending on the individual's venous vascular anatomic disposition, rerouting of venous blood via the transcerebral or the cortical venous system may produce symptoms far away from the actual location of the nidus. This has practical implications, as it means that if one is faced with the clinical presentation of intracranial hemorrhage or ischemia, the possibility of a venous cause needs to be excluded, and external carotid angiograms should be performed as part of the angiographic protocol.

Variations of the venous vascular anatomy (developmental venous anomalies) have been recognized as representing compensation for a poorly developed deep or superficial venous system. They therefore do not represent a true vascular malformation and are perceived to not produce symptoms. We now know that under certain circumstances (venous outflow obstruction or associated micro-arteriovenous fistulas), these normal variations of the veins in the region can be associated with clinical symptoms.

The purpose of this book is to emphasize the importance of the neurovascular anatomy in the daily practice of neurointerventional therapists and impress on the readers that knowledge of neurovascular anatomy will, in a significant way, enable one to practice more safely.

# Contributors

Ronit Agid, MD, FRCPC
Staff Neuroradiologist and Associate Professor of Radiology
Division of Neuroradiology
University of Toronto, Toronto Western Hospital
Toronto, Ontario, Canada

Karel G. terBrugge, MD, FRCPC
The David Braley and Nancy Gordon Chair in Interventional
    Neuroradiology
Professor of Radiology and Surgery
Head, Division of Neuroradiology
University of Toronto, Toronto Western Hospital
Toronto, Ontario, Canada

Juan Pablo Cruz, MD
Staff Neuroradiologist and Assistant Professor
Department of Radiology
Hospital Clínico de la Pontifica Universidad Católica de Chile
Santiago, Chile

Richard I. Farb, MD, FRCPC
Staff Neuroradiologist and Associate Professor of Radiology
Division of Neuroradiology
University of Toronto, Toronto Western Hospital
Toronto, Ontario, Canada

Sasikhan Geibprasert, MD
Staff Neurointerventionalist and Lecturer
Department of Radiology
Ramathibodi Hospital, Mahidol University
Bangkok, Thailand

Pakorn Jiarakongmun, MD
Staff Neuroradiologist and Associate Professor
Department of Radiology
Ramathibodi Hospital, Mahidol University
Bangkok, Thailand

Timo Krings, MD, PhD, FRCPC
Professor of Radiology and Surgery
Director, Neuroradiology Program
University of Toronto, Toronto Western Hospital
Toronto, Ontario, Canada

Pradeep Krishnan MD
Clinical and Research Fellow - Pediatric Neuroradiology
Hospital for Sick Children
Toronto, Ontario, Canada

Emanuele Orrù, MD
Endovascular Surgical Neuroradiology Fellow
The Russell H. Morgan Department of Radiology
Division of Interventional Neuroradiology
The Johns Hopkins Hospital
Baltimore, Maryland

Vitor Mendes Pereira, MD MSc
Staff Interventional Neuroradiologist and Associate Professor
    of Radiology and Surgery
Division of Neuroradiology
University of Toronto, Toronto Western Hospital
Toronto, Ontario, Canada

Sirintara Pongpech, MD
Professor and Head of Radiology
Ramathibodi Hospital, Mahidol University
Bangkok, Thailand

Sarah Power, MB, PhD, FFR (RCSI)
Diagnostic and Interventional Neuroradiology Fellow
University of Toronto, Toronto Western Hospital
Toronto, Ontario, Canada

Tiago Rodrigues, MD
Assistant Professor
Neuroradiology Department
Centro Hospitalar do Porto
Porto, Portugal

Robert A. Willinsky, MD, FRCPC
Staff Neuroradiologist and Professor of Radiology
Division of Neuroradiology
University of Toronto, Toronto Western Hospital
Toronto, Ontario, Canada

Christopher D. Witiw, MD
Neurosurgery Resident
Department of Neurosurgery
University of Toronto
Toronto, Ontario, Canada

# Section I

## Aortic Arch

# 1 The Common Origin of the Brachiocephalic and Left Common Carotid Artery

## 1.1 Case Description

### 1.1.1 Clinical Presentation

A 33-year-old woman with a prior history of head and neck lymphoma in infancy treated with radiation and chemotherapy developed bilateral common carotid stenosis postradiation. She underwent bilateral common carotid artery (CCA) stenting after a left-sided transient ischemic attack (TIA)-like episode at an outside institution. Several months later, she had episodes of visual loss. Magnetic resonance imaging (MRI) demonstrated artifactual signal loss in the right CCA (RCCA) in the region of the stent and diffuse multifocal narrowing of the left CCA (LCCA).

## 1.1.2 Radiologic Studies

See ▶ Fig. 1.1.

## 1.1.3 Diagnosis

Multifocal postradiation stenosis in a patient with a common supra-aortic trunk that gives rise to the brachiocephalic trunk and the LCCA.

## 1.2 Embryology and Anatomy

Development of the aortic arch and great vessels results from formation and selective involution of paired vascular arches

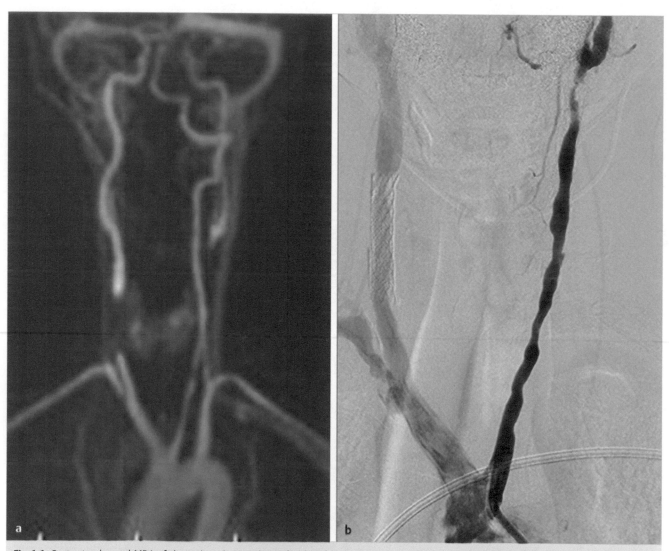

**Fig. 1.1** Contrast-enhanced MRA of the arch and cervical vessels (a) and LCCA angiogram in anteroposterior (AP) view at the arch and neck (b) demonstrate the common origin of the brachiocephalic trunk and the LCCA from the aortic arch — the so-called "bovine arch." There are multifocal stenoses of the LCCA. Reflux of contrast from the origin of the LCCA into the common trunk and into the RCCA is observed. Note the signal gap in the MRA resulting from local field inhomogeneity related to the stent (within the RCCA).

connecting the embryonic aortic sac (ventral aorta) with the paired dorsal aortae.

Between the second and seventh week of gestation, branchial apparatus development occurs, with formation of six paired branchial arches in the wall of the foregut, numbered from cephalad to caudad. The embryonic aortic vascular arches arise in a cranial to caudal sequence, forming primitive arterial arcades around the pharyngeal arches. Regression or disappearance of some vascular arch segments, with persistence and remodeling of others, results in the formation of the thoracic aorta and its major branches. The first and second pair of vascular arches appear by days 24 and 26, respectively; the third and fourth by day 28; and the sixth by day 29. The fifth arch never fully develops or appears briefly and then involutes. By the time of appearance of the sixth arch, the first and second arches have largely regressed.

The ascending thoracic aorta is formed from the truncus arteriosus proximally and the aortic sac/ventral aorta distally. The aortic sac forms right and left horns. The right horn subsequently gives rise to the brachiocephalic artery, whereas the left forms the proximal portion of the aortic arch between the brachiocephalic arteries and LCCAs. The ventral aorta and the third vascular arches form paired primitive carotid arteries from which intracranial blood flow during early development is primarily derived. The CCAs are derived from the proximal portions of these primitive vessels.

The segment of the dorsal aorta between the third and fourth arches obliterates, and the fourth and sixth vascular arches undergo asymmetric remodeling. On the left side, the fourth arch and dorsal aorta form the definitive aortic arch (between the LCCA and left subclavian arteries) and the most proximal portion of the descending thoracic aorta. On the right side, the fourth arch and part of the dorsal aorta constitute the proximal portions of the right subclavian artery, with gradual loss of connection to the midline descending aorta. The ventral portions of the sixth vascular arches give rise to the pulmonary arteries. The dorsal contribution of the sixth arch regresses on the right while persisting on the left side as the ductus arteriosus.

In the neck, the vertebral arteries (VAs) develop from plexiform longitudinal anastomoses between seven pairs of embryonic cervical intersegmental arteries initially connected to the paired dorsal aortae. The seventh cervical intersegmental arteries enlarge bilaterally into the developing limb buds and migrate to form the bilateral subclavian arteries, retaining their connection with the dorsal aortae and ultimately receiving blood supply through the brachiocephalic trunk on the right and aortic arch on the left. Connections between the first six cervical intersegmental arteries and the dorsal aortae bilaterally usually regress completely.

Usual anatomy of the human aorta is the origin of three major branches from the superior aspect of the arch, which in order of origin are the brachiocephalic trunk, the LCCA, and the left subclavian artery. However, variations of branching pattern are common, with a typical branching pattern found in only approximately two-thirds of cases. The most common variant branching pattern is a shared origin of the brachiocephalic trunk and the LCCA, occurring in approximately 25% of cases. This variation occurs if, during arch development, the proximal part of the third aortic arch (which is normally absorbed into the left horn of the aortic sac) instead becomes absorbed into

the right horn of the aortic sac. It has been erroneously termed a "bovine arch" and is an incidental finding on imaging or angiographic studies. The true bovine arch has no resemblance to any aortic arch variations encountered in humans, as it is constituted by a single vessel arising from the arch that will give rise to the right subclavian artery, a bicarotid trunk, and the left subclavian artery.

## 1.3 Clinical Impact

Although asymptomatic, the presence of a common origin of brachiocephalic and LCCAs can introduce an additional challenge to procedures requiring selective catheterization of the LCCA. Recognition of the variant anatomy can be achieved during diagnostic angiography or from preprocedural computed tomographic angiography or magnetic resonance angiography (MRA) if performed. If selective engagement of the LCCA cannot be achieved using a standard (multipurpose or straight) catheter, it may be achieved with a complex curve catheter (e.g., sidewinder), the curve of which is conventionally reformed in the left subclavian artery. In the situation of a common brachiocephalic and LCCA trunk, a reverse or figure eight curve may be required for LCCA access, in which case the catheter curve can be formed in the brachiocephalic artery. Because of an often acute angulation of the LCCA from the common trunk, insertion of a long shuttle sheath into the vessel for interventional procedures may not be a viable option, and a more pliable guiding catheter may be required instead (such as an 8F Sidewinder Guide). A right radial or brachial approach for LCCA access and intervention may also be considered.

## 1.4 Additional Information and Cases

In approximately 9% of cases with a common origin, the LCCA originates from the brachiocephalic artery more distally, i.e. between 1 and 2.5 cm from the aortic arch (▶ Fig. 1.2).

Other variant branching patterns of the aortic arch include formation of a left brachiocephalic trunk with combined origin of the LCCA and left subclavian arteries, which occurs in approximately 1–2% of cases, and a direct origin of the left VA from the aortic arch, occurring in approximately 0.5–1% of cases (▶ Fig. 1.3; ▶ Fig. 1.4).

Congenital anomalies or malformations of the aortic arch can be explained by persistence of embryological vascular arch segments that normally regress, disappearance of vascular arch segments that normally remain, or a combination of both. The more common congenital arch anomalies include left arch with aberrant right subclavian artery (0.4–2%), right arch with aberrant left subclavian artery, right aortic arch with mirror image branching, and double aortic arch.

| Pearls and Pitfalls |
| --- |
| • A common origin of the brachiocephalic artery and LCCA is a common asymptomatic finding related to abnormal embryonic arch development. |
| • It may pose a challenge during catheterization of the LCCA. |

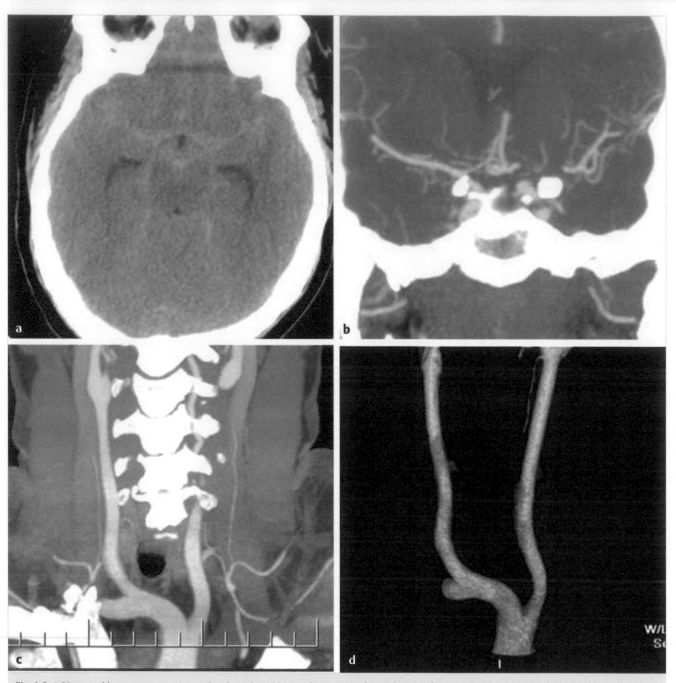

**Fig. 1.2** A 39-year-old woman presenting with subarachnoid hemorrhage. Nonenhanced CT (a) shows acute blood in the subarachnoid basal cisterns. Contrast-enhanced CT in coronal reformats (b,c) shows a 3-mm anterior communicating artery aneurysm. There is a long-segment common supra-aortic trunk giving rise to both the brachiocephalic trunk and the LCCA. 3D CTA reconstruction of the common carotids (d) shows the anatomy of this anatomical variation better.

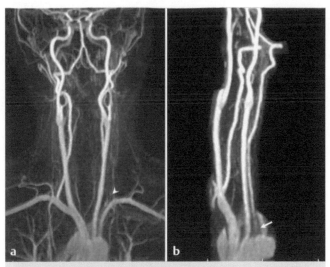

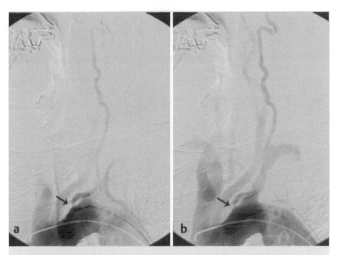

**Fig. 1.3** A 48-year-old woman being worked up for occipital headaches and vertigo after neck manipulation. Contrast-enhanced MRA (a,b) demonstrates the absence of the left VA origin at the expected proximal left subclavian artery on AP images (*short white arrow*). The oblique projection shows that the left VA arises directly from the aortic arch (*white arrow*) between the LCCA and the left subclavian artery.

**Fig. 1.4** (a,b) Arch aortogram reveals a direct origin of the left VA, with stenosis at the origin of the left VA, related to atherosclerotic disease (*black arrows*).

## Further Reading

[1] Kau T, Sinzig M, Gasser J et al. Aortic development and anomalies. Semin Intervent Radiol 2007; 24: 141–152

[2] Layton KF, Kallmes DF, Cloft HJ, Lindell EP, Cox VS. Bovine aortic arch variant in humans: clarification of a common misnomer. AJNR Am J Neuroradiol 2006; 27: 1541–1542

[3] Müller M, Schmitz BL, Pauls S et al. Variations of the aortic arch – a study on the most common branching patterns. Acta Radiol 2011; 52: 738–742

[4] Osborn AG. The aortic arch and great vessels. In: Diagnostic Cerebral Angiography. 2nd ed. Philadelphia, PA: Lippincott Williams & Wilkins; 1999:3–29

[5] Sadler TW. Cardiovascular system. In: Langman's Medical Embryology. 11th ed. Philadelphia, PA: Wolters Kluwer/Lippincott Williams & Wilkins; 2010:165–196

[6] Shaw JA, Gravereaux EC, Eisenhauer AC. Carotid stenting in the bovine arch. Catheter Cardiovasc Interv 2003; 60: 566–569

[7] Stojanovska J, Cascade PN, Chong S, Quint LE, Sundaram B. Embryology and imaging review of aortic arch anomalies. J Thorac Imaging 2012; 27: 73–84

# 2 The Aberrant Subclavian Artery

## 2.1 Case Description

### 2.1.1 Clinical Presentation

A 6-year-old boy with a history of aortic coarctation underwent a thoracic CTA for diagnostic workup.

### 2.1.2 Radiologic Studies

See ▸ Fig. 2.1.

### 2.1.3 Diagnosis

Aberrant right subclavian artery with an aortic coarctation.

## 2.2 Embryology and Anatomy

Development of the aortic arch and great vessels results from the formation and selective involution of paired vascular arches connecting the embryonic aortic sac (ventral aorta) with paired dorsal aortae, as discussed in Case 1. Congenital aortic arch anomalies result from errors in the embryological development of the vascular arches and can be explained by abnormal persistence of arch segments that usually regress, involution of segments that usually remain, or both. A left aortic arch with an aberrant right subclavian artery (ARSA) is the most common congenital arch anomaly, occurring in approximately 0.4 to 2% of cases.

During normal arch development, the segment of the dorsal aorta between the third and fourth arches obliterates, and the fourth vascular arches undergo asymmetric remodeling. On the right side, the fourth arch forms the most proximal portion of right subclavian artery, maintaining its connection to the definitive aortic arch through the brachiocephalic artery formed from the right horn of the aortic sac/ventral aorta. The subclavian artery more distally is formed from a segment of the right dorsal aortic arch and the right seventh intersegmental artery.

The portion of the right dorsal aorta between the origin of the seventh intersegmental artery and the junction with the left dorsal aorta involutes. An ARSA occurs when there is abnormal obliteration of the right fourth vascular arch and the portion of the right dorsal aorta cranial to the seventh intersegmental artery. As a result, the right subclavian artery forms from the seventh intersegmental artery and the distal part of the right dorsal aorta. There is, therefore, interruption of the primitive arch segment between the right common carotid artery (RCCA) and right subclavian arteries, and the right subclavian artery arises directly off the aorta. As development proceeds, the origin of the right subclavian artery shifts cranially to lie just below the left subclavian origin. Therefore, the ARSA is the last branch of the aortic arch, arising distal to the left subclavian origin. Because its origin is derived from the right dorsal aorta, it must cross the midline posterior to the esophagus to perfuse the right upper extremity. Commonly, but not in all cases, a diverticular outpouching is present at the origin of the ARSA. Known as a diverticulum of Kommerell, this outpouching is thought to represent a remainder of the primitive right dorsal aorta (▸ Fig. 2.2).

## 2.3 Clinical Impact

An ARSA is usually asymptomatic, as the trachea and esophagus are not completely encircled by vascular structures. However, in some patients, tortuosity and dilatation of the aberrant artery or aneurysmal dilatation of the Kommerell diverticulum can result in compression of the esophagus, with resultant dysphagia: so-called dysphagia lusoria. Nonspecific thoracic pain, dyspnea related to tracheal compression, and development of arterioesophageal or arteriotracheal fistulas with hematemesis or hemoptysis can also occur. Aneurysm formation in the aberrant vessel or diverticulum is, however, possible. Subclavian steal syndrome caused by stenosis or occlusion of the aberrant right subclavian proximal to the right vertebral origin is a rare clinical entity. Occasionally, the anomaly can be associated with

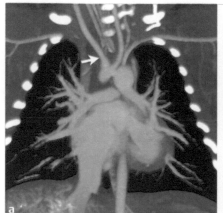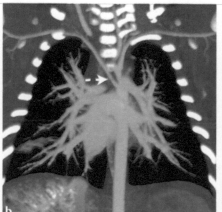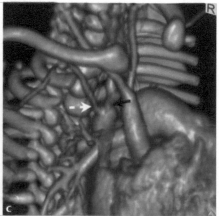

**Fig. 2.1** (a,b) Coronal reformats and (c) 3D volume reconstruction of a thoracic CTA. The RCCA arises as a single vessel from the aortic arch (*white arrow*). The right subclavian artery has an aberrant origin and arises as a single trunk (*dashed arrow*) from the arch, distal to the left subclavian artery. The aortic coarctation is located between the left subclavian and the aberrant right subclavian (*black arrow* in c).

other congenital abnormalities, such as hypoplastic left heart syndrome, coarctation of the aorta, and atrioventricular canal defects.

The presence of an ARSA increases the difficulty of interventional procedures requiring catheterization of the right subclavian artery or right vertebral artery (VA). It can be readily identified on cross-sectional studies, such as CTA and magnetic resonance angiography. Its presence can also be inferred from barium swallow studies performed for dysphagia, in which findings include anterior displacement of the esophagus with an abnormal indentation on the posterior wall of the esophagus in the upper mediastinum. On catheter angiography, the absence of filling of the right subclavian artery on right brachiocephalic injection should raise the suspicion of an ARSA if it has been not already identified from diagnostic cross-sectional imaging. The origin of the vessel distal to the left subclavian artery can then be sought, and an arch aortogram can be performed if necessary.

In the setting of an ARSA, where possible, posterior circulation endovascular procedures may have to be performed through the left VA, as right vertebral catheterization from a femoral approach can be problematic. Alternatively, a right radial or brachial approach can be considered for VA catheterization; however, this approach can cause difficulties for coronary catheterization. For example, the angular course of the aberrant vessel to the aorta can impose difficulty in passing a guidewire into the ascending aorta.

Treatment of the anomaly is not required in asymptomatic patients. However, in symptomatic patients or in the setting of aneurysm formation, intervention may be considered with various surgical or combined surgical and endovascular approaches. One possible combined approach is the endovascular occlusion of the aortic origin of the aberrant artery combined with surgical subclavian artery transposition and distal prevertebral occlusion. Occlusion of the proximal right subclavian artery without subclavian artery reconstruction can result in right arm ischemia or subclavian steal syndrome.

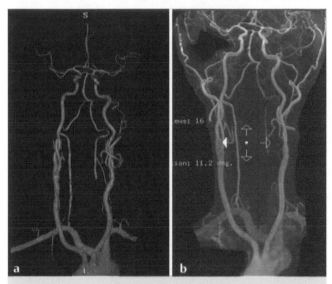

**Fig. 2.2** MRA in anteroposterior (AP) view (a) and coronal MRA (b) demonstrate an aberrant right subclavian artery resulting from formation from the C7 segmental artery. Note the separate origins of the RCCA and LCCA in this case, rather than a common origin.

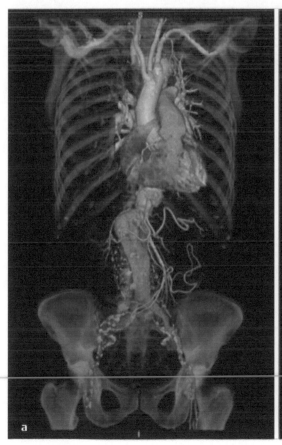

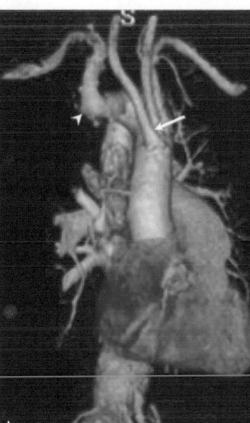

**Fig. 2.3** 3D CTA reformats of the thoracoabdominal aorta in AP (a) and oblique (b) views in a 73-year-old woman being worked up for an abdominal aortic aneurysm. In this case, the first vessel to arise from the aortic arch is the RCCA (*white arrow*). The right subclavian artery is the last vessel to arise from the aortic arch (*white arrowhead*), after the left subclavian. The aberrant subclavian artery will cross the midline behind the thoracic esophagus, after which it will resume its normal path (not shown).

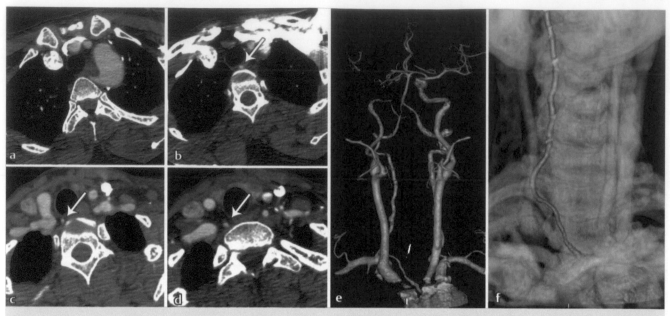

**Fig. 2.4** Contrast-enhanced axial CT (a–d) and 3D CTA reconstruction images in AP (e) and oblique (f) views demonstrating an aberrant right VA (*white arrows*), originating directly from the aortic arch (lusoria origin), related to development of the right VA from the C8 segmental artery, rather than the C6 or C7 levels.

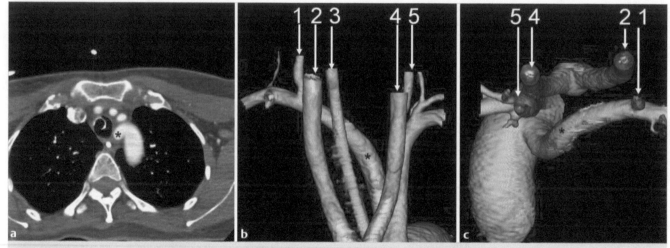

**Fig. 2.5** CTA in axial cut (a) and 3D reformats in AP (b) and superior (c) views demonstrating an aberrant subclavian artery (*asterisks* in a,b,c). 1, right VA; 2, RCCA; 3, nasogastric tube; 4, LCCA; 5, left VA.

## 2.4 Additional Information and Cases

Occasionally, an ARSA arises from a common trunk with the left subclavian artery. This can occur in combination with a shared origin of the CCAs, forming an uncommon type of vascular ring, sometimes called a bitruncus arch. Only two great vessels arise from the arch, and compression of the trachea by the bicarotid truncus in front and the bisubclavian truncus behind may cause stridor.

Isolation of the right subclavian artery occurs when there are two breaks in the primitive aortic arch, leaving the subclavian artery separated from the aortic arch. Patients with this anomaly can present with subclavian steal syndrome as a result of retrograde VA flow supplying the upper limb. This anomaly generally occurs on the side contralateral to the arch and so is more commonly associated with a right aortic arch (▶ Fig. 2.3; ▶ Fig. 2.4; ▶ Fig. 2.5; ▶ Fig. 2.6).

### Pearls and Pitfalls

- The presence of an aberrant right subclavian artery is usually asymptomatic; however, tortuosity and dilatation of the aberrant artery or aneurysmal dilatation of the Kommerell diverticulum can result in compression of the esophagus, resulting in dysphagia (known as dysphagia lusoria in some patients).
- Endovascular procedures involving the right VA and right subclavian artery may be difficult in patients with an ARSA.

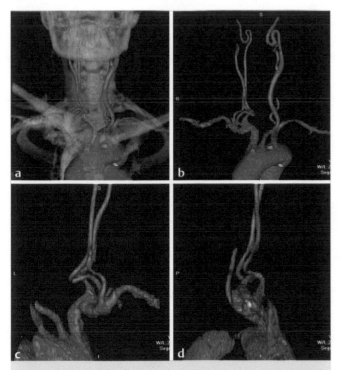

**Fig. 2.6** CTA 3D reconstructions in AP (a,b), posterior-anterior (c), and oblique (d) views demonstrate separate origins of the right external and internal carotid arteries related to persistence of the ductus caroticus, with complete involution of the third aortic arch, resulting in absent migration of the external carotid artery toward the carotid axis.

## Further Reading

[1] Kau T, Sinzig M, Gasser J et al. Aortic development and anomalies. Semin Intervent Radiol 2007; 24: 141–152

[2] Müller M, Schmitz BL, Pauls S et al. Variations of the aortic arch – a study on the most common branching patterns. Acta Radiol 2011; 52: 738–742

[3] Osborn AG. The aortic arch and great vessels. In: Diagnostic Cerebral Angiography. 2nd ed. Philadelphia, PA: Lippincott Williams & Wilkins; 1999:3–29

[4] Sadler TW. Cardiovascular system. In: Langman's Medical Embryology. 11th ed. Philadelphia, PA: Wolters Kluwer/Lippincott Williams & Wilkins; 2010:16;5–196

[5] Shaw JA, Gravereaux EC, Eisenhauer AC. Carotid stenting in the bovine arch. Catheter Cardiovasc Interv 2003; 60: 566–569

[6] Stojanovska J, Cascade PN, Chong S, Quint LE, Sundaram B. Embryology and imaging review of aortic arch anomalies. J Thorac Imaging 2012; 27: 73–84

# Section II

**Internal Carotid Artery**

# 3 The Carotid Segments, the Aberrant ICA, and the Persistent Stapedial Artery

## 3.1 Case Description

### 3.1.1 Clinical Presentation

A 32-year-old man presented with pulsatile tinnitus and a retrotympanic vascular mass.

### 3.1.2 Radiologic Studies

See ▶ Fig. 3.1; ▶ Fig. 3.2.

### 3.1.3 Diagnosis

Aberrant right internal carotid artery (ICA).

## 3.2 Anatomy

The aberrant ICA occurs as a hemodynamic response to a segmental agenesis of the first (i.e., cervical) segment of the ICA secondary to disturbed differentiation of the third branchial arch. It represents a collateral pathway between the external carotid artery (ECA) and the petrous ICA via the ascending pharyngeal artery (APhA).

The ICA segments have been classified by various methods, most of which are based on anatomic or surgical criteria. However, to understand the occurrence of specific variations like the one described in the present case, a model based on embryologic considerations, such as that proposed by Santoyo-Vazquez and Lasjaunias, may be more helpful. In this model, the ICA is formed by seven segments, the boundaries of which are defined by transient embryonic vessels.

As previously described, during formation of the craniocervical vessels and the arch, the ventral aorta and both dorsal aortas (DAos) are connected by six aortic arches (AAs). The lower three arches (IV–VI) participate in the development of the aortic arch and supra-aortic trunks, whereas arches I–III are involved in ICA development. Cranial to the AA I, at this stage, the DAo will also give origin to other embryonic vessels. In caudocranial order, these are the primitive maxillary artery (PMI), the dorsal ophthalmic artery (DO), and the ventral ophthalmic artery.

Bearing these considerations in mind, the future segments of the adult ICA are defined by the following embryonic vessels:

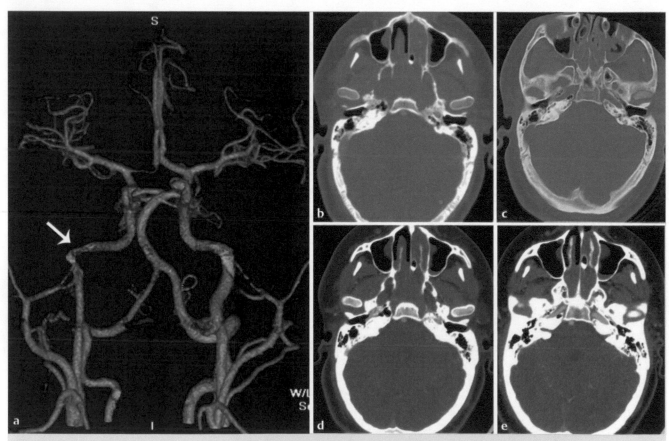

**Fig. 3.1** 3D CTA in anteroposterior (AP) view (a) demonstrates an aberrant course of the right ICA (*white arrow*), running more laterally compared with the contralateral left side. Contrast-enhanced axial CT images in bone (b,c) and soft tissue (d,e) windows reveal a vascular structure corresponding to the right ICA within the right middle ear.

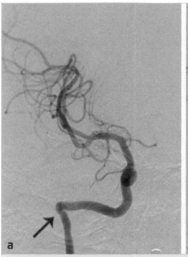
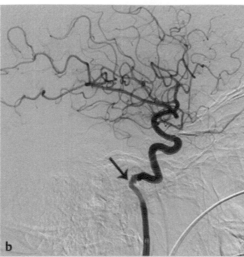
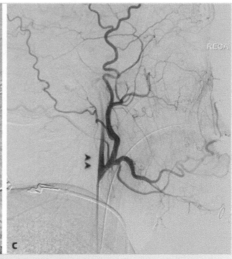

**Fig. 3.2** Right ICA angiogram in AP (a) and lateral (b) views confirms the lateral course of the right ICA. The right ECA angiogram in lateral view (c) reveals the ascending pharyngeal origin of the right ICA (*double arrowheads*). Note the focal narrowing of the "aberrant ICA" as it enters the skull base, marking the entry point into the inferior tympanic canaliculus (arrows).

- segment 1: AA III,
- segment 2: the DAo between AAs III and II,
- segment 3: the DAo between AAs II and I,
- segment 4: the DAo between AA I and the PMI,
- segment 5: the DAo between the PMI and the DO,
- segment 6: the DAo between the DO and the opening of the ophthalmic artery (OA), and
- segment 7: the DAo between the opening of the OA and the bifurcation of the ICA into a rostral (telencephalic) and a caudal division.

Cranially to the seventh segment, there are no additional ICA segments, as all other future arteries that will develop further distally will have a different temporal or phylogenetic origin. During embryonic life, the aortic arches and the embryonic vessels will undergo regression and significant modifications that will give shape to the ICA as it is seen in adults.

However, the remnants of these embryonic vessels will be relevant in defining the boundaries of the different ICA segments: AA III will persist and evolve into the cervical ICA distal to the carotid bulb. The carotid bulb is, from an embryological point of view, therefore a separate structure from the ICA. AA II regresses rapidly, and the only portion remaining forms the stapedial and hyoid arteries. These will be annexed by the ventral pharyngeal artery (originating from the ventral aorta) to form the future ECA and internal maxillary artery. The remnant of AA II is the caroticotympanic artery (CTymA). AA I will regress and contribute to the development of the ECA, together with the ventral aorta. The remnant of AA I will be the mandibulovidian artery. The PMI will regress to form the posterior hypophyseal artery and contribute to form the meningohypophyseal trunk. In most adults, the DO will regress and contribute to form the inferolateral trunk. The caudal division of the ICA reaches the cephalic end of the ipsilateral ventral neural artery to constitute the future PcomA. The rostral or telencephalic division will evolve initially into the anterior choroidal artery and anterior cerebral artery, which later will give rise to the middle cerebral arteries.

In cases of segmental agenesis of the ICA, each of these embryonic vessels represents the potential point of vascular reconstitution of flow into the other distally preserved ICA segments. Most of these unusual flow patterns have been improperly described as aberrant courses of the ICA. After a complex process of regression and annexation of the different vascular structures involved, the ICA develops into its final appearance, resembling a continuous vessel, with its characteristic path and curves. Still, the seven embryonic segments can be distinguished by the origin of the embryonic arteries' remnants:

1. cervical segment: immediately distal to the bulb to the entry point of the of the carotid canal,
2. ascending intrapetrous segment: from the entry point of the carotid canal to the origin of the CTymA,
3. horizontal intrapetrous segment: from the origin of the CTymA to the origin of the mandibulovidian artery,
4. segment ascending foramen lacerum: from the origin of the mandibulovidian artery to the origin of the meningohypophyseal trunk,
5. horizontal cavernous segment: from the origin of the meningohypophyseal trunk to the origin of the inferolateral trunk,
6. clinoid segment: from the origin of the inferolateral trunk to the origin of the OA, and
7. supraclinoid ICA segment: from the origin of the OA.

Each of the segments, because of their phylogenetic differences, has a different heritage and vulnerability, which explains the specific involvement of certain segments and the preservation of adjacent ones in certain disease processes.

In normal subjects, the ICA enters the petrous bone medial to the styloid process via the carotid canal. The vertical petrous segment runs anterior to the cochlea and is separated from the middle ear by a thin plate of bone. Then, the ICA turns anteriorly to run inferior and posteromedial to the Eustachian tube, traverses through the foramen lacerum, and enters the cavernous sinus.

In patients with an aberrant ICA, the inferior tympanic branch of the APhA enlarges in response to segmental ICA agenesis and anastomoses with the CTymA (remnant of the hyoid artery) to reconstitute the ICA in the horizontal petrous segment. The inferior tympanic artery enters the skull through the inferior tympanic canaliculus (Jacobsen canal), which explains the focal narrowing of the ICA seen on digital subtraction angiography and computed tomographic angiography at this level.

Therefore, in cases of an aberrant course of the ICA, the "cervical ICA" is actually composed of the APhA, its inferior tympanic branch, and the caroticotympanic branch of the ICA, and not by the first ICA segment.

Clinical diagnosis of aberrant ICA is difficult because symptoms and signs are often nonspecific or absent. Symptoms like pulsatile tinnitus, conductive hearing loss, and a pulsatile retrotympanic mass can be seen. The clinical picture can be interpreted as otosclerosis, glomus tumor, or other vascular malformation. To avoid an arterial injury during surgery, a temporal bone computed tomography (CT) scan should be performed when dealing with a "vascular" retrotympanic mass.

On CT, the aberrant ICA runs posterior to the jugular bulb, with a focal stenosis as it enters the skull base. There will be a deficient bony plate along the tympanic portion of the ICA, and the vertical segment of the carotid canal will be absent. On digital subtraction angiography, the aberrant ICA will show a characteristic lateral swing beyond the vestibular line (also called the line of Lapayowker) within the petrous bone and will then turn medially into the middle ear cavity.

The stapedial artery is a transient embryonic vessel that arises at 4 to 5 weeks of fetal life. It is a branch of the hyoid artery, which derives from the second branchial arch. It extends cranially and passes through the mesenchymal primordium of the stapes to form the obturator foramen. The stapedial artery gives rise to two intracranial arteries: the upper or supraorbital branch, which later becomes the middle meningeal artery (MMA), and the lower or maxillomandibular division, which divides into two branches (a mandibular branch and an infraorbital branch) that will later become the inferior alveolar and infraorbital arteries, respectively. The maxillomandibular division

leaves the cranial cavity through the foramen spinosum and anastomoses with the ventral pharyngeal artery at this level. This anastomosis triggers the involution of the stapedial artery, which occurs during the 10th week of fetal life. The hyoid artery persists as the caroticotympanic branch of the ICA. If the stapedial artery persists (PSA), the connection between the inferior division is annexed by the ventral pharyngeal artery, and the superior division is supplied by the PSA. As the connection between both divisions is through the foramen spinosum, in cases of PSA, this foramen is absent or hypoplastic. The end result will be that the MMA will be supplied by the ICA via the PSA.

The PSA has a prevalence of ~0.5% in the general population and presents as a pulsatile mass in the middle ear cavity, with or without pulsatile tinnitus. Occasionally, it may show conductive hearing loss as a result of stapes ankylosis. A PSA can be seen as an isolated variant or in association with an aberrant ICA. In the latter cases, it arises from the petrous ICA, enters the anteromedial hypotympanum via the Jacobsen canal, crosses over the cochlear promontory, passes between the crura of the stapes (obturator foramen) to enter the facial nerve (fallopian) canal, or runs parallel to it in its own canal. Then the PSA continues superiorly, as an enlarged superior tympanic or superficial petrosal artery, to form the MMA. When the PSA occurs in isolation, the abnormal artery is formed by enlargement of the more distal caroticotympanic artery arising from the vertical petrous ICA and then follows the same course as described earlier. Therefore, the foramen spinosum is absent or hypoplastic, as the MMA does not arise from the proximal internal maxillary artery, as typically seen.

In cases with a PSA, CT findings include a small canaliculus exiting the carotid canal (in cases of isolated PSA), a linear soft tissue density structure crossing the middle ear over the promontory, an enlarged facial nerve canal, or a separate parallel bony canal. The foramen spinosum will be absent, as previously mentioned. Of note, ~3% of the population may have an absent foramen spinosum without a PSA, so it is an indirect sign of PSA, and the diagnosis has to be made based on the other CT findings.

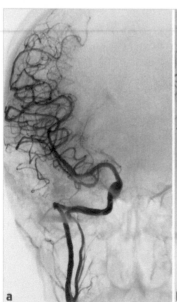
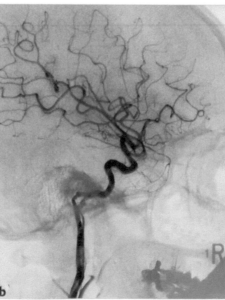

Fig. 3.3 A 28-year-old woman presented with conductive hearing loss and retrotympanic mass. Right ICA angiograms in AP (a) and lateral (b) views demonstrate a double origin of the right ICA. The cervical segment of the "normal" right ICA appears hypoplastic and joins the "ascending pharyngeal origin" ICA at the petrous segment.

## 3.3 Clinical Impact

The aberrant ICA is a well-recognized although rare vascular anomaly. Clinically it can mimic glomus tumors, other vascular malformations (such as aneurysms and hemangiomas), or otosclerosis. Misdiagnosis of this anomaly may lead to serious morbidity resulting from massive bleeding or stroke. If there is uncontrolled bleeding, endovascular treatment has to be performed and may require parent vessel sacrifice, stent grafts, or overlapping flow diverters.

## 3.4 Additional Information and Cases

An important clinical differential diagnosis is the tympanic or jugulotympanic paraganglioma, the most common middle ear vascular tumor. Although clinically it may be challenging to differentiate between an aberrant ICA, PSA, or paraganglioma, temporal bone CT will easily distinguish these entities. It will show a small soft tissue mass over the promontory in cases of tympanic paragangliomas, and a permeative vascularized mass centered in the jugular foramen, extending into the middle ear, in cases of jugulotympanic paragangliomas. Another differential diagnosis is the dehiscent jugular bulb, for which temporal bone CT will show a focal dehiscence of the bony plate covering the jugular bulb, with a small portion of the internal jugular vein protruding into the middle ear (▶ Fig. 3.3; ▶ Fig. 3.4; ▶ Fig. 3.5; ▶ Fig. 3.6).

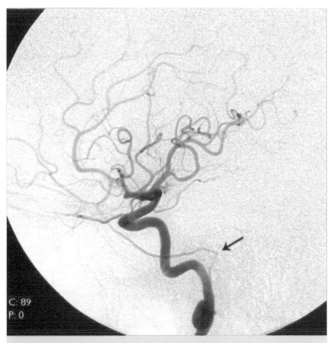

**Fig. 3.4** A 27-year-old man presented with pulsatile mass seen during otoscopy. Left ICA angiogram reveals a vessel arising from the petrous ICA (*black arrow*), supplying the MMA, which is the classic angiographic appearance of a PSA.

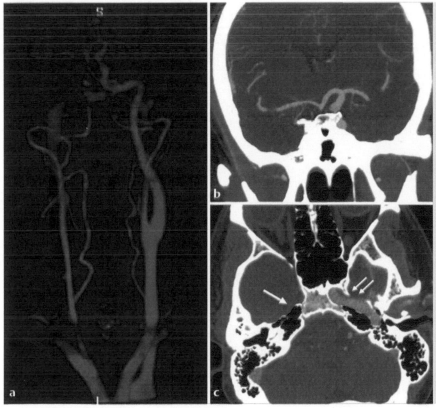

**Fig. 3.5** 3D CTA (a) and contrast-enhanced CT in coronal (b) and axial (c) images demonstrate a congenital absent right ICA. Note the absence of the right carotid canal (white arrow) and prominent size of the left ICA (*white double arrows*) supplying the right cerebral hemisphere through the anterior communicating artery.

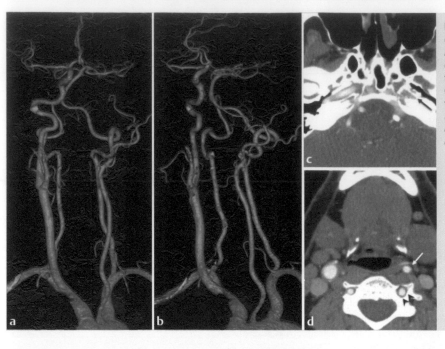

**Fig. 3.6** 3D CTA in AP (a) and oblique (b) views demonstrates the absence of the left ICA. The left ACA is supplied through the anterior communicating artery and the left middle cerebral artery through the left posterior communicating artery. Contrast-enhanced axial CT (c,d) images show the absence of the left carotid canal (*black arrow*) and the prominent sizes of the left ECAs (*white arrow*) and left vertebral arteries (*double black arrowheads*).

## Pearls and Pitfalls

- In the "aberrant ICA," there is agenesis of the first ICA segment (cervical segment).
- The "aberrant ICA" actually is composed by the APhA, its inferior tympanic branch, and the caroticotympanic branch of the ICA, which serve as a collateral route to reconstitute the ICA in the horizontal petrous segment.
- The PSA may occur in isolation or associated with an aberrant ICA. In either case, the foramen spinosum will be absent or hypoplastic and the MMA will originate from the PSA and not from the ECA.

## Further Reading

[1] Lasjaunias P, Santoyo-Vazquez A. Segmental agenesis of the internal carotid artery: angiographic aspects with embryological discussion. Anat Clin 1984; 6: 133–141

[2] Roll JD, Urban MA, Larson TC, III, Gailloud P, Jacob P, Harnsberger HR. Bilateral aberrant internal carotid arteries with bilateral persistent stapedial arteries and bilateral duplicated internal carotid arteries. AJNR Am J Neuroradiol 2003; 24: 762–765

[3] Sauvaget E, Paris J, Kici S et al. Aberrant internal carotid artery in the temporal bone: imaging findings and management. Arch Otolaryngol Head Neck Surg 2006; 132: 86–91

[4] Silbergleit R, Quint DJ, Mehta BA, Patel SC, Metes JJ, Noujaim SE. The persistent stapedial artery. AJNR Am J Neuroradiol 2000; 21: 572–577

[5] Thiers FA, Sakai O, Poe DS, Curtin HD. Persistent stapedial artery: CT findings. AJNR Am J Neuroradiol 2000; 21: 1551–1554

[6] Willinsky R, Lasjaunias P, Berenstein A. Intracavernous branches of the internal carotid artery (ICA). Comprehensive review of their variations. Surg Radiol Anat 1987; 9: 201–215

# 4 Persistent Carotid-Vertebrobasilar Anastomoses

## 4.1 Case Description

### 4.1.1 Clinical Presentation

A 48-year-old man was evaluated for right-sided weakness with sudden onset 1 week before admission to our hospital.

### 4.1.2 Radiologic Studies

See ► Fig. 4.1; ► Fig. 4.2.

### 4.1.3 Diagnosis

Left primitive hypoglossal artery (HA) supplying the posterior circulation with an acute anterior medullary ischemia.

## 4.2 Embryology and Anatomy

Carotid–vertebrobasilar anastomoses exist briefly in the earlier stages of embryonic development to supply the developing hindbrain. The understanding of the complex and sophisticated

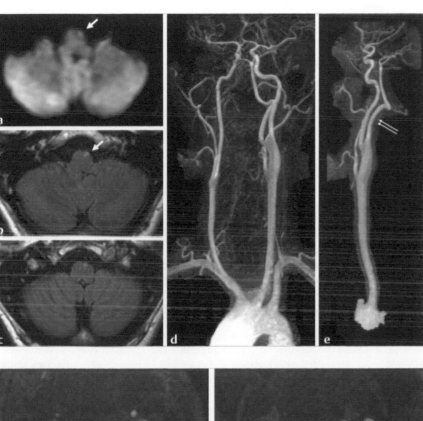

Fig. 4.1 Diffusion-weighted MRI (a) and fluid-attenuated inversion recovery (b,c) weighted images demonstrate a tiny focus of hypersignal in the left anterior medulla oblongata just cranial to the pyramids consistent with recent ischemic stroke. Contrast-enhanced MRA in anteroposterior (AP) (d) and lateral (e) views demonstrates hypoplasia of both VAs in the cervical portion. The basilar artery (BA) is fed by a congenital carotid–vertebrobasilar anastomosis that arises from the left ICA beyond the left common carotid bifurcation and connects to the intradural segment of the VA. This segmental anastomosis is the primitive HA.

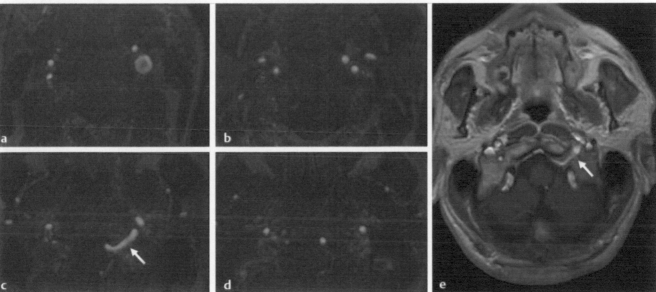

Fig. 4.2 Source images (a–d) and a contrast-enhanced T1-weighted MRI (e) reveal the course of the primitive HA through the hypoglossal canal to form the BA (*white arrows*).

developmental anatomy of the craniocervical vasculature has its foundation in the seminal works by Congdon and Padget.

The primordial vascular system is organized into a series of three bilateral longitudinal systems: two ventral ones, the ventral and dorsal aortas that were discussed previously, and a dorsal one, located on the midline ventral to the neural tube, the longitudinal neural arteries. These longitudinal vessels are interconnected by transverse segmental arteries.

When the embryo is 4 mm long (28 ± 1 days; Padget stage I), the posterior circulation and the vertebrobasilar system as such do not exist yet. The caudal division of the ventral aorta courses over the midbrain, whereas the nourishment for the hindbrain comes through bilateral paired branches arising from the dorsal aortas that are usually transitory. At the cervical level, these branches are the first six segmental arteries.

The first and second of these arteries are called proatlantal arteries (PaAs) type 1 and type 2. At the intracranial level, two vessels bridge the dorsal aortas and the longitudinal neural arteries: the HA and, more cranially, the trigeminal artery (TA). Between the HA and the TA, Padget identified a third anastomosis, the otic artery (OtA), a finding that was not replicated in other works and is discussed in greater detail later.

These anastomoses persist for less than 1 week, and then they usually involute at the same time as the posterior circulation is developing. At 29 ± 1 days, the internal carotid artery (ICA) is better defined, and its caudal extremity anastomoses with the cranial longitudinal neural artery, giving origin to a primordial posterior communicating artery (PcomA). At the same time, the vertebrobasilar system begins to acquire its definitive architecture when the bilateral longitudinal neural arteries partially merge on the midline, constituting a primitive basilar artery (BA); at this point, the TA and HA start to disappear. Caudally, the definitive vertebral artery (VA) takes form through a series of longitudinal anastomoses linking the first six cervical intersegmental arteries. The ventral and dorsal portions of the segmental arteries regress, except for the PaA, which links to the BA by its cranial branch. At Padget stage III (31 ± 1 days, 10 mm), the collateral caudal branch of the sixth segmental artery connects with the cranial branch of the seventh segmental artery, which will become the adult subclavian artery, reversing the flow in a caudocranial direction. At this point, the BA blood supply no longer comes from the carotid system but, instead, via the VA, thus establishing the vertebrobasilar system. At this stage, the segmental embryonic vessels have disappeared, although some of them may persist in the adult.

Different studies have reported the general incidence of carotid-vertebrobasilar anastomoses between 0.1% and 1.25%. Probably for hemodynamic reasons, the persistence of these vessels is associated with aberrations in vascular embryogenesis, and thus they are often observed with other abnormalities of the vertebrobasilar circulation or of the circle of Willis.

The following section describes these vessels in the embryonic period and in their persistent form (adult configuration) from caudal to cranial.

## 4.2.1 Proatlantal Arteries

Proatlantal arteries (PaAs) are the last to disappear in the embryo and are related to the two most cranial intersegmental cervical segmental arteries. Persistence of a PaA has been reported in fewer than 50 cases.

PaA type 2 corresponds to the second intersegmental artery. It arises from the external carotid artery (ECA) and accompanies the second cervical nerve root. It courses posterior to the second cervical space to the vertebral canal. This artery usually regresses to the C2 occipitovertebral anastomosis. When the vessel does not involute, it originates from the ECA shortly after its origin, runs superoposteriorly as a vascular loop, and then ascends and pierces the dura at the C1 level, passing through the transverse foramen of the atlas. It then anastomoses with the contralateral VA V3 segment to form the BA ventral to the medulla.

PaA type 1 corresponds to the first intersegmental artery and is associated with the first cervical nerve. Because it maintains supply to the posterior circulations until the VAs are fully developed, this intersegmental artery is the last to disappear, typically at the 10–12-mm stage of the embryo, when it forms the intracranial part of the VA. If it regresses, the proximal remnant of this artery is, in the adult vasculature, the occipital artery, with its C1 occipitovertebral anastomosis. Persistence of this vessel is rarer than persistence of type 2 PaA. When still present in the postembryonic period, it originates from the posterior wall of the ICA between the C2–C4 level, runs dorsally to the first cervical space, passes in the occipitocervical space, and perforates the dura without ever running in the cervical canal. It joins the V3 segment of the VA in the suboccipital area before penetrating the foramen magnum. The persistent PaA is more often positioned laterally to the ICA in its course and makes a sharp curve dorsally and above the atlas, entering into the cranial cavity. Usually, there are no branches arising from the PaA, and only rarely does the occipital artery arise from the PaA. The ipsilateral, contralateral, or both VAs are hypoplastic or absent in around 50% of cases of persistent PaA (▸ Fig. 4.3; ▸ Fig. 4.4).

## 4.2.2 Hypoglossal Artery

This artery is the first to disappear in the embryo. It is the second most common persisting carotid vertebrobasilar anastomosis, with a prevalence of 0.02–0.1% in angiographic series. In the embryo, the vessel originates on the primitive ICA and enters the hypoglossal canal ventrally of the 12th cranial nerve rootlets, keeping its central position in this canal to join the ipsilateral VA ventral to the brain stem. According to Padget, the vessel normally involutes at 29 ± 1 days. When the vessel persists in the postdevelopmental age, it usually arises from the posterior wall of the ICA between C1 and C2 or at the C2 level. Similar to its embryological course, it joins the 12th cranial nerve and passes through the hypoglossal canal to anastomose with the VA. In rare cases, the HA may arise from the posterior surface of the ECA, immediately opposite the lingual artery. It then courses rostrally and posteriorly behind the ICA in its cervical segment as the occipital branch of the ECA. After making a loop opposite the atlantooccipital region, it enters the hypoglossal canal. Persistence of this vessel is usually associated with hypoplasia or aplasia of the ipsilateral VA and PcomA. The persistent HA can be associated with neural compression symptoms regarding either the 12th or the 11th cranial nerve. Although this vessel is usually present as an incidental and asymptomatic finding during a carotid angiographic exam, it has also been reported that the HA is the persisting carotid–vertebrobasilar anastomosis that is most often associated with additional vas-

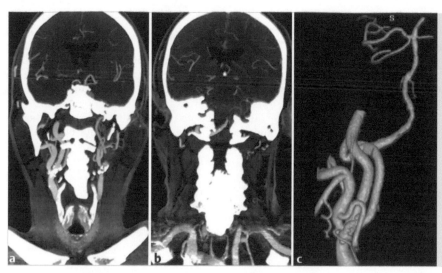

**Fig. 4.3** CTA in coronal views (a,b) and 3D reconstruction in oblique view (c) demonstrate a right PaA type 1 supplying the posterior fossa.

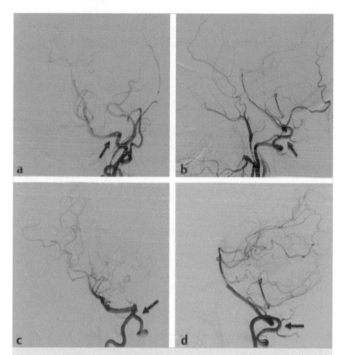

**Fig. 4.4** Left ECA (a,b) and left VA (c,d) angiograms in AP (a,c) and lateral (b,d) views demonstrate a prominent remnant of the proatlantal type 1 anastomosis (i.e., the C1 occipitovertebral anastomosis) between the occipital and VA at the C1 level. Vasospasm of the left ECA is observed related to catheterization.

cular pathology, especially aneurysms of both the HA and the intracranial vessels and, in particular, the BA.

## 4.2.3 Otic Artery

There continues to be controversy about the existence of the otic artery. According to Lie's guidelines on diagnosing persistent carotid-vertebrobasilar anastomoses, the persistent OtA should rise from the ICA petrosal segment in the lateral portion of the petrous carotid canal, close to the medial turn. It should then run through the internal acoustic meatus with the facial and vestibulocochlear nerves before connecting with the BA at

a caudal point. In the limited literature available, no definitive evidence of a true persistent OtA was found, and the vessels described thus far were in fact low-originating TAs or stapedial artery remnants. Lasjaunias concluded that this artery does not exist as a distinct vascular system separate from the TA, based on the assumption that as the eighth cranial nerve remains in the petrous bone, there are no phylogenetic or recent acquisitions that justify anastomosis of the paired longitudinal neural arterial plexus with the dorsal aorta or its remnant across the skull base at that level. The TA, HA, and PaAs, in contrast, are all segmental arteries related to the metameric embryonic structure of the diencephalon, rhombencephalon, and spinal cord and their related nerves. The otic structures are not segmental and develop mainly from the otic placode. Thus, there is no reason to expect a segmental communication at this level. Unlike the other three carotid–vertebrobasilar anastomoses, there is no evidence for the existence of an otic artery in lower animals.

## 4.2.4 Trigeminal Artery

The TA is the most common persistent carotid–vertebrobasilar anastomosis; it accounts for 85% of these persisting vessels, and its presence has been reported in 0.1 to 0.6% of angiograms. When it persists, the TA usually takes origin from the posterior wall of the ICA in the cavernous part, after leaving the carotid canal. The artery can also originate from the lateral or anterior walls of the ICA at that level. Other possible sites of origin include but are not limited to the distal part of the petrosal segment, the carotid siphon, and the presellar portion of the ICA. In the cavernous sinus, the artery is located superior to the oculomotor, trochlear, and abducens nerves, and medial to the ophthalmic branch of the trigeminal nerve and the trigeminal ganglion. The TA emanates from the posterior wall of the cavernous sinus, following either a para- or an intrasellar course. It then reaches the posterior cranial fossa in two ways: In about 50% of the cases, the TA penetrates the sella turcica, runs in its own groove, and perforates the dura mater near the clivus; in the other half of the cases, it runs extradurally after leaving the cavernous sinus, between the sensory trigeminal root and the lateral side of the sella, in a groove of the posterior clinoid process. The roof of this groove is formed by the petroclinoid ligament. It then joins the BA, usually between the origins of the anterior inferior cerebellar arteries (AICAs) and of the superior cerebellar arteries (SCAs). TAs can be further classified into the following types:

- TA Saltzman type 1: this subtype joins the BA between the SCA and the AICA. The BA proximal to the junction is usually hypoplastic and the PcomAs are absent or poorly opacified. The TA supplies both posterior cerebral arteries (PCAs) and SCAs (▶ Fig. 4.5; ▶ Fig. 4.6).
- TA Saltzman type 2: this subtype also joins the BA between the SCAs and the AICAs, but a PcomA is present and supplies at least one PCA (▶ Fig. 4.7; ▶ Fig. 4.8).

- TA Saltzman type 3 is referred to the TA variant when it directly joins with a cerebellar artery without anastomosing with the BA. It can anastomose with the SCA (Saltzman type 3a), with the AICA (Saltzman type 3b, the most common type), or with the posterior inferior cerebellar artery (Saltzman type 3c) (▶ Fig. 4.9).

As with the other carotid-vertebrobasilar anastomoses, the BAs and VAs caudal to the anastomosis may show hypoplasia in varying degrees.

## 4.3 Clinical Impact

Most carotid-vertebrobasilar anastomoses are incidental findings. However, they may be associated with intracranial vascular anomalies, most commonly aneurysms (▶ Fig. 4.10), and cranial nerve symptoms.

The role of these vessels is particularly important in the general configuration of the blood supply to the brain. They can constitute the only, or main, feeder to the posterior circulation and can therefore explain otherwise unexpected infarct locations, as microembolic phenomena from a common lesion, such as a common carotid artery or ICA atherosclerotic plaque, can lead to infarctions in territories normally fed by the posterior circulation.

Of note is that the persistent TA occurs with a much higher frequency among children with PHACE syndrome (posterior fossa, hemangioma, arterial lesions, cardiac abnormalities/aortic coarctation, and eye abnormalities; 12–16%).

## 4.4 Additional Information

The carotid-vertebrobasilar anastomoses are rarely encountered in clinical practice, and they constitute an exceptional finding during angiographic exams of the intracranial circulation, but they may be more frequently encountered with increased use of noninvasive vascular imaging of the head and neck region.

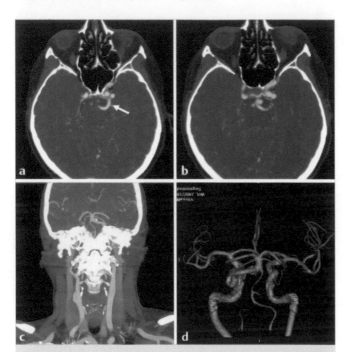

**Fig. 4.5** CTA in axial (a,b) and coronal (c) reconstructions demonstrates an anomalous artery traversing the left prepontine cistern, connecting the left cavernous ICA to the BA. The 3D CTA reconstruction (d) in posterior-anterior view confirms the presence of a left trigeminal artery.

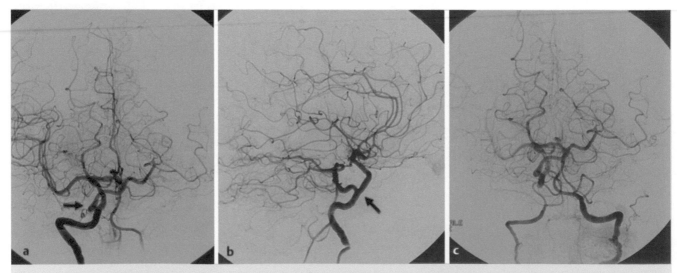

**Fig. 4.6** Right ICA angiogram in AP (a) and lateral (b) views and left VA angiogram in AP view reveal a right trigeminal artery arising from the right petrous-cavernous ICA joining the upper third of the BA.

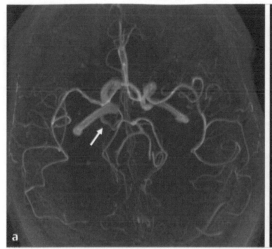

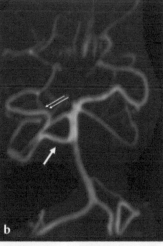

**Fig. 4.7** Time-of-flight MRA in craniocaudal view (a) and AP view (b) demonstrates a Saltzman type 2 trigeminal artery (*white arrow*), given the presence of a right-sided fetal-type PCA (*double arrows*).

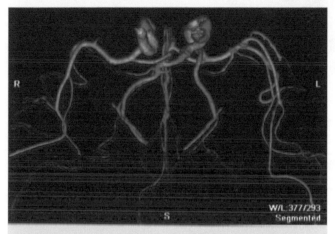

**Fig. 4.8** CTA 3D reconstruction in a basal view demonstrates the presence of a left trigeminal artery and a fetal type origin of the left PCA from the left ICA.

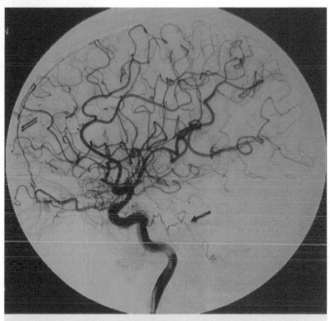

**Fig. 4.9** Right ICA angiogram in lateral view in a patient sent for investigation of subarachnoid hemorrhage demonstrates a trigeminal artery supplying the right posterior inferior cerebellar artery territory (*black arrow*). Note the prominent size of the anterior falcine artery (*double arrows*) arising from the ophthalmic artery without any arteriovenous shunt, likely as a result of the meningeal irritation.

Differential diagnosis between the aforementioned persisting vessels should be carried out considering both the origin of the abnormal vessel and the route or the point of entry in the skull base. The diagnosis of a persistent PaA requires the vessel to originate from the ICA (type 1) or ECA (type 2) and enter the skull through the foramen magnum. Further distinction between types 1 and 2 can be made on the basis of the fact that type 2 vessels pass through the transverse foramen of the atlas, whereas type 1 does not. The persistent HA arises from the ICA at the level between C1 and C2 and enters the skull through the hypoglossal canal, the BA is filled beyond the point where the HA joins it, and the posterior communicating arteries are absent or not visible on angiograms. The TA usually originates in the cavernous ICA and then anastomoses with the BA with two possible routes through the skull base: a medial and a lateral one. It is important to differentiate this vessel from other vessels that can arise in or near this portion of the ICA; these arteries do not feed the posterior circulation. They typically are the marginal artery of the tentorium and the meningohypophyseal trunk, and other variants are far less common (i.e., persisting maxillary artery, middle meningeal artery with a cavernous carotid origin, etc.).

### Pearls and Pitfalls

- The most common carotid-vertebrobasilar anastomosis is the TA, followed by the HA and the PaAs. The existence of the OtA is controversial.
- The differentiation of the carotid-vertebrobasilar anastomoses should be based on origin of the vessel and point of entry through the skull base.
- The HA appears to be more commonly associated with intracranial aneurysms compared with other carotid-vertebrobasilar anastomoses.

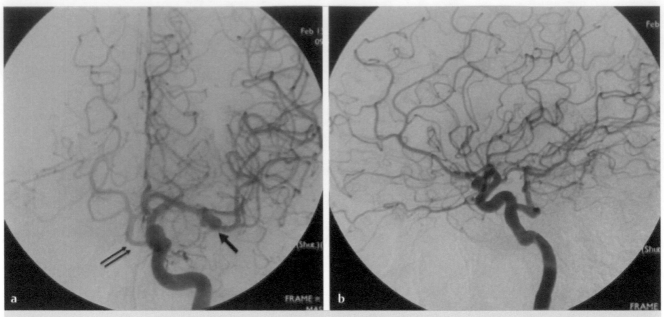

**Fig. 4.10** Left ICA angiogram in AP (a) and lateral (b) views shows a saccular aneurysm at the left middle cerebral artery bifurcation (*black arrow*) in a patient who was sent for further investigation for multiple aneurysms. There is an incidental finding of a left trigeminal artery (*double arrows*).

# Further Reading

[1] Agnoli AL. Vascular anomalies and subarachnoid haemorrhage associated with persisting embryonic vessels. Acta Neurochir (Wien) 1982; 60: 183–199

[2] Congdon ED. Transformation of the aortic-arch system during the development of the human embryo. Contrib Embryol 1922; 68: 47–110

[3] Lasjaunias P, Berenstein A. Surgical Neuroangiography. Vol 3. Berlin: Springer-Verlag; 1990: 197

[4] Lie AA. Congenital Anomalies of the Carotid Arteries. Amsterdam: Excerpta Medica Foundation 1968: 70–75

[5] Luh GY, Dean BL, Tomsick TA, Wallace RC. The persistent fetal carotid-vertebrobasilar anastomoses. AJR Am J Roentgenol 1999; 172: 1427–1432

[6] Padget DH. The development of the cranial arteries in the human embryo. Contrib Embryol 1948; 212: 205–261

[7] Saltzman GF. Patent primitive trigeminal artery studied by cerebral angiography. Acta Radiol 1959; 51: 329–336

[8] Siddiqui AH, Chen PR. Intracranial collateral anastomoses: relevance to endovascular procedures. Neurosurg Clin N Am 2009; 20: 279–296

[9] Vasović L, Jovanović I, Ugrenović S, Vlajković S, Jovanović P, Stojanović V. Trigeminal artery: a review of normal and pathological features. Childs Nerv Syst 2012; 28: 33–46

[10] Vasović L, Milenković Z, Jovanović I, Cukuranović R, Jovanović P, Stefanović I. Hypoglossal artery: a review of normal and pathological features. Neurosurg Rev 2008; 31: 385–395, discussion 395–396

[11] Vasović L, Mojsilović M, Andelković Z et al. Proatlantal intersegmental artery: a review of normal and pathological features. Childs Nerv Syst 2009; 25: 411–421

# 5 The Inferolateral and the Meningohypophyseal Trunk

## 5.1 Case Description

### 5.1.1 Clinical Presentation

A 53-year-old woman presented with left ptosis 4 months before admission and subsequently developed swelling of the left eye and proptosis. Investigation demonstrated a dural arteriovenous fistula involving the cavernous sinus region on the left side with drainage toward the superior ophthalmic vein on the left. Arterial supply was through the inferolateral trunk (ILT) from the left internal carotid artery (ICA). A previous transvenous attempt to treat this fistula was unsuccessful, as the compartment that harbored the shunt and opened into the superior ophthalmic vein could not be reached.

### 5.1.2 Radiologic Studies

See ▶ Fig. 5.1.

### 5.1.3 Diagnosis

Dural arteriovenous fistula of the cavernous sinus fed by the ILT.

## 5.2 Anatomy

A variable number of arterial branches arise from the cavernous ICA, the most consistent of which are the meningohypophyseal trunk (MHT) and the ILT. The MHT projects posteriorly and laterally from its origin at the posterior genu of the cavernous ICA and subdivides into four branches: the tentorial marginal artery (or artery of Bernasconi and Cassinari), the dorsal meningeal artery (also known as the dorsal or lateral clival artery), the basal tentorial artery, and the inferior hypophyseal artery. The tentorial artery courses posteriorly along the roof of the cavernous sinus, toward the free margin

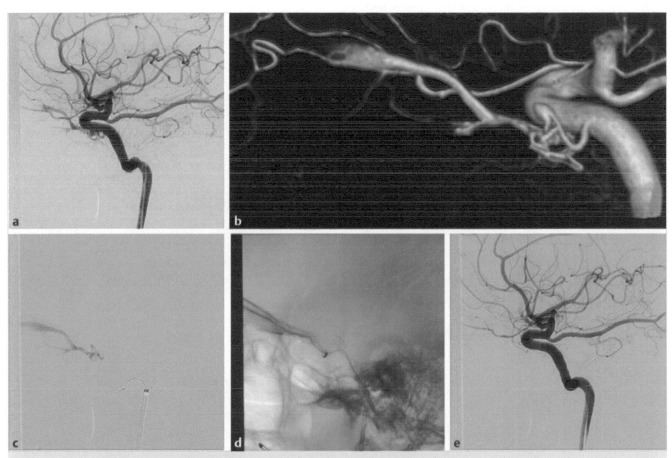

**Fig. 5.1** Left ICA angiogram in lateral view (a) and 3D rotational reconstruction (b) demonstrates the left cavernous sinus dural AV fistula. The sole arterial supply identified was through an enlarged left ILT from the left ICA. There was early venous drainage through the left superior ophthalmic vein, as well as some early filling of the proximal aspect of the inferior ophthalmic vein. Although the superior ophthalmic vein filled early, flow through the vein was slow, with delayed emptying and contrast stasis. A microcatheter was advanced into the proximal portion of the left ILT. Microcatheter injection (c) confirmed stable position proximally in the left ILT and demonstrated filling of the fistula. Flow through the fistula was slow, presumably as the microcatheter was partially occlusive in the ILT. Despite multiple attempts with different microcatheter and microguidewire combinations, no distal position of the microcatheter could be obtained. As the security margin was perceived to be small, no liquid embolic material was used, and instead, the single low-flow fistulous-type dural arteriovenous fistula was treated with a transarterial ligation approach, using electrolytically detachable coils that were deployed via the ILT (d) into the distal fistulous segment of the ILT, which led to angiographic obliteration of the fistula. Control angiographies obtained 1 year later in both the ECA and the ICA (e) did not demonstrate fistula recurrence.

of the tentorium. The dorsal meningeal artery runs superolateral to the abducens nerve into Dorello's canal and supplies the dura of the clivus, where it anastomoses with the clival branches of the ascending pharyngeal artery. The basal tentorial artery runs along the roof of the petrous bone laterally along the border between the tentorium and the petrous ridge. The inferior hypophyseal artery supplies the medial wall of the cavernous sinus.

The ILT arises from the horizontal segment of the cavernous ICA and also harbors three major branches: a superior, anterior, and posterior branch (► Fig. 5.2).

The superior branch supplies the roof of the cavernous sinus, and therefore the proximal portions of the oculomotor and trochlear nerves. Both the anterior and the posterior branch are subdivided into medial and lateral rami. The anteromedial branch courses toward the superior orbital fissure, supplying distal portions of the oculomotor, trochlear, and abducens nerves and anastomoses (as the deep recurrent ophthalmic artery) with the intraorbital ophthalmic artery. The lateral ramus of the anterior branch enters the foramen rotundum, thereby anastomosing with the external carotid artery (ECA; via the artery of the foramen rotundum, which arises from the maxillary artery). The posteromedial branch of the ILT runs toward the foramen ovale, where it anastomoses with the accessory meningeal artery of the ECA. This portion of the ILT supplies the abducens nerve, the gasserian ganglion, and the motor root of the fifth cranial nerve. The posterolateral branch of the ILT also supplies the gasserian ganglion. This branch anastomoses with the middle meningeal artery (MMA) at the level of the foramen spinosum.

## 5.3 Clinical Impact

Although the cranial nerve supply and the potential ECA–ICA anastomoses are covered in various chapters, we think that the ILT and MHT deserve special attention, as they exemplify the prototype of "dangerous" vessels that can still be embolized safely once their anatomy is understood. The ILT and MHT are important pathways for ECA–ICA anastomoses and play a major role in the supply of the cranial nerves of the cavernous sinus region. The major anastomoses to keep in mind when working in this region are between the anterolateral branch of the ILT and the artery of the foramen rotundum at the foramen rotundum, between the posteromedial branch of the ILT and the accessory meningeal artery at the foramen ovale, between the posterolateral branch of the ILT and the MMA at the foramen spinosum, and between the lateral clival artery of the MHT and the clival branch of the ascending pharyngeal artery at the level of the foramen lacerum. The cranial nerve supply to remember when treating lesions supplied by ILT and MHT includes:

- cranial nerve III: superior branch of ILT;
- cranial nerve IV: superior and anteromedial branch of ILT, tentorial artery of MHT;
- cranial nerve V: posteromedial and posterolateral branch of ILT; and
- cranial nerve VI: anteromedial and posteromedial branch of ILT, tentorial artery of MHT, and lateral clival artery of MHT.

To protect the small vasa nervorum in cases of particle embolization (e.g., to devascularize meningiomas), we advocate the use of particles that are larger than 150 μm in these vessels. In cases of dural arteriovenous (AV) fistulas fed by these arteries,

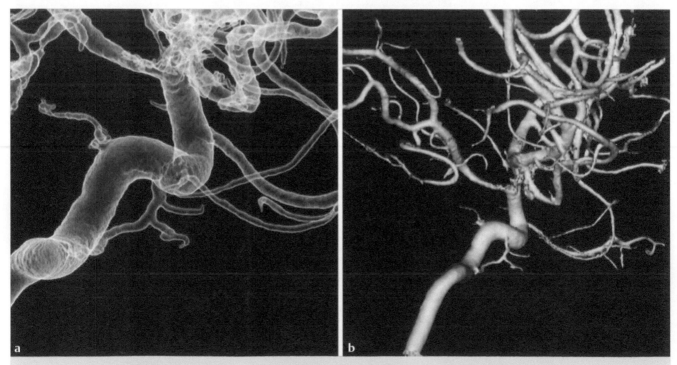

**Fig. 5.2** ICA angiogram 3D rotational reconstruction images (a,b) demonstrate the three major branches of the ILT: the superior, anterior, and posterior branches that extend toward the roof of the cavernous sinus, to the foramen rotundum, and to the foramen ovale, respectively.

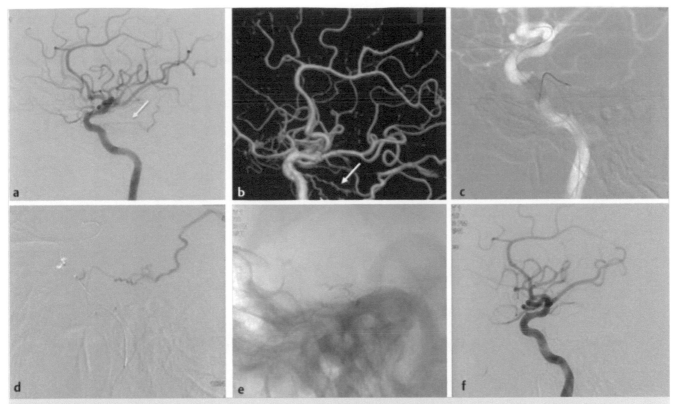

**Fig. 5.3** A right ICA angiogram in lateral view (a) and 3D reconstruction (b) demonstrate a tentorial dural arteriovenous fistula supplied solely by the artery of the free margin of the tentorium that arose from the MHT (*white arrows*). As this vessel formed a sharp angle with the ICA, the microguidewire could only enter the orifice but was unable to penetrate deeply. A balloon was placed just distal to the MHT and inflated, thereby allowing the microcatheter to be placed distal into the feeding artery (c,d). Before liquid embolic embolization, the position of the balloon was readjusted to cover the orifice of the MHT so as to stabilize the microcatheter and avoid reflux to the ICA. Plain radiography (e) reveals the glue cast. Complete obliteration of the fistula was achieved (f).

transvenous approaches (especially for cavernous sinus dural fistulas) may be more desirable than transarterial approaches. For the transarterial approaches, liquid embolic materials that penetrate deeply or wedge-type injections carry the risk of opening the collaterals and anastomoses, and therefore carry a higher risk for inadvertent embolization of the intracranial circulation and interference with the cranial nerve supply.

# 5.4 Additional Information and Cases

The superselective arterial navigation of a microcatheter into these small vessels (MHT and ILT) can be challenging, as the catheter has to be guided from a significantly larger-size artery into a much smaller one, and this smaller artery arises either close to a curve or at an acute angle. In these instances, the microcatheter is likely to protrude into the larger parent vessel when forward pressure is applied, rather than advancing into the smaller feeding artery. In these instances, temporary inflation of a nondetachable balloon in the parent vessel during microcatheterization can facilitate superselective distal microcatheterization, as the inflated balloon not only prevents prolapse of the microcatheter into the parent artery but also redirects the trajectory of the applied forward pressure toward the MHT or ILT. Once a distal position is achieved, the balloon can be used to prevent reflux and to further stabilize the position of the microcatheter (▶ Fig. 5.3; ▶ Fig. 5.4).

## Pearls and Pitfalls

- There are considerable variations in the anatomy of the ILT and the MHT, and the different arteries arising from these trunks can only rarely be identified, as they are very small under normal circumstances.
- Conditions in which these arteries are enlarged include arteriovenous shunting lesions (especially dural AV fistulas of the tentorium and the cavernous sinus, but also maxillofacial arteriovenous malformations [AVMs]), meningiomas (especially if hypervascularized), cavernous hemangiomas of the cavernous sinus, juvenile angiofibromas, and paragangliomas.
- Navigation into these arteries may be made easier by using a balloon both to prevent protrusion of the catheter into the parent vessel (i.e., ICA) and to stabilize the position in the artery once selected.

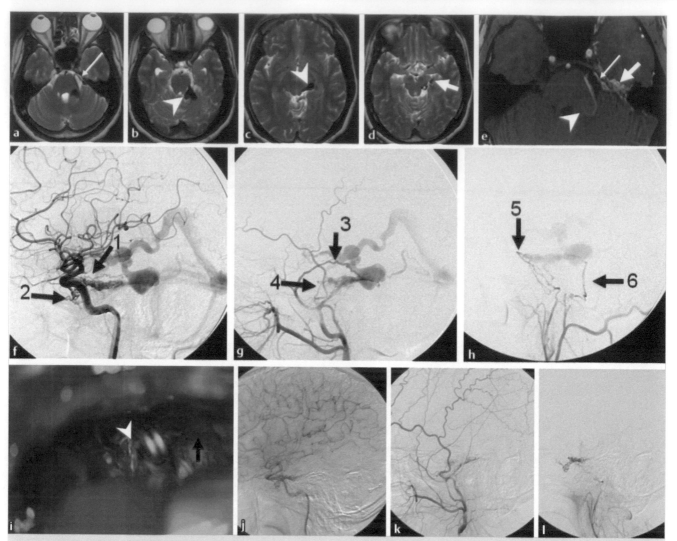

**Fig. 5.4** A 36-year-old patient presented with a bruit in his left ear that led to further investigation with MRI. Axial T2-weighted scans at various levels (a–d) and time-of-flight MRA source data (e) revealed a dilated lateral mesencephalic vein (arrowheads in a–e) draining toward the basal vein of Rosenthal (arrow in d). The vein was filled from a superior petrosal vein (small arrow in a and e) originating from the petrous apex to enter the mesencephalic vein at the lateral surface of the pons. The shunting zone was suspected to be located in the petrous apex, given the significant flow signals in this region (white arrow in e). Conventional angiography of the left ICA (lateral view in f), internal maxillary artery (g), and the common trunk of the occipital artery and the ascending pharyngeal artery (h) revealed a dural arteriovenous fistula that was fed by the artery of the free margin of the tentorium (1) of the MHT and by the posterior division of the ILT (2) that anastomoses with the MMA (3), via its lateral branch and with the accessory meningeal artery (4) via its medial branch. The ascending pharyngeal artery contributes to the shunt via the lateral clival anastomosis with the MHT (5). Note the stylomastoid branch of the occipital artery (6) that anastomoses with the petrosal branch of the MMA to supply the facial nerve in the facial arcade. Given the rich anastomotic network and the close relationship to the facial nerve supply, a surgical approach with surgical disconnection of the petrosal vein was favored over an endovascular approach. The surgical view (i) shows the clip on the petrosal vein (the arrowhead is pointing to the deflated remnant of this vein). The clip was placed at the dural piercing of the petrosal vein (the arrow points to the dura covering the petrous apex). Postsurgical conventional angiography of the left ICA (lateral view in j), the internal maxillary artery (k), and the common trunk of the occipital artery and the ascending pharyngeal artery (l) revealed complete exclusion of the cortical venous reflux

# Further Reading

[1] Capo H, Kupersmith MJ, Berenstein A, Choi IS, Diamond GA. The clinical importance of the inferolateral trunk of the internal carotid artery. Neurosurgery 1991; 28: 733–737, discussion 737–738

[2] Lasjaunias P, Moret J, Mink J. The anatomy of the inferolateral trunk (ILT) of the internal carotid artery. Neuroradiology 1977; 13: 215–220

[3] Marinkovic S, Gibo H, Vucevic R, Petrovic P. Anatomy of the cavernous sinus region. J Clin Neurosci 2001; 8 Suppl 1: 78–81

[4] Reisch R, Vutskits L, Patonay L, Fries G. The meningohypophyseal trunk and its blood supply to different intracranial structures. An anatomical study. Minim Invasive Neurosurg 1996; 39: 78–81

[5] Robinson DH, Song JK, Eskridge JM. Embolization of meningohypophyseal and inferolateral branches of the cavernous internal carotid artery. AJNR Am J Neuroradiol 1999; 20: 1061–1067

[6] Zhao WY, Krings T, Yang PF et al. Balloon-assisted superselective microcatheterization for transarterial treatment of cranial dural arteriovenous fistulas: technique and results. Neurosurgery 2012; 71 Suppl Operative: ons269–ons273, discussion ons273

# 6 The Dural Ring and the Carotid Cave

## 6.1 Case Description

### 6.1.1 Clinical Presentation

In a 33-year-old woman with a long-standing history of migraines, an incidental aneurysm was discovered during routine MRI.

### 6.1.2 Radiologic Studies

See ▸ Fig. 6.1.

### 6.1.3 Diagnosis

Unruptured aneurysms of the superior hypophyseal artery above the distal dural ring.

## 6.2 Anatomy

The anatomy surrounding the area of the anterior clinoid process (ACP) and the so-called paraclinoid internal carotid artery (ICA) region is complex. The ACP connects medially to the planum sphenoidale via the roof of the optic canal and to the sphenoid body via the optic strut. The optic strut separates the optic canal (medially) from the superior orbital fissure (laterally). There are three dural folds in this region: the falciform ligament, the distal dural ring, and the proximal dural "ring," also called the carotid-oculomotor membrane (COM).

The falciform ligament is the most cranial of the three dural folds. It lies above the optic nerve just proximal to the optic canal entry point, where the nerves enter into the optic canal. This ligament blends medially with the dura that covers the

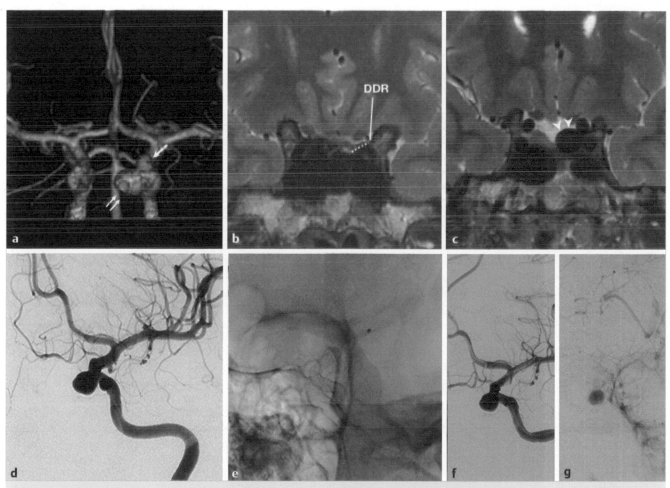

**Fig. 6.1** Computed tomographic angiography three-dimensional reconstruction (a) shows a medially oriented aneurysm (*double arrows*) in the clinoid segment of the ICA, arising below the origin of the ophthalmic artery (arrow). MRI coronal high-resolution T2-weighted images (b,c) show the location of the distal dural ring (DDR on b). The neck of the aneurysm is above the DDR, and the dome is therefore exposed to the subarachnoid space (arrowheads). Left ICA angiogram in oblique view before treatment (d) shows the clinoid segment medially oriented aneurysm before treatment. Plain radiography in oblique view (e) after deployment of two telescoping flow diverter stents demonstrates overlapping of the stents at the neck of the aneurysm. The left ICA angiogram after treatment in arterial (f) and venous (g) phases shows contrast stasis within the aneurysm sac, reflecting a satisfactory flow effect.

planum sphenoidale. The falciform ligament is an important landmark at the time of microneurosurgical approach to aneurysms in this region.

The proximal dural "ring" or COM marks the transition of the cavernous to the clinoid segment of the ICA. The COM lines the lower margin of the ACP. It separates the ACP from the oculomotor nerve, extending from the oculomotor nerve medially to surround the ICA, forming a distinct ring only on the anterior and lateral margins of the artery. The ring is incomplete on the medial side of the ICA.

The distal dural ring (DDR) is formed by dura extending medially from the upper surface of the ACP, posteriorly from the upper surface of the optic strut, laterally from the distal end of the carotid sulcus, and anteriorly from the upper surface of the diaphragma sellae and posterior clinoid process. The carotid collar is a thin dural layer between the COM and DDR that surrounds the clinoid ICA. The carotid collar is loosely attached to the ICA except at the DDR, where it blends into a continuous dural layer. The DDR and COM join together to form a single layer at the posterior tip of the ACP, which will blend with the diaphragma sellae.

The clinoid segment of the ICA is the portion of the artery located between the proximal and distal dural ring. The DDR is the anatomical landmark that separates the extradural from the intradural ICA, or the clinoid segment from the ophthalmic segment of the ICA.

The DDR is firmly attached to the lateral wall of the ICA, but medially, the dura turns downward before attaching to the ICA wall and creating a focal recess. This recess between the DDR and medial ICA wall was called the "carotid cave" by Kobayashi and colleagues in 1989. The importance of this recess lies in the fact that the arachnoid can push through to create a subarachnoid space below the level of the DDR. These recesses can be present in ~75% of individuals, according to anatomic studies in cadavers.

There are two large ICA branches arising in the region of the carotid cave: the ophthalmic artery (OA) and the superior hypophyseal artery complex.

The OA originates more frequently from the intradural ICA, distal to the DDR, below the optic nerve. However, there are cases when the origin of the artery is in the clinoid segment (i.e., below the DDR), having a short extradural component before it becomes intradural—the so-called interdural origin (~7%). In addition, the OA may originate from the cavernous segment, as the dorsal OA, or less frequently, from the A1 segment, the so-called primitive ventral OA (see Case 7).

The superior hypophyseal artery complex is a group of one to five small branches that arise from the medial wall of the ICA in the vicinity of the OA ("paraclinoid" ICA). They can be located above or below the DDR and are considered the vessels involved in the development of carotid cave aneurysms.

## 6.3 Clinical Impact

Determining the correct location of an aneurysm in this region is important when assessing its risk of rupture and, therefore, choosing the appropriate management strategies. Aneurysms located below the DDR are, in general, considered extradural, thus representing lesions with virtually no risk of subarachnoid hemorrhage. Extradural lesions will present clinically with symptoms related to mass effect, and asymptomatic small aneurysms are, in our practice, managed conservatively. In contrast, lesions distal to the DDR are intradural and, therefore, have a risk for subarachnoid hemorrhage and may warrant treatment.

Carotid cave aneurysms, considered by some to be the most proximal intradural ICA aneurysms, present a unique challenge. These lesions can be located below the level of the DDR but still have their dome exposed to the subarachnoid space, as the carotid cave may contain an arachnoid membrane recess. This is more probable if the aneurysm is anteromedially oriented, where the carotid cave is deeper and can even go down to the level of the COM.

Direct visualization of the DDR and the carotid cave can be challenging. Surrogate bone landmarks have been suggested on unsubtracted angiography, including the base of the ACP, the superior surface of the ACP, and the tuberculum sellae. These markers may not suffice, as the anatomy of the DDR is more variable than that of the bony structures.

The origin of the OA has also been suggested as a marker for the location of the DDR. Aneurysms proximal to the OA would be considered extradural, and those at or distal to the OA would be considered intradural. This approach has two main flaws. First, up to 15% of patients will have an "atypical" origin of the OA, as discussed previously. Second, the approach does not account for aneurysms that arise from the superior hypophyseal arteries located in the carotid cave.

On computed tomography, the optic strut (posterior root of the ACP), which forms the floor of the optic canal, has been suggested as a surrogate marker for the DDR. As discussed before, the DDR may turn downward before attaching to the medial wall of the ICA and, therefore, may be located below the level of the optic strut.

Attempts to directly visualize the DDR have been performed with high-field MR studies using high-resolution coronal T2-weighted fast spin-echo (T2W-FSE) as well as fusion MR angiography with 3D steady-state T2-weighting. These are promising techniques and will likely help in the understanding of the complex anatomy of the region, but large samples with surgical correlation to fully validate these methods are still lacking.

Carotid cave aneurysms carry the potential risk for a subarachnoid hemorrhage, but no cohort has separated this subtype of aneurysm from other paraclinoid aneurysms, so their natural history remains poorly understood. Treatment decisions regarding carotid cave aneurysms should be done on a case-by-case basis and require a thorough understanding of the local anatomy. MRI may help in better defining the anatomy of the dural folds, specially the DDR.

## 6.4 Additional Information and Cases

See ▶ Fig. 6.2, ▶ Fig. 6.3.

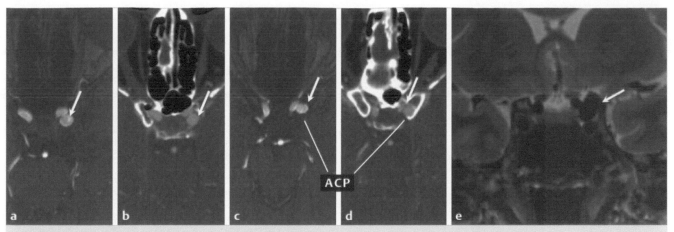

**Fig. 6.2** Composite panel (a–d) with source images of a 3-T time-of-flight MRA (a,c) and CTA (b,d) show a laterally oriented clinoid ICA aneurysm (*arrows*). The neck is located at the posterolateral wall of the artery, and the dome points laterally with remodeling the bone of the ACP. A MRI coronal high-resolution T2-weighted image (e) shows the sac pointing laterally, below the expected location of the DDR. This aneurysm, given that is pointing laterally, where the DDR is firmly attached, is therefore completely extradural and carries no risk for subarachnoid hemorrhage at this stage. Conservative management was recommended.

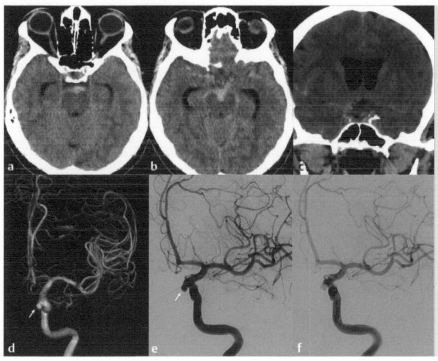

**Fig. 6.3** Unenhanced axial (a,b) and coronal (c) CT reveals diffuse hyperdensity within the basal cisterns and bilateral Sylvian fissures, representing subarachnoid hemorrhage. Blood is seen, in particular, in the carotid cave on the left. Left ICA angiogram (d,e) revealed a solitary left-sided carotid cave aneurysm (*white arrows*) that, given its location, the blood distribution, and the fact that no other culprit lesion was found, was deemed as the culprit lesion and subsequently coiled (f).

## Pearls and Pitfalls

- The DDR is the anatomical landmark that marks the transition from the extradural to the intradural ICA.
- The DDR has a narrow depression medially called the carotid cave, in which an arachnoid recess may be seen. This depression is deeper in the anteromedial region.
- Carotid cave aneurysms may have an intradural component even though they may be located below the level of surrogate bony markers for the DDR (i.e., the optic strut).
- Laterally oriented clinoid segment aneurysms are extradural, and their dome has no relation with the carotid cave.
- High-resolution MRI sequences may be helpful in directly visualizing the dural folds in this region, especially the DDR.

## Further Reading

[1] Beretta F, Sepahi AN, Zuccarello M, Tomsick TA, Keller JT. Radiographic imaging of the distal dural ring for determining the intradural or extradural location of aneurysms. Skull Base 2005; 15: 253–261, discussion 261–262

[2] Joo W, Funaki T, Yoshioka F, Rhoton AL, Jr. Microsurgical anatomy of the carotid cave. Neurosurgery 2012; 70 Suppl Operative: 300–311, discussion 311–312

[3] Kobayashi S, Koike G, Orz Y, Okudera H. Juxta-dural ring aneurysms of the internal carotid artery. J Clin Neurosci 1995; 2: 345–349

[4] Kobayashi S, Kyoshima K, Gibo H, Hegde SA, Takemae T, Sugita K. Carotid cave aneurysms of the internal carotid artery. J Neurosurg 1989; 70: 216–221

[5] Rhoton AL, Jr. Aneurysms. Neurosurgery 2002; 51 Suppl: S121–S158

[6] Thines L, Lee SK, Dehdashti AR et al. Direct imaging of the distal dural ring and paraclinoid internal carotid artery aneurysms with high-resolution T2 turbo-spin echo technique at 3-T magnetic resonance imaging. Neurosurgery 2009; 64: 1059–1064, discussion 1064

[7] Watanabe Y, Nakazawa T, Yamada N et al. Identification of the distal dural ring with use of fusion images with 3D-MR cisternography and MR angiography: application to paraclinoid aneurysms. AJNR Am J Neuroradiol 2009; 30: 845–850

# 7 The Dorsal and Ventral Ophthalmic Arteries

## 7.1 Case Description

### 7.1.1 Clinical Presentation

A 22-year-old man imaged before retreatment of a facial arteriovenous malformation (AVM).

### 7.1.2 Radiologic Studies

See ▶ Fig. 7.1.

### 7.1.3 Diagnosis

Dorsal ophthalmic artery supplying the orbital component of a facial AVM.

## 7.2 Embryology and Anatomy

The orbit contains structures derived from different embryonic layers: the neuroectoderm (optic nerve [ON], retina, ciliary bodies), the paraxial mesoderm (musculoaponeurotic system, bone, cartilage), and the surface ectoderm (lens, lacrimal gland, eyelids). In humans, there are three arterial systems that potentially participate in the supply to the orbit: the primitive ventral ophthalmic artery (PVOA), the dorsal ophthalmic artery (DOA), and the orbital artery, a branch of the stapedial artery that constitutes the future middle meningeal artery (see Case 3). As such, the final appearance of the ophthalmic artery (OA) and the blood supply to the orbit in the adult are the result of multiple regressions and anastomoses that occur early in embryonic life.

The PVOA arises from what will become the A1 segment of the anterior cerebral artery (ACA). This artery supplies the structures derived from the neuroectoderm and will follow the path of the ON, which is an "orbital extension" of the central nervous system. This artery enters the orbit through the optic canal, inferior and medial to the ON, and gives rise to the central retinal artery and the nasal ciliary artery.

The DOA arises from the cavernous (or fifth) segment of the internal carotid artery (ICA), enters the orbit through the superior orbital fissure, and courses inferior and lateral to the ON. This artery gives off the temporal ciliary artery.

The orbital artery (branch of the future middle meningeal artery) enters the orbit via the superior orbital fissure. It then divides into a medial ethmoidonasal branch and a lateral lacrimal branch. Both vessels will follow the various rami of the ophthalmic division of the trigeminal nerve (V1), providing supply to the musculoaponeurotic system and the eyelids.

According to Lasjaunias et al, in the embryo, the PVOA and the DOA anastomose in the orbit near the ON. In a process that is not predictable, the proximal part of the PVOA and DOA regresses and a new anastomosis develops between the supraclinoid ICA and the PVOA, forming the origin of the future OA. The remnant of the DOA is part of the inferolateral trunk (ILT). At the 20-mm stage, the ethmoidonasal (medial) branch of the orbital artery (branch of the future middle meningeal artery) crosses from lateral to medial over the ON to anastomose with what will become the orbital segment of the OA. At this stage, a true ON anastomotic ring has formed. The OA starts to assimilate the orbital artery, and at the 40-mm stage of the embryo, this process is completed and the configuration of the "adult" OA becomes apparent.

Multiple variations in the regression pattern of these primitive vessels and transient anastomoses may occur, which will give rise to different configurations in the origin of the OA and the orbital supply:

- If the PVOA regresses and no annexation from the supraclinoid ICA occurs, the supply to the orbit will be taken over by the DOA (the so-called persistent DOA). In this case, the OA will originate from the cavernous ICA in the region of the ILT and will enter the orbit through the superior orbital fissure.

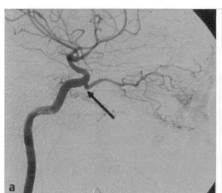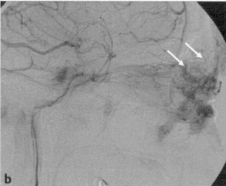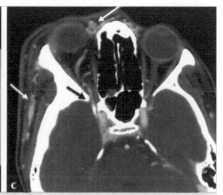

**Fig. 7.1** Left ICA angiogram in lateral view in early (a) and late (b) phases shows that the ophthalmic artery originates at the junction between the horizontal cavernous and the clinoid segment (*arrow*), within the region of the ILT, and supplies the facial compartment of a diffuse AVM (*white arrows* in b). Contrast-enhanced computed tomography (c) demonstrates the abnormal vessels over the roof of the nose and along the right side of the face (*white arrows*). The ophthalmic artery enters the orbit through the superior orbital fissure (*black arrow* in c).

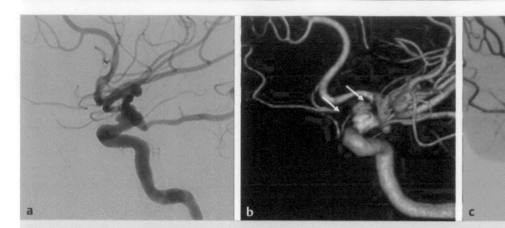

**Fig. 7.2** Left ICA angiogram in lateral view (a) shows a broad-necked aneurysm in the distal supraclinoid segment in a 54-year-old man who presented with subarachnoid hemorrhage. Note the absence of an OA in the expected location at the junction of the clinoid and supraclinoid ICA segments. Left ICA 3D rotational reconstruction (b) and maximum-intensity projection image (c) demonstrate an artery arising from the proximal left A1 segment (*white arrows*) coursing inferiorly, entering the orbit and supplying the orbital components, corresponding to a primitive ventral ophthalmic artery.

- A DOA may coexist with an adult-type OA (i.e., dual origin of the OA) or, less frequently, a PVOA. If an intraorbital anastomosis between both branches exists, both arteries will supply the oculosensory structures. In the absence of an intraorbital anastomosis, the central retinal artery will arise from the most distal (ventral) vessel.
- If the PVOA is not annexed by the supraclinoid ICA, the former will represent the main supply to the oculosensory structures (the so-called persistent PVOA). In this case, the retinal artery will be supplied by the PVOA, which will originate from the A1 segment of the ACA and enter the orbit through the optic canal. This variant can be seen with both an adult-type OA or a DOA, which will supply the rest of the orbital elements. Rarely, a persistent PVOA will be present as the sole supply to the orbit.
- In cases in which the A1 segment disappears, the PVOA may give rise to the ACA in a variant known as the infraoptic course of the ACA (see Case 10).

## 7.3 Clinical Impact

In patients with a DOA and a normal or PVOA, it will be the most distal artery that will supply the oculosensory structures. In the setting of coexistence of the DOA with a normal OA or PVOA, embolization through the DOA can be performed safely, if there are no anastomoses between the DOA and the PVOA or OA.

## 7.4 Additional Information and Cases

See ▸ Fig. 7.2; ▸ Fig. 7.3; ▸ Fig. 7.4; ▸ Fig. 7.5; ▸ Fig. 7.6; and ▸ Fig. 7.7.

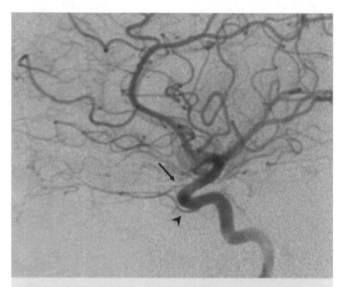

**Fig. 7.3** Left ICA angiogram in lateral view demonstrates the persistence of the dorsal ophthalmic artery (*arrowhead*) with an adult-type ophthalmic artery (arrow) or so-called dual origin of the ophthalmic artery. In this case, the central retinal artery arises from the supraclinoid ophthalmic artery (the more distal or ventral artery).

### Pearls and Pitfalls

- The remnant of the DOA in the adult is the ILT.
- If there is a DOA, it will enter the orbit through the superior orbital fissure and not through the optic canal, so all of its trajectory is extradural.
- A PVOA may be seen arising from the A1 segment. This artery will enter the orbit through the optic canal.
- In cases of a dual origin of the OA (i.e., a DOA and a PVOA or a normally located OA), it is the most distal vessel that provides the arterial supply to the oculosensory structures.

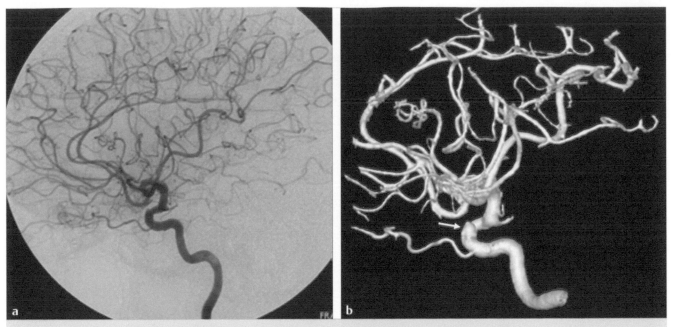

**Fig. 7.4** Left ICA angiogram in lateral view (a) and 3D rotational reconstruction (b) demonstrate persistence of the dorsal ophthalmic artery, as the supraclinoid ICA has failed to annex the primitive ventral ophthalmic artery, which has regressed. Note the presence of a carotico-ophthalmic aneurysm (*white arrow*) in this patient, who presented with subarachnoid hemorrhage.

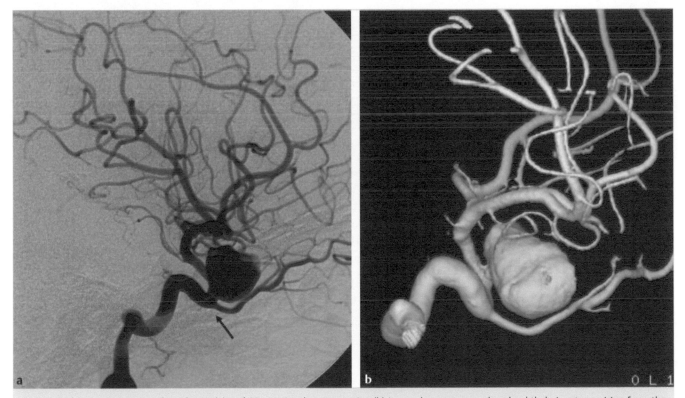

**Fig. 7.5** Right ICA angiogram in lateral view (a) and 3D rotational reconstruction (b) image demonstrate a dorsal ophthalmic artery arising from the right ILT region (*arrow*) in a patient with a large carotico-ophthalmic aneurysm.

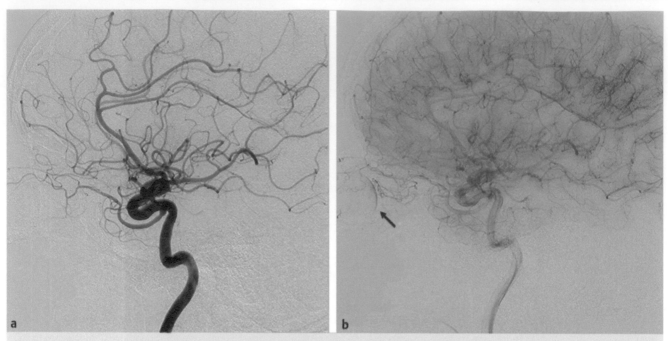

**Fig. 7.6** Left ICA angiogram in lateral view in arterial (a) and capillary (b) phases shows a dorsal ophthalmic artery arising from the ILT region of the cavernous left ICA. The choroidal blush seen on the capillary phase (*arrow*) is an indicator of the origin of the central retinal artery.

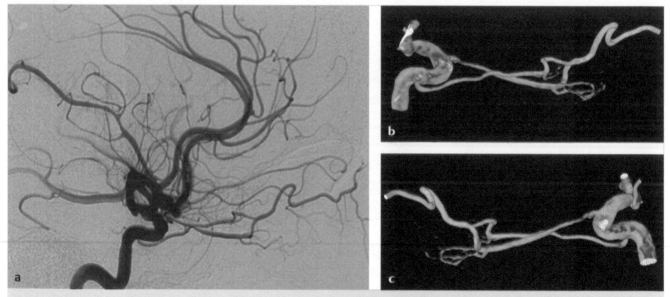

**Fig. 7.7** Right ICA angiogram in lateral view (a) and 3D rotational reconstruction (b,c) images demonstrate a case with persistence of the dorsal ophthalmic artery and an adult-type ophthalmic artery or the so-called dual origin of the ophthalmic artery.

# Further Reading

[1] Agarwal N, Singh PL, Karimi RJ, Gandhi CD, Prestigiacomo CJ. Persistent vestige of dorsal ophthalmic artery: a case report. J Neurointerv Surg 2013; 5: e25

[2] Hayreh SS. Orbital vascular anatomy. Eye (Lond) 2006; 20: 1130–1144

[3] Komiyama M. Letter to the editor – embryology of the ophthalmic artery: a revived concept. Interv Neuroradiol 2009; 15: 363–368

[4] Lasjaunias P, Berenstein A, ter Brugge KG. Surgical Neuroangiography. Vol. 1. 2nd ed. Berlin: Springer; 2006

[5] Willinsky R, Lasjaunias P, Berenstein A. Intracavernous branches of the internal carotid artery (ICA). Comprehensive review of their variations. Surg Radiol Anat 1987; 9: 201–215

# 8 The Branches of the Ophthalmic Artery

## 8.1 Case Description

### 8.1.1 Clinical Presentation

A 54-year-old man presented with a long-standing pulsatile mass in the left medial periorbital region.

### 8.1.2 Radiologic Studies

See ► Fig. 8.1.

### 8.1.3 Diagnosis

Medial orbital arteriovenous malformation (AVM) with main supply derived from the ophthalmic artery (OA).

## 8.2 Anatomy

The blood supply of the orbit depends mainly on the OA, with minor contributions from the external carotid artery (ECA). The intraorbital segment of the OA gives rise to numerous arterial branches that supply the orbital structures. The branching pattern of the OA shows a high variability in the order and site of origin of the different branches. Conceptually, these branches can be divided into four groups: the ocular group (central retinal and ciliary arteries), the orbital group (lacrimal and muscular arteries), the extraorbital group (ethmoidal, supraorbital, supratrochlear, palpebral, and dorsal nasal arteries), and the dural group (recurrent deep and superficial arteries). Typically, these branches are annexed by the OA and form the "adult" pattern of the OA.

### 8.2.1 Ocular Group

The ocular group originates from the embryonic internal carotid artery (ICA), via the ventral OA (hyoid branch) and shows little variability in its branching pattern. The order in which the ocular group branches originate is independent of the OA origin but depends on whether the artery courses over (83% of cases) or under (17% of cases) the optic nerve (ON). When the OA courses over the ON, the first branch is the central retinal artery (CRA), followed by a long posterior ciliary artery. When the OA courses under the ON, the first branch is the long lateral posterior ciliary artery and the second is the CRA. The CRA is a terminal branch, with no well-established anastomoses. Therefore, compromising this artery during embolization procedures will invariably result in retinal ischemia and monocular blindness. The long posterior ciliary arteries may arise separately or as part of a musculociliary trunk. They supply the choroid and are responsible for the choroidal blush, which serves as a surrogate marker for the CRA, as the ciliary arteries and the CRA arise closely together from the OA.

### 8.2.2 Orbital Group and Lacrimal Artery

The third branch typically corresponds to the lacrimal artery. The lacrimal artery typically arises from the first bend, lateral to the ON, and follows an oblique lateral course along the lacrimal nerve to reach a superior and medial position with respect to the lateral rectus to finally reach the lacrimal gland. The recurrent meningeal branch of the middle meningeal artery joins the lacrimal artery through the superior orbital fissure, serving as a potential anastomosis between ECA and ICA. Alternatively, the lacrimal artery can arise from the middle meningeal artery (meningolacrimal variant; see Case 25) and enter the orbit through the Hyrtl foramen. The lacrimal artery finally divides into muscular, zygomatic, and glandular branches. The latter gives rise to the lateral palpebral artery (see following).

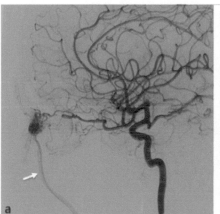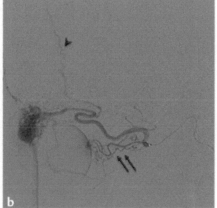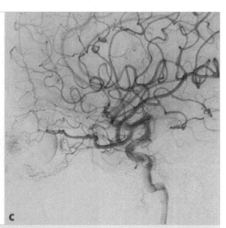

**Fig. 8.1** Left ICA angiogram in lateral view (a) shows an AVM nidus in the medial orbit, supplied mainly by the medial palpebral arteries, draining via the angular vein to the common facial vein (*white arrow*). Superselective microcatheter injection in the OA (b) proximal to the characteristic OA bend shows opacification of the long ciliary arteries (*black double arrows*) and the choroidal blush, meaning the catheter is proximal to the CRA, which is thus an unsafe position for embolization (see following). Note the anterior falcine artery (*black arrowhead*), which is a distal branch of the anterior ethmoidal artery. After a more distal catheterization and liquid embolic embolization, the left ICA angiogram in lateral view (c) shows no residual AV shunting and persistent that choroidal blush, indicating that the CRA was preserved.

### 8.2.3 Extraorbital Group

The ethmoidal arteries supply blood to the ethmoid sinuses, nasal cavity, and nasal septum. The anterior ethmoidal artery courses medial and inferior to the superior oblique muscle and enters the skull through the anterior ethmoidal foramen to become the anterior falcine artery. The size of this artery will depend on the extent of dural supply to the falx and anterior cranial fossa, which is highly variable. The posterior ethmoidal artery is an inconstant branch. It enters the skull through the posterior ethmoidal foramen and gives variable dural supply to the posterior and medial third of the anterior cranial fossa. At least one of the ethmoidal arteries will invariably be involved in the supply to anterior fossa meningiomas or dural AV fistulas. Nasal septal supply can be prominent and can explain failed ECA embolizations for treatment of refractory epistaxis.

The supraorbital artery usually arises from the third segment of the OA (after the bend around the ON). It courses under the roof of the orbit to exit through the supraorbital foramen and supplies the upper eyelid and scalp, where it anastomoses with superficial temporal artery branches.

The palpebral arteries are composed of the medial group (superior and inferior), distal branches of the OA, and the lateral palpebral branch of the lacrimal artery. There is a rich anastomotic network between these arteries within the eyelids.

The supratrochlear and dorsal nasal arteries are terminal branches of the OA. They leave the orbit at the medial corner of the orbit. The supratrochlear artery has a rich anastomotic network with its contralateral homolog and with multiple ECA branches that supply the skin in this region. The dorsal nasal artery anastomoses with its contralateral homologue over the root of the nose and with the angular branch of the facial artery (▶ Table 8.1).

## 8.3 Clinical Impact

Knowing the anatomy of the orbital segment of the OA is fundamental for performing a safe embolization of orbital lesions. The distal branches of the OA are safe to embolize, as long as the microcatheter tip is located beyond the origin of the CRA (arterial bend seen in lateral angiograms) and reflux is avoided.

**Table 8.1** Summary of the major anastomoses between the OA and ECA.

| OA Branch | Connecting Artery | ECA Branch |
|---|---|---|
| Lacrimal Artery | Recurrent Meningeal Artery | Middle Meningeal Artery |
| | Transverse Facial Artery | Superficial Temporal Artery |
| Ethmoidal Arteries | Nasal Septal Arteries | Sphenopalatine Artery (Internal Maxillary Artery) |
| Supraorbital Artery | Frontal Branch | Superficial Temporal Artery |
| Palpebral Arteries | Zygomatic Branch | Superficial Temporal Artery |
| | Infraorbital Artery | Internal Maxillary Artery |
| | Angular Artery | Facial Artery |
| Supratrochlear Artery | Frontal Branch | Superficial Temporal Artery |
| Dorsal Nasal Artery | Angular Artery | Facial Artery |
| | Lateral Nasal Artery | Facial Artery |

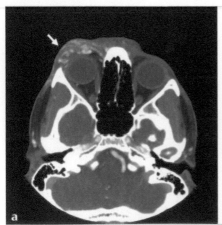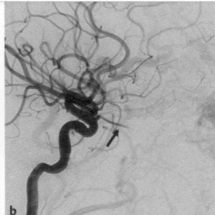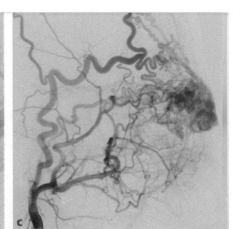

**Fig. 8.2** A 19-year-old man presented with a partially treated large orbital AVM. Axial CTA image (a) shows a superior palpebral mass with multiple tortuous vessels; pathognomonic findings for a facial region AVM (*white arrow*). Right ICA angiogram in lateral view (b) shows prior OA ligation (*black arrow*) with a preserved choroidal blush (not shown). Right ECA angiogram in lateral view (c) shows how the AVM has recruited supply from various superficial temporal artery and internal maxillary artery branches.

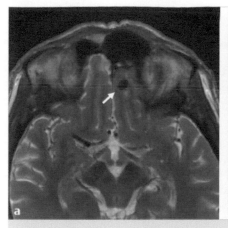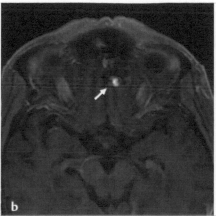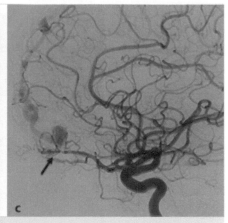

**Fig. 8.3** A 70-year-old man presented with nonspecific headaches. Axial T2-weighted (a) and contrast-enhanced T1-weighted (b) MRI show an enhancing flow-void in the left anterior fossa that corresponds to a venous pouch (*white arrows*), which raises the possibility of a dural arteriovenous fistula (DAVF). Left ICA angiogram in lateral view (c) shows a Borden type III ethmoidal DAVF, supplied by dural branches of the anterior ethmoidal artery (*black arrow*).

## Pearls and Pitfalls

- The OA serves as an anastomotic hub between various ECA branches.
- The CRA is a terminal branch with no documented anastomoses, and compromising this artery during embolization procedures will result in monocular blindness.
- There is dural supply from ethmoidal branches of the OA, which invariably will be involved in the supply to anterior fossa dural AV fistulas.
- The ethmoidal arteries' supply to the nasal septum is highly variable in its extent. In patients with failed ECA embolization for epistaxis, these branches can then be targeted surgically.

In addition, understanding the importance of documenting the choroidal blush (which depends on the ciliary arteries from the ocular group) before ECA and/or OA embolization is critical. If these safeguards are not followed, monocular blindness may result as a consequence of retinal infarct.

## 8.4 Additional Information and Cases

See ▶ Fig. 8.2, ▶ Fig. 8.3.

## Further Reading

[1] Agid R, ter Brugge K, Rodesch G, Andersson T, Söderman M. Management strategies for anterior cranial fossa (ethmoidal) dural arteriovenous fistulas with an emphasis on endovascular treatment. J Neurosurg 2009; 110: 79–84

[2] Hayreh SS. Orbital vascular anatomy. Eye (Lond) 2006; 20: 1130–1144

[3] Lasjaunias P, Berenstein A, ter Brugge KG. Surgical Neuroangiography. Vol. 1. 2nd ed. Berlin: Springer; 2006

[4] Perrini P, Cardia A, Fraser K, Lanzino G. A microsurgical study of the anatomy and course of the ophthalmic artery and its possibly dangerous anastomoses. J Neurosurg 2007; 106: 142–150

[5] Willems PW, Farb RI, Agid R. Endovascular treatment of epistaxis. AJNR Am J Neuroradiol 2009; 30: 1637–1645

# 9 The Anterior Choroidal Artery

## 9.1 Case Description

### 9.1.1 Clinical Presentation

A 50-year-old woman presented to the emergency department with acute onset of headache. CT demonstrated a subarachnoid hemorrhage, and digital subtraction angiography was performed.

### 9.1.2 Radiologic Studies

See ▶ Fig. 9.1.

### 9.1.3 Diagnosis

Anterior choroidal artery (AChoA) aneurysm in the setting of a duplicated AChoA.

## 9.2 Embryology and Anatomy

In its developmental anatomy, the internal carotid artery (ICA) ends with a bifurcation into a rostral (cranial) and a caudal branch. In adult life, the rostral branch will give rise to the ICA distal to the posterior communicating artery (PcomA), the AChoA, the anterior cerebral artery (ACA), and the middle cerebral artery. The caudal branch will form the PcomA, parts of the basilar artery, and the posterior cerebral artery (PCA). The cranial division gives rise to a prominent ACA and AChoA at the "choroidal" stage of development (roughly 5 weeks), which supply the choroid plexus and anastomose at the interventricular foramen with each other via their respective choroidal branches. In addition, both vessels also give rise to perforating diencephalic and telencephalic branches that course toward the

vesicles (i.e., the later hemispheres), with the AChoA supplying the more posterior aspect of the vesicle.

At this stage, the caudal division gives rise to the posterior choroidal artery that anastomoses with the AChoA at the atrium. As a result of hemispheric growth and increased antegrade flow of the basilar system that connects to the caudal division of the ICA, the telencephalic branches of the posterior choroidal artery will annex the telencephalic territory previously supplied by the AChoA and will form the later PCA. Thereby, the posterior choroidal branch adopts the hemispheric supply from the AChoA. As the hemispheres grow further, the volume of brain supplied by the AChoA diminishes in favor of the PCA. However, many variations in the territories of the ACA, PCA, and the AChoA exist and can be explained by the aforementioned embryological considerations. As the AChoA provides the main blood supply to the posteromedial aspects of the growing cortex during the early stages of development, it is conceivable that when the telencephalic branches of the embryonic posterior choroidal artery fail to take over this territory, cortical branches of the AChoA may persist as the main supply to the temporal, parietal, and occipital lobes. In fact, a spectrum of variations exists, ranging from a single cortical branch originating from the AChoA to complete replacement of the PCA by branches of the AChoA.

The AChoA typically originates distal to the PcomA as the first branch of the cranial division of the embryonic ICA from its posterior wall. Although "duplications" of the AChoA have been reported, they are presumably related to separate origins of the uncal (or telencephalic) branch and the diencephalic or choroidal branch of the AChoA from the ICA.

The typical course of the AChoA can be divided into the cisternal and intraventricular segments. In most instances, the AChoA courses through the perimesencephalic cistern, along

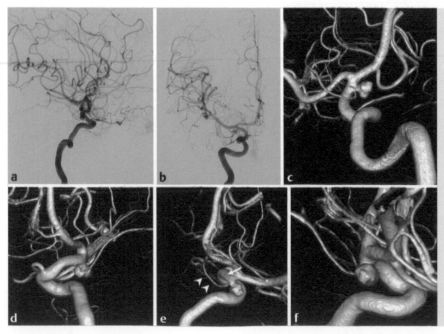

**Fig. 9.1** Right ICA angiograms in lateral (a) and anteroposterior (b) views and 3D rotational reconstruction (c–f) demonstrate a 4-mm narrow-necked inferolaterally directed aneurysm that is situated cranial to the origin of the AChoA. The AChoA appears duplicated, with the superior smaller branch (*white arrow*) having a short medial course toward the uncus and the larger branch (*arrowheads*) extending to the choroidal fissure.

the cerebral peduncles, and is in close proximity to the basal vein of Rosenthal and the optic tract. Anterolateral to the lateral geniculate body, the AChoA enters the choroidal fissure to reach the choroidal plexus of the temporal horn. The point of entry into the ventricle has been termed the plexal or choroidal point and is important, as no further brain-supplying vessels are derived from the AChoA beyond this point. It can be identified by the characteristic bend the artery makes (steep downward course for a few millimeters, followed by a sharp posterior turn) when entering the choroidal fissure (▶ Fig. 9.2).

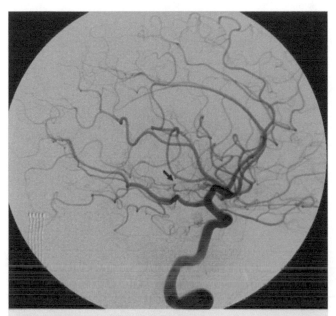

**Fig. 9.2** Right ICA angiogram in lateral view demonstrates the AChoA arising cranial to the PcomA and coursing posteriorly toward the choroid fissure. The plexal (or choroidal point) is marked by a sharp curve, followed by a posterior turn (*arrow*). Note the prominent pituitary blush in this patient.

The AChoA supplies the uncus, the amygdala, and the piriform cortex, as well as the anterior hippocampus. In addition, it will give rise to supply to the globus pallidum and the posterior limb of the internal capsule. Further posterior, it will give branches to the optic tract, the lateral geniculate body, the ventrolateral thalamus, and the mesencephalon (including red nucleus, substantia nigra, and subthalamic nucleus). After its plexal point, it will only supply the choroid plexus.

## 9.3 Clinical Impact

Given the extensive potential supply of the AChoA to "eloquent" brain structures, occlusion of this artery can have a significant effect on the patient. The most common neurological deficit in AChoA territory infarcts is hemiplegia, caused by the involvement of the pyramidal tract in the posterior limb of the internal capsule. However, hemisensory loss resulting from the involvement of the ventrolateral thalamus, or homonymous hemianopia, caused by the involvement of the lateral geniculate body or of the geniculocalcarine tract, may also be present. Hemineglect or aphasia can occur. This wide variety of symptoms is related to the anatomical variations in the extent of its territory and the presence of potential collateral supply. Infarctions in these regions can be related to small-vessel disease. However, they have also been described in patients with atrial fibrillation or atherosclerotic disease. Iatrogenic infarctions may be related to arterial dissections.

## 9.4 Additional Information and Cases

See ▶ Fig. 9.3, ▶ Fig. 9.4, ▶ Fig. 9.5, ▶ Fig. 9.6, ▶ Fig. 9.7, ▶ Fig. 9.8, ▶ Fig. 9.9, and ▶ Fig. 9.10.

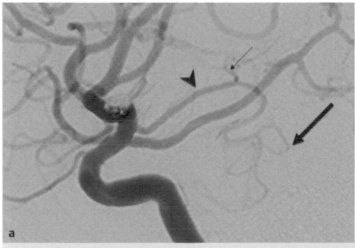
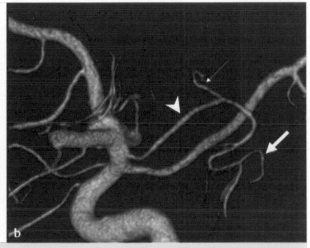

**Fig. 9.3** Left ICA injection, lateral view (a) and 3D reconstruction (b). Persistent neocortical anterior temporal lobe supply (*arrow*) from a dominant AChoA (*arrowhead*). Normally, the anterior temporal lobe is, on its inferior portion, supplied by the anterior inferior temporal branch of the PCA and, on its lateral portion, by the anterior temporal branch of the inferior division of the middle cerebral artery. In the present case, there is incomplete regression of the telencephalic AChoA branches because of incomplete annexation of the PCA of the anterior temporal lobe territory.

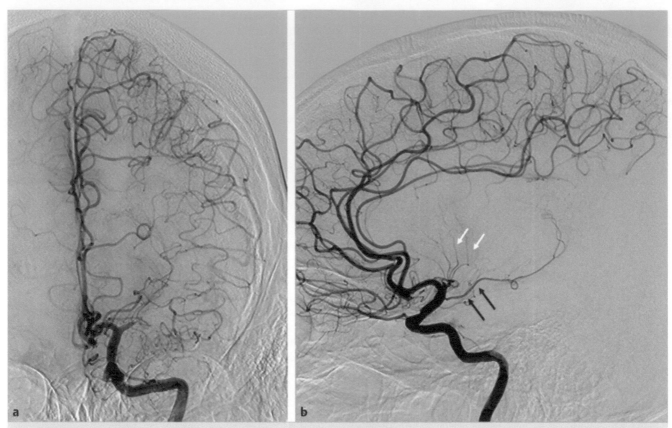

**Fig. 9.4** Left ICA angiogram in a patient with acute stroke and distal middle cerebral artery occlusion in anteroposterior (a) and lateral (b) views demonstrates the AChoA with its basal supply (*black arrows*) to the uncus, the amygdala, and piriform cortex, as well as the anterior hippocampus and, more posteriorly, the globus pallidum and the posterior limb of the internal capsule. Also note its spatial relation to the lenticulostriate arteries (*white arrows*).

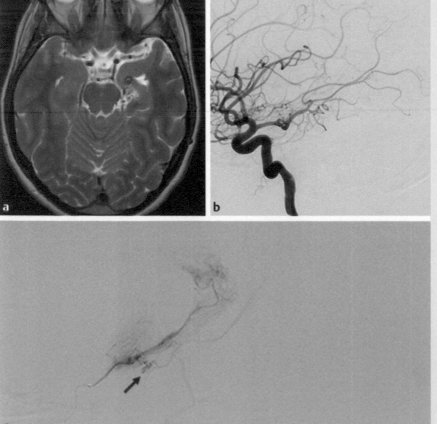

**Fig. 9.5** A 23-year-old patient was seen on follow-up after radiosurgery of a left mesial temporal lobe arteriovenous malformation (AVM) that had previously bled into the hippocampus. T2-weighted MRI follow-up after 4 years (a) demonstrated a small residual nidus of vessels as confirmed by left ICA angiogram in lateral view (b), with superselective injections (c). After injection into the AChoA, the AVM is seen to arise just proximal to the choroidal point and is fed by tiny perforating branches of the distal segment of the AChoA (*arrow*) before entering the choroid fissure.

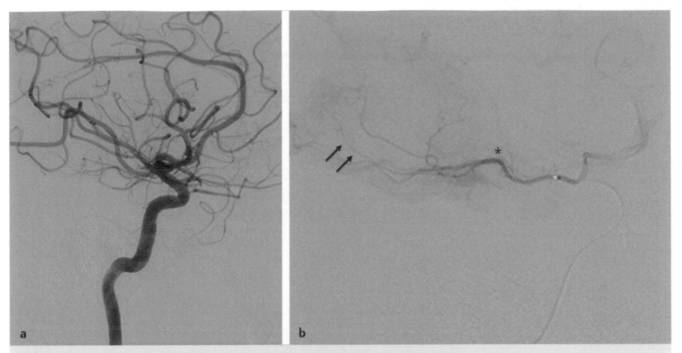

**Fig. 9.6** Right ICA angiogram in lateral view (a) with microcatheter injection (b) demonstrates the microanatomy of an AChoA with persistent telencephalic supply to the occipital lobe. Distant to the choroidal point (asterisk) in this patient, a telencephalic vessel can be appreciated that has retained supply to the occipital lobe (arrows).

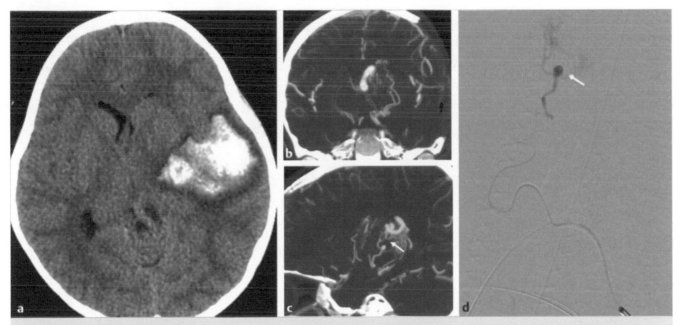

**Fig. 9.7** This 14-year-old child presented with acute onset of headaches and dense hemiplegia on the right, followed by loss of consciousness. Unenhanced axial CT (a) demonstrated a left basal ganglia hemorrhage, and emergency craniotomy was performed. CTA in coronal (b) and sagittal (c) reformats after this procedure demonstrated an AVM that was fed predominantly by lenticulostriate and choroidal arteries. A pseudoaneurysm (*white arrows*) arising from a dilated perforating branch of the AChoA was seen and deemed the culprit for this patient's hemorrhage. It was subsequently catheterized (d) and excluded with glue embolization to avoid early rebleeding.

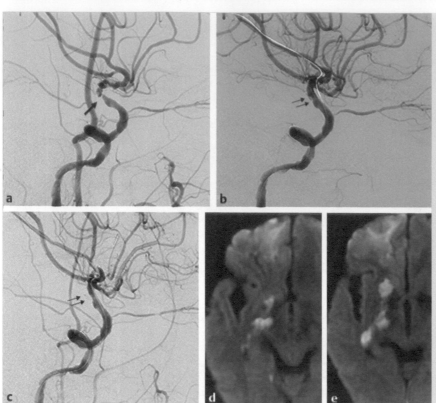

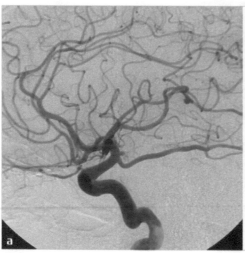

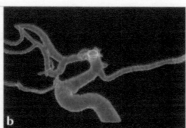

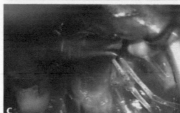

Fig. 9.8 A 71-year-old patient presented with multiple episodes of ischemia, the last of which had left her with a moderate hemiparesis despite best medical treatment. CT perfusion demonstrated hypoperfusion of her entire right hemisphere, and the patient experienced worsening of her symptoms when she had low blood pressure. Right ICA angiogram in lateral view (a) demonstrated a high degree of intradural ICA stenosis (*arrow*). Given her significant symptoms and failure of medical therapy, balloon angioplasty was attempted despite the close proximity between the stenotic plaque and the AChoA. After angioplasty (b,c), a dissecting flap (thin double arrows) was seen that, during mounting the stent over the exchange wire, had proceeded to occlude the AChoA. Diffusion-weighted MRI (d,e) after the procedure demonstrated an acute infarction in her AChoA territory involving the uncus, the hippocampus, and the cerebral peduncle.

Fig. 9.9 Left ICA angiograms in lateral view (a) and 3D rotational reconstruction (b) demonstrate a small AChoA aneurysm in this patient, who presented with an acute subarachnoid hemorrhage. The patient underwent surgical clipping (c).

## Pearls and Pitfalls

- During embryologic development, the AChoA transiently supplies an extensive cortical territory that is usually transferred later to the PCA. Therefore, the territory of this artery can vary tremendously between patients.
- As there is an absence of branches of the AChoA to the brain once it has pierced the ventricular wall, embolization past this plexal point is deemed safe.
- The AChoA anastomoses at the level of the plexus with posterior choroidal arteries of the PCA and at the interventricular foramen with the ACA.

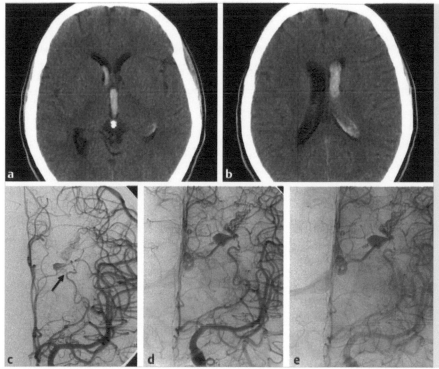

**Fig. 9.10** Unenhanced axial CT (a,b) in a patient presenting with headaches demonstrates a purely intraventricular hemorrhage that was related to a deep-brain AVM seen on the left ICA angiogram in anteroposterior view (c,d,e). The AVM was fed by both the perforating leptomeningeal vessels and the AChoA. The choroidal artery harbored an intranidal outpouching, which was regarded as the source of hemorrhage. The transition from a ventriculopetal to a ventriculofugal course (*arrow*) marks the entry of the AChoA into the lateral ventricle.

# Further Reading

[1] Hupperts RM, Lodder J, Heuts-van Raak EP, Kessels F. Infarcts in the anterior choroidal artery territory. Anatomical distribution, clinical syndromes, presumed pathogenesis and early outcome. Brain 1994; 117: 825–834

[2] Hussein S, Renella RR, Dietz H. Microsurgical anatomy of the anterior choroidal artery. Acta Neurochir (Wien) 1988; 92: 19–28

[3] Lasjaunias P, Berenstein A, ter Brugge KG. Surgical Neuroangiography. Vol. 1. 2nd ed. Berlin: Springer; 2006:563–575

[4] Rhoton AL, Jr, Fujii K, Fradd B. Microsurgical anatomy of the anterior choroidal artery. Surg Neurol 1979; 12: 171–187

[5] Rosner SS, Rhoton AL, Jr, Ono M, Barry M. Microsurgical anatomy of the anterior perforating arteries. J Neurosurg 1984; 61: 468–485

# Section III

## Anterior Circulation

# 10 The Infraoptic Course of the Anterior Cerebral Artery

## 10.1 Case Description

### 10.1.1 Clinical Presentation

A 34-year-old man presented with anxiety-related episodic hypertension. On physical examination, he was found to have a heart murmur and congenital absence of the ring and little finger of his left hand. He was subsequently diagnosed with having a bicuspid aortic valve and postductal coarctation of the aorta, which was treated successfully with aortic stenting. Screening cerebral magnetic resonance angiography showed an infraoptic course of bilateral anterior cerebral arteries (ACAs) and a 7.5-mm incidental anterior communicating artery (AcomA) aneurysm.

### 10.1.2 Radiological Studies

See ▶ Fig. 10.1.

### 10.1.3 Diagnosis

Left AcomA aneurysm with infraoptic course of bilateral ACAs.

## 10.2 Embryology and Anatomy

During normal embryogenesis, the rostrolateral portion of the perioptic arterial plexus gives rise to the terminal segment of the internal carotid artery (ICA) and the primitive ophthalmic artery. The middle cerebral, anterior cerebral, posterior communicating, anterior choroidal, and temporary dorsal and ventral ophthalmic arteries arise at this site.

The embryogenesis of an infraoptic ACA is still controversial. Some of the hypotheses proposed in the literature are that:

1. the embryonic anastomosis between the primitive maxillary artery and the ACA may persist;
2. an anomalous vessel may arise from the persistent enlarged embryonic anastomotic loop between primitive dorsal arteries and ventral ophthalmic arteries;
3. the primitive prechiasmal anastomosis between the branches of the ICA, ophthalmic artery, and ACAs may persist.

The error in embryogenesis is likely to occur in the early stages of cranial arterial development at the level of the perioptic arterial plexus.

The characteristic features of an infraoptic course of the A1 are that the artery arises from the ICA at the level of the ophthalmic origin and is located underneath the optic nerve to supply distally the territorial distribution of a normal ACA via an anastomotic segment in the vicinity of the ACA. Approximately 75% of infraoptic ACAs are seen on the right side, 15% on the left side, and 10% bilaterally.

The configurations of proximal ACAs in the presence of an infraoptic A1 have been classified into four types, as demonstrated in ▶ Fig. 10.2.

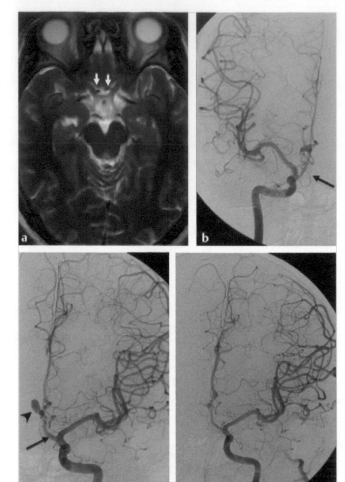

Fig. 10.1 T2-weighted MRI (a) shows an infraoptic course of the A1 segments of the ACAs bilaterally, with an abnormal medial course of the A1 segments relative to the optic nerves (*white arrows*). Right (b) and left ICA (c) angiograms in anteroposterior views show the infraoptic course of the A1 segments of bilateral ACAs (*arrows*). There is an outpouching at the left A1–A2 junction, representing a left AcomA aneurysm (*arrowhead*). Left ICA angiogram postcoiling in anteroposterior view (d) reveals complete occlusion of the left AcomA aneurysm after coiling.

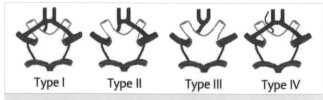

Fig. 10.2 The four different types of an infraoptic A1 as modified after Wong et al. Type 1: infraoptic anastomotic branch between the ICA and ACA in the presence of a normal anatomy around the ICA. Of note is that this type is not commonly associated with aneurysms. Type 2: infraoptic A1 with the bifurcation at the level of the ophthalmic origin but no supraoptic A1. Type 3: similar to type 2 except for the absence of contralateral A1. Type 4: an accessory ACA variant.

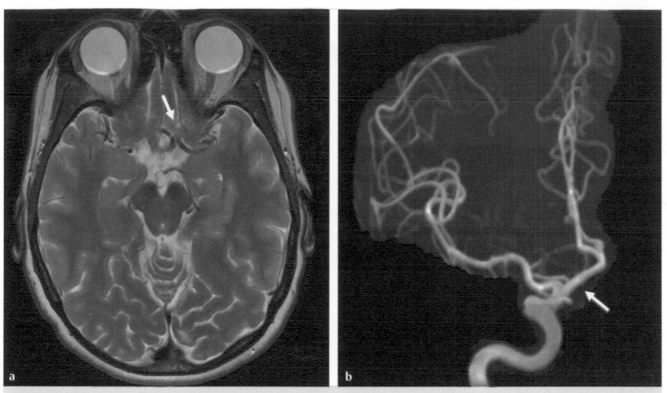

**Fig. 10.3** T2-weighted MRI (a) and time-of-flight MRA (b) demonstrate the infraoptic course of the A1 segment of the left ACA (*white arrows*).

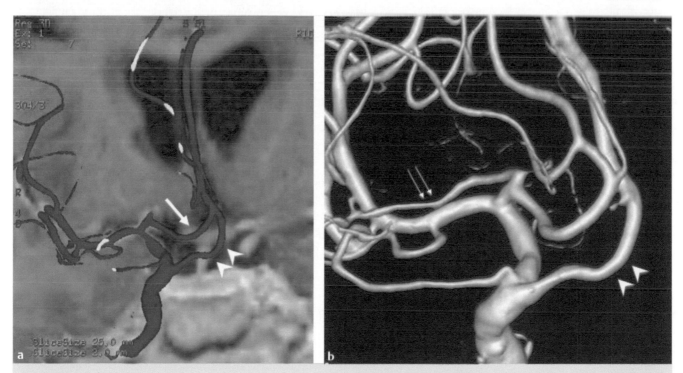

**Fig. 10.4** T1-weighted MRI in coronal view with angiogram fusion (a) and right ICA angiogram three-dimensional rotational reconstruction (b) demonstrate a dual origin of the ACA, with a normal ACA originating from the bifurcation (*white arrows*) and an infraoptic ACA arising from the cavernous right ICA (*white arrowheads*). A prominent right recurrent artery of Huebner is also noted (*thin white double arrows*), supplying the right middle cerebral artery cortical territory.

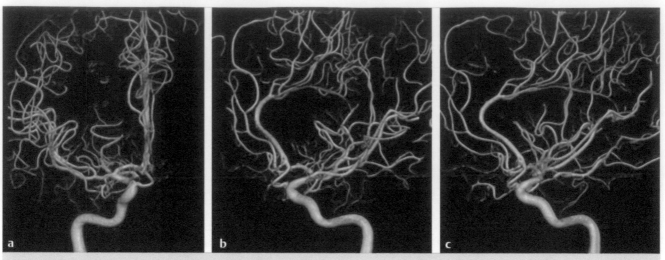

**Fig. 10.5** Right ICA rotational 3D angiogram in anteroposterior (a), oblique (b), and lateral (c) views in another patient also demonstrates a "double" right A1 segment (or type 1 infraoptic ACA).

## 10.3 Clinical Impact

Treatment of aneurysms associated with this variation will vary depending on the type of infraoptic course. In type 1, the presence of both an infraoptic A1 and a supraoptic A1 provides an additional access route for endovascular intervention. In type 2 configurations (with infraoptic A1), the aneurysms may be approached surgically via an anterior interhemispheric or subfrontal approach if endovascular options are not deemed possible. In cases with a proximal aneurysm of the infraoptic A1, however, the aneurysm may be obscured by the optic nerve during craniotomy. Because these types of aneurysms are usually in close proximity to the cavernous sinuses and the cranial nerves, they may be more difficult to treat surgically. Proximal control of the parent vessel may require an extended skull-base approach. In type 3, the absence of contralateral A1 limits the time allowed for temporary clipping. These considerations highlight why in our practice endovascular options are the method of first choice in patients presenting with an aneurysm and this peculiar variation.

including inherited connective tissue disorders, intrinsic structural factors such as medial defects, and acquired factors such as hypertension and hemodynamic stress. In 10% of cases, tumors (prolactinomas and craniopharyngiomas) have been present. Rarely, an infraoptic ACA is associated with congenital cranial abnormalities, such as abnormal gyral segmentation and craniofacial anomalies (▶ Fig. 10.3; ▶ Fig. 10.4; ▶ Fig. 10.5).

> **Pearls and Pitfalls**
>
> - An infraoptic segment of the A1 should be diagnosed if the A1 arises from the ICA at the level of the ophthalmic artery and if the vessel courses underneath the optic nerve.
> - Most infraoptic ACAs are right-sided, but they can occur bilaterally.
> - Proximal A1 aneurysms may be obscured during surgery by the optic nerve in patients with an infraoptic course of the A1.

## 10.4 Additional Information and Cases

Many anatomic variations associated with an infraoptic ACA have been described in the literature. They include association with a fused pericallosal artery, agenesis of the contralateral ICA, ectopic origin of the sylvian artery, azygous A2, carotid–vertebrobasilar artery anastomoses, plexiform AcomA, ophthalmic artery arising from the middle meningeal artery, and absent ACA associated with coarctation or Moyamoya. The infraoptic A1 s are frequently associated with intracranial aneurysms, according to the literature, in more than 50% of cases. Approximately two-thirds of the aneurysms are seen in the AComA. The pathogenesis of the aneurysms involves several factors,

## Further Reading

[1] Chakraborty S, Fanning NF, Lee SK, ter Brugge KG. Bilateral infraoptic origin of anterior cerebral arteries: a rare anomaly and its embryological and clinical significance. Interv Neuroradiol 2006; 12: 155–159

[2] Lasjaunias P, Berenstein A, ter Brugge KG. Surgical Neuroangiography. Vol. 1. 2nd ed. Berlin: Springer; 2006

[3] Mercier P, Velut S, Fournier D et al. A rare embryologic variation: carotid-anterior cerebral artery anastomosis or infraoptic course of the anterior cerebral artery. Surg Radiol Anat 1989; 11: 73–77

[4] Spinnato S, Pasqualin A, Chioffi F, Da Pian R. Infraoptic course of the anterior cerebral artery associated with an anterior communicating artery aneurysm: anatomic case report and embryological considerations. Neurosurgery 1999; 44: 1315–1319

[5] Wong ST, Yuen SC, Fok KF, Yam KY, Fong D. Infraoptic anterior cerebral artery: review, report of two cases and an anatomical classification. Acta Neurochir (Wien) 2008; 150: 1087–1096

# 11 The Anterior Communicating Artery Complex

## 11.1 Case Description

### 11.1.1 Clinical Presentation

A 37-year-old woman with long-standing chronic hydrocephalus presented with an incidental unruptured anterior communicating artery (AComA) aneurysm.

### 11.1.2 Radiologic Studies

See ▶ Fig. 11.1.

### 11.1.3 Diagnosis

AComA aneurysm.

## 11.2 Anatomy

The most widely used classification of anterior cerebral artery (ACA) anatomy to date is the one proposed in 1938 by Fischer. It defines five segments: A1, the precommunicating segment; A2, the segment that runs below the genu of the corpus callosum; A3, the segment that runs around the genu of the corpus callosum; and A4 and A5, which are considered the terminal portions of the ACA. Given that it has become common language in the neurovascular anatomy, this nomenclature is used in this section.

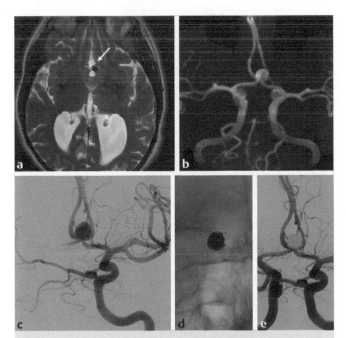

**Fig. 11.1** Axial T2-weighted MRI (a) shows dilated ventricles and a prominent flow void in the AComA region (*white arrow*). Time-of-flight magnetic resonance angiography (b) and left internal carotid artery (ICA) angiogram in working projection (c) reveal a broad-necked AComA aneurysm. Plain radiography (d) and simultaneous bilateral carotid injections (d) after X-stenting and coiling show complete occlusion of the aneurysm. The decision to perform an X-stent-assisted coiling was made to preserve the patency of the AComA.

The right and left A1 segments join to form the AComA in the midline in the lamina terminalis region, above the optic chiasm (70%) or, less frequently, above the cisternal segment of the optic nerves (30%). The "classic" anatomy, in which two equal-sized A1 segments form the AComA, is seen in only 20% of cases. Most commonly, one A1 segment will be dominant and bifurcate into the two A2 segments. In these cases, the AComA will be defined by the entry point of the hypoplastic A1. Complete absence of the A1 segment does not occur.

The AComA complex gives rise to small perforating vessels that are highly variable. Most commonly, these arteries will arise from the medial part of the AComA when the A1 segments are symmetrical, and ipsilateral to the dominant A1 when the segments are unequal. In cases of fenestrated or duplicated AComA, both limbs will have perforators arising from each limb. Three major groups of perforators have been described: the hypothalamic arteries that supply the lamina terminalis, the anterior hypothalamus, and the infundibulum of the pituitary; the chiasmal branches; and the subcallosal branches, which supply the rostrum and genu of the corpus callosum, the anterior cingulate gyrus, the septum pellucidum, and both columns of the fornix. The subcallosal artery is usually the largest, and often it is a single branch, whereas the other groups of perforators often consist of multiple small branches.

The anatomy of the medial lenticulostriate arteries arising from the ACA and of the recurrent artery of Heubner is discussed in Case 14. Multiple variations of the AcomA complex and its adjacent vessels can be identified.

### 11.2.1 A1 Segment Fenestration

Fenestrations of the A1 segment are rare, with an estimated prevalence of 0 to 4% in anatomic studies and less than 0.1% in angiographic studies (▶ Fig. 11.2). These fenestrations may be caused by the optic nerve coursing through the fenestration, which can be explained by the same considerations used to explain the infraoptic course of the A1, as outlined in the previous chapter; in most instances, though, a fenestration of the A1 segment is related to incomplete obliteration of anastomoses of a primitive vascular network. An association between A1 fenestrations and proximal A1 aneurysms has been proposed, but it is mostly based on isolated case reports.

### 11.2.2 AComA Fenestration

The AComA develops from a multichanneled vascular network during the embryologic stage that coalesces in various degrees by the time of birth. This process is responsible for the wide variety of AcomAs.

Fenestrations of the AComA are common, with large autopsy and surgical series reporting single, double, or even triple fenestrations of the AComA in up to 40% of specimens. The prevalence of these variations in imaging literature will vary, depending on the technique used. At this time, the gold standard is considered to be 3D rotational catheter angiography, given its highest spatial resolution and postprocessing capabilities. With this technique, variations can be seen in about 5% of cases. The

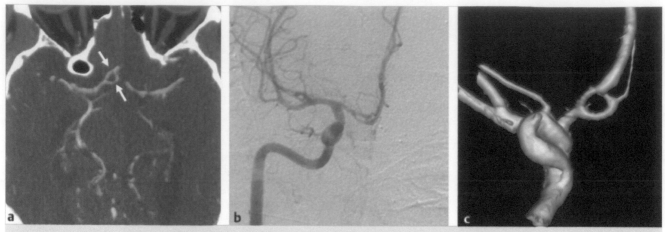

**Fig. 11.2** A 60-year-old man presented for postoperative arteriovenous malformation assessment. Axial CTA (a) reveals a fenestrated supraoptic A1 segment (*arrows*). Right ICA angiogram in anteroposterior view (b) and 3D rotational reconstruction (c) better depict the anatomic variation.

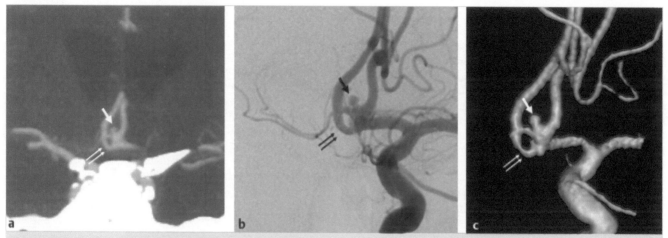

**Fig. 11.3** A 63-year-old woman presented with a subarachnoid hemorrhage. CTA in coronal reformat (a) shows an AComA fenestration (*double arrows*) with a small aneurysm arising from the upper limb (arrow). Left ICA angiograms in working projection (b) and 3D rotational reconstruction (c) better depict the findings.

difference from the surgical literature can be explained because in current practice, not all vessels are studied with 3D angiography, and competing flow from the contralateral A1 can preclude the opacification of smaller fenestrated limbs. In addition, in many fenestrations, bridging arteries are too thin (0.1–0.3 mm) and are beyond the spatial resolution of 3D angiography.

There is a proposed association between AComA fenestrations and aneurysms that is highlighted by the fact that about 8% of patients with AComA aneurysms harbor visible AComA fenestrations (▶ Fig. 11.3; ▶ Fig. 11.4).

## 11.2.3 Persistent Primitive Olfactory Artery

A persistent primitive olfactory artery is a rare, but well-known, variant of the proximal ACA, with an estimated prevalence of 0.14%. The ACA begins to develop as a secondary branch of the primitive olfactory artery at 5 weeks' gestation. Normally, the primitive olfactory artery regresses and becomes the recurrent artery of Heubner. If the normal regression of the

proximal primitive olfactory artery does not occur, the ACA or some of the ACA branches may arise from this persistent embryonic vessel (▶ Fig. 11.5). The persistent primitive olfactory artery courses along the straight sulcus and makes a characteristic hairpin turn to give rise to the distal ACA. Angiography in these cases may demonstrate an absent recurrent artery of Heubner. The incidence of ruptured aneurysms in patients with a persistent primitive olfactory artery has been reported to be high.

## 11.3 Clinical Impact

The main effect on the endovascular treatment that variations of the AComA anatomy have is in deciding the approach for the treatment of AComA aneurysms. Symmetric A1 segments may not tolerate two endovascular devices in them, so a bilateral approach with two femoral accesses should be considered. In addition, the angle in which the aneurysm arises from the AComA complex may make one side more favorable for endovascular approach than the other.

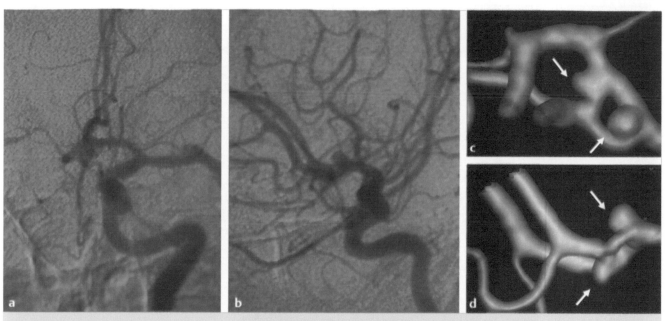

**Fig. 11.4** Left ICA angiograms in anteroposterior (a) and lateral (b) views and 3D rotational reconstruction (c,d) demonstrate a fenestrated A1 with aneurysms arising at both the proximal and the distal aspect of the fenestration (*arrows*).

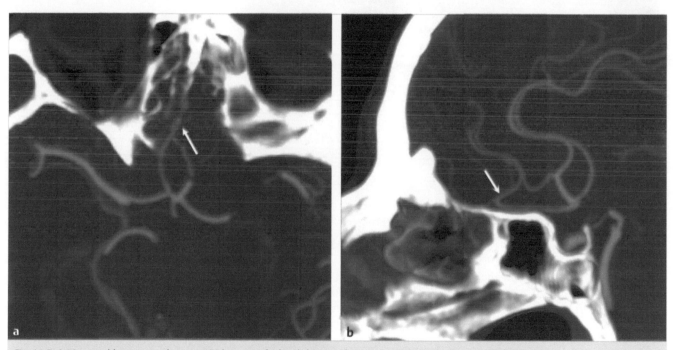

**Fig. 11.5** A 62-year-old woman underwent CTA because of a family history of aneurysms. CTA axial (a) and sagittal (b) projection images show a large branch arising from the AComA complex region that follows the path of the olfactory bulb. It has a distal sharp hairpin curve (*arrows*), after which it gives rise to the frontopolar and anterior internal frontal arteries. This corresponds to a persistent primitive olfactory artery.

It is also important to be aware of the local arterial anatomy and the branches arising from this region. Efforts should always be made to preserve the AcomA complex branches, as they supply highly eloquent brain regions. The operator should be familiar with the potential neurological syndromes related to ischemia from these territories (▶ Fig. 11.6; ▶ Fig. 11.7). Temporary occlusion with balloon catheters should be kept to a minimum during balloon assisted coiling, even if distal flow to the ACA is seen from the contralateral A1.

## 11.4 Additional Information and Cases

See ▶ Fig. 11.8.

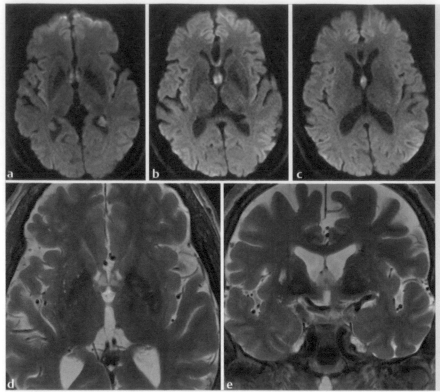

**Fig. 11.6** A 56-year-old previously healthy male patient experienced sudden onset of anterograde amnesia (Korsakoff syndrome) and inappropriate affect. Magnetic resonance diffusion-weighted imaging (a,b,c) and axial (d) and coronal (e) T2-weighted images revealed acute ischemia in the genu of the corpus callosum and the fornices bilaterally (i.e., in the arterial territory of the subcallosal artery that arises from the AComA complex).

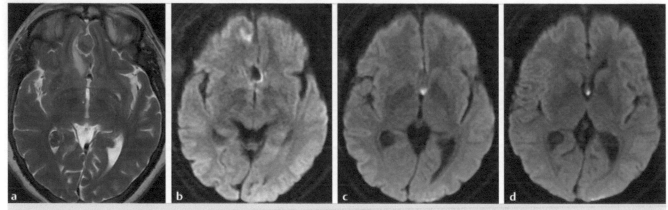

**Fig. 11.7** T2-weighted MRI (a) and diffusion-weighted images (b,c,d) of a patient who experienced altered affect and severe anterograde amnesia after removal of an olfactory groove meningioma and concomitant surgical clip ligation of an AComA demonstrate ischemia in the territory of the subcallosal artery, similar to the case in ▶ Fig. 11.6.

## Pearls and Pitfalls

- The anatomy of the AComA complex region is highly variable. This can be explained by persistence of anastomotic channels from a primitive vascular network of this region.
- There are several small arteries that arise from the anterior communicating artery and supply highly eloquent brain tissue, the most prominent of which is the subcallosal artery.
- Fenestrations may be associated aneurysm formation.

## Further Reading

[1] Aktüre E, Arat A, Niemann DB, Salamat MS, Başkaya MK. Bilateral A1 fenestrations: Report of two cases and literature review. Surg Neurol Int 2012; 3: 43

[2] Avci E, Fossett D, Aslan M, Attar A, Egemen N. Branches of the anterior cerebral artery near the anterior communicating artery complex: an anatomic study and surgical perspective. Neurol Med Chir (Tokyo) 2003; 43: 329–333, discussion 333

[3] de Gast AN, van Rooij WJ, Sluzewski M. Fenestrations of the anterior communicating artery: incidence on 3D angiography and relationship to aneurysms. AJNR Am J Neuroradiol 2008; 29: 296–298

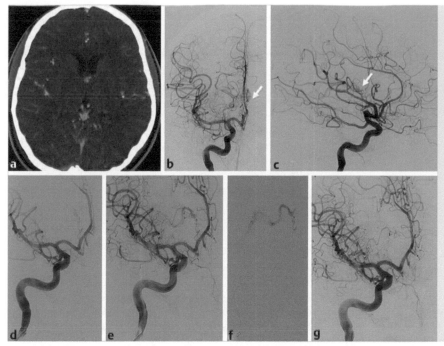

**Fig. 11.8** Contrast-enhanced CT (a) demonstrates a small subcallosal arteriovenous malformation in a 16-year-old boy who presented initially with a septal and intraventricular hemorrhage. Right ICA angiogram in anteroposterior (b) and lateral (c) views reveals a small arteriovenous malformation at the level of the foramen of Monro (*white arrows*), supplied by the subcallosal artery of the AComA, best seen on oblique view (d,e). The branch could be catheterized distally (f), and the arteriovenous malformation was occluded (g).

[4] Dimmick SJ, Faulder KC. Fenestrated anterior cerebral artery with associated arterial anomalies. Case reports and literature review. Interv Neuroradiol 2008; 14: 441–445

[5] Dimmick SJ, Faulder KC. Normal variants of the cerebral circulation at multidetector CT angiography. Radiographics 2009; 29: 1027–1043

[6] Fischer E. Die Lageabweichungen der vorderen Hirnarterie im Gefäßbild. Zentralbl Neurochir 1938; 3: 300–313

[7] Hernesniemi J, Dashti R, Lehecka M et al. Microneurosurgical management of anterior communicating artery aneurysms. Surg Neurol 2008; 70: 8–28, discussion 29

[8] Kwon WK, Park KJ, Park DH, Kang SH. Ruptured saccular aneurysm arising from fenestrated proximal anterior cerebral artery: case report and literature review. J Korean Neurosurg Soc 2013; 53: 293–296

[9] Serizawa T, Saeki N, Yamaura A. Microsurgical anatomy and clinical significance of the anterior communicating artery and its perforating branches. Neurosurgery 1997; 40: 1211–1216, discussion 1216–1218

[10] van Rooij SB, van Rooij WJ, Sluzewski M, Sprengers ME. Fenestrations of intracranial arteries detected with 3D rotational angiography. AJNR Am J Neuroradiol 2009; 30: 1347–1350

# 12 The Azygos Anterior Cerebral Artery

## 12.1 Case Description

### 12.1.1 Clinical Presentation

A 54-year-old woman was investigated for recurrent migraines. Unenhanced computed tomography at an outside institution had revealed an aneurysm.

### 12.1.2 Radiographic Studies

See ▶ Fig. 12.1.

### 12.1.3 Diagnosis

Azygos anterior cerebral artery (ACA) with a callosomarginal bifurcation aneurysm.

## 12.2 Embryology and Anatomy

The azygos ACA is a relatively uncommon vascular anomaly, with a prevalence ranging between 0.2% and 4%. Embryologically, the azygos vessel appears to form via fusion of the A2 segment, which originates either from the medial branch of the olfactory artery at the 16-mm stage of embryogenesis (40 days of gestation) or from the continuation of the median artery in the corpus callosum at the 20–24-mm stage. According to the Baptista classification, the azygos ACA is type 1 when there is a single unpaired ACA, as in the present case description. In type 2, there are bihemispheric ACAs, one of which is dominant and supplies both hemispheres. Finally, in type 3, there is an accessory ACA in the presence of a median artery that arises from the anterior communicating artery. Type 2 has an estimated prevalence of 2 to 7%. It can be differentiated from the azygos ACA by the presence of a hypoplastic A2 segment. Its main clinical relevance is that occlusion of the dominant A2 segment will result in bilateral ACA territory infarcts. Type 3 has also been termed ACA trifurcation. The ACA trifurcation is defined by three A2 segments arising from the anterior communicating artery. It has an estimated prevalence of 2 to 13%. This normal variant may be explained by persistence and/or enlargement of the median callosal artery (▶ Fig. 12.2).

Azygos ACAs are associated with other malformations, including midline anomalies, such as corpus callosum agenesis, holoprosencephaly, hydranencephaly, and defects of septum pellucidum. There appears to be an association with arteriovenous malformations (▶ Fig. 12.3), saccular aneurysms, defects of olfactory bulbs and tracts, and polycystic kidney disease.

Among these, the presence of saccular aneurysms is the most significant association. The incidence of aneurysm formation ranges from 13 to 71% in azygos ACA. These aneurysms are usually located at distal bifurcations of the unpaired ACA, generally at the callosomarginal bifurcation. Augmentation of hemodynamic stress is implicated as one of the probable mechanisms in aneurysm formation; another possible factor is ectasia of the azygos vessel resulting from mural degenerative changes.

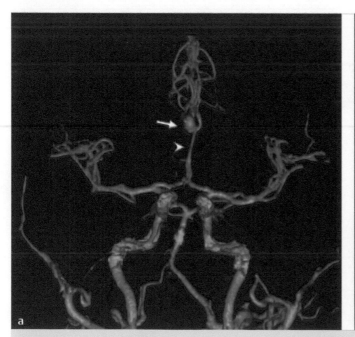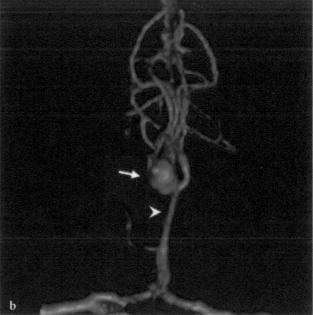

**Fig. 12.1** 3D CTA reconstructions (a,b) demonstrate an azygos ACA (*arrowheads*) with a distal aneurysm in the callosomarginal artery bifurcation (*arrows*).

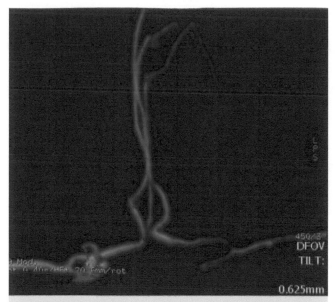

**Fig. 12.2** A 76-year-old woman presented with left watershed territory strokes. CTA 3D volume reconstruction in anteroposterior (AP) view shows three branches coming out of the anterior communicating artery complex region, in keeping with an ACA "trifurcation."

## 12.3 Clinical Impact

In a patient harboring an azygos ACA who presents with subarachnoid hemorrhage, careful evaluation of the distal azygos ACA has to be performed, given the significant association with saccular aneurysms. Because it is a single vessel supplying both frontal hemispheres, occlusion of the azygos ACA by thromboembolic events, vasospasm, or accidental surgical clipping may be disastrous.

## 12.4 Additional Information and Cases

See ▶ Fig. 12.4, ▶ Fig. 12.5, ▶ Fig. 12.6, and ▶ Fig. 12.7.

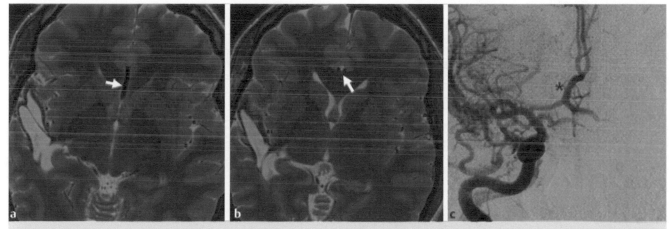

**Fig. 12.3** A 25-year-old woman was sent for postoperative assessment of an arteriovenous malformation. Axial T2-weighted MRIs (a,b) show a single prominent flow void in the anterior interhemispheric fissure that bifurcates in two branches in front of the genu of the corpus callosum (*arrows*). Right internal carotid artery angiogram in AP view (c) shows a single A2 segment (*asterisk*), which is the characteristic of the azygos configuration of the ACA.

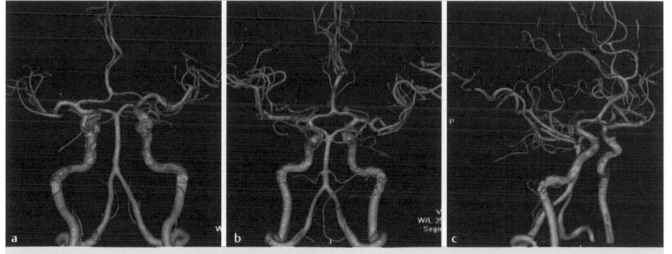

**Fig. 12.4** 3D CTA reconstructions in AP (a,b) and oblique (c) views of two different cases demonstrate an azygos A2 segment of the ACAs.

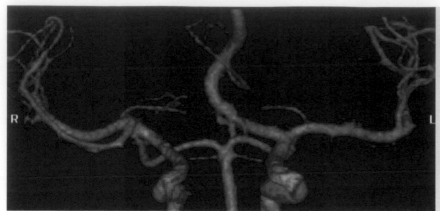

**Fig. 12.5** 3D CTA reconstruction in AP view in a patient with a azygos ACA and an hypoplastic/aplastic right A1 segment.

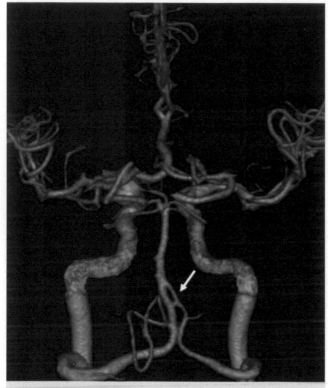

**Fig. 12.6** 3D CTA reconstruction in AP view in a patient with an azygos ACA associated with an unfused basilar artery (*arrow*).

## Pearls and Pitfalls

- Azygos ACA may be associated with distal aneurysms at its first bifurcation.
- Azygos ACA may be associated with midline anomalies, such as corpus callosum agenesis, holoprosencephaly, hydranencephaly, and defects of septum pellucidum.

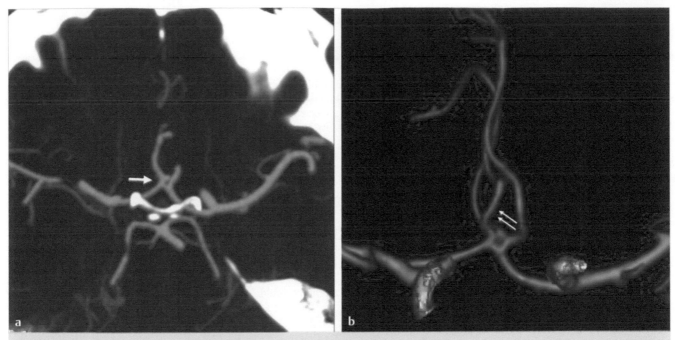

**Fig. 12.7** A 37-year-old woman presented with headaches to the emergency department. A CTA axial maximum-intensity projection image (a) shows an anterior communicating artery duplication (*arrow*). CTA 3D reconstruction (b) shows three A2 segments arising from the anterior communicating artery region; the middle one corresponds to the persistent median callosal artery (*thin double arrows*).

## Further Reading

[1] Auguste KI, Ware ML, Lawton MT. Nonsaccular aneurysms of the azygos anterior cerebral artery. Neurosurg Focus 2004; 17: E12

[2] Baptista AG. Studies on the arteries of the brain. II. The anterior cerebral artery; some anatomic features and their clinical implications. Neurology 1963; 13: 825–835

[3] Baykal S, Ceylan S, Dinç H, Soylev E, Usul H, Akturk F. Aneurysm of an azygos anterior cerebral artery: report of two cases and review of the literature. Neurosurg Rev 1996; 19: 57–59

[4] Huh JS, Park SK, Shin JJ, Kim TH. Saccular aneurysm of the azygos anterior cerebral artery: three case reports. J Korean Neurosurg Soc 2007; 42: 342–345

[5] Kanemoto Y, Tanaka Y, Nonaka M, Hironaka Y. Giant aneurysm of the azygos anterior cerebral artery—case report. Neurol Med Chir (Tokyo) 2000; 40: 472–475

[6] Lasjaunias P, Berenstein A, ter Brugge KG Surgical Neuroangiography. Vol. 1. 2nd ed. Berlin: Springer, 2006

# 13 The Cortical Branches of the Anterior Cerebral Artery

## 13.1 Case Description

### 13.1.1 Clinical Presentation

A 53-year-old man had a sudden onset of headaches and left-sided hemiparesis and was brought to the emergency department.

### 13.1.2 Radiologic Studies

See ▸ Fig. 13.1, ▸ Fig. 13.2, and ▸ Fig. 13.3.

### 13.1.3 Diagnosis

Ruptured arteriovenous malformation (AVM) fed by the inferior parietal branch of the distal anterior cerebral artery (ACA).

## 13.2 Embryology and Anatomy

Similar to the anatomy of the cortical branches of the middle cerebral artery (MCA), which are discussed in Case 16, there is considerable variation in the cortical branches of the ACA. Their nomenclature is primarily based on the cortical territory they supply. The distal ACA supplies the medial aspect of the frontal and parietal lobes and extends to a variable degree over the convexity in equilibrium with the distal MCA branches. Given its interhemispheric central supply, occlusion of the ACA is commonly associated with contralateral lower extremity weakness. After the anterior communicating artery, the A2 courses under the lamina terminalis and the genu of the corpus callosum to ascend in the interhemispheric fissure. The vessel continues as the pericallosal artery in the epicallosal cistern and gives rise to multiple branches that are named according to their vascular supply. Posteriorly, the pericallosal artery will be in hemodynamic balance with the pericallosal branch of the posterior cerebral artery at the level of the splenium. Via this anastomosis, the ACA can take part in the supply to the medial posterior choroidal arteries. The cortical branches of the ACA are, in order of appearance, the orbitofrontal, frontopolar, internal frontal (anterior, middle, and posterior), paracentral, superior parietal, and inferior parietal arteries. The largest branch of the A2 is the callosomarginal artery, which lies superior to the peri-

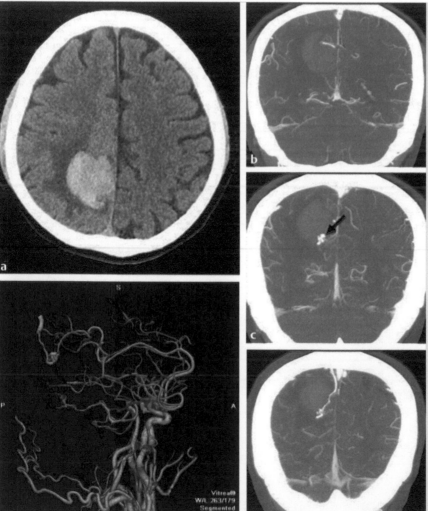

**Fig. 13.1** Unenhanced CT (a) demonstrates a right apical frontoparietal hemorrhage. CTA (coronal reformats: b,c,d; 3D reconstruction: e) revealed, as the source for the hemorrhage, an AVM fed by the distal ACA (inferior parietal branch) with a focal intranidal outpouching (*arrow*) that was held responsible for the bleed. Drainage of this monocompartmental AVM was directed into a median parietal vein. Case is continued in ▸ Fig. 13.2.

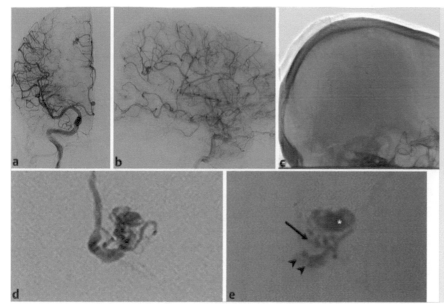

**Fig. 13.2** (a–e) Angiography with right internal carotid artery injection (anteroposterior and lateral) confirmed the diagnosis. A microcatheter was advanced into the distal inferior parietal branch (c), and the subsequent microcatheter injection (d) demonstrated the AVM, the intranidal aneurysm, and the drainage. The glue cast after liquid embolic embolization demonstrates occlusion of the intranidal aneurysm (asterisk), the distal feeding artery (*arrow*), and the proximal draining vein (*arrowheads*). Case is continued in ▶ Fig. 13.3.

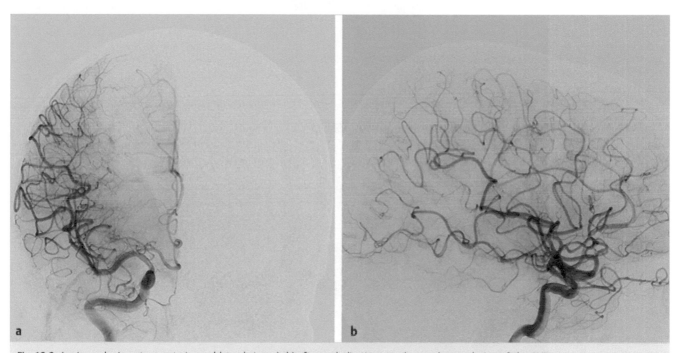

**Fig. 13.3** Angiography in anteroposterior and lateral views (a,b) after embolization reveals complete occlusion of the AVM.

callosal artery and from which some of the aforementioned branches may originate (▶ Fig. 13.4). In addition to these cortical branches, the pericallosal artery also supplies the corpus callosum via short radially oriented callosal arteries that traverse the corpus callosum to supply the septum and the fornix.

## 13.3 Clinical Impact, Additional Information and Cases

See ▶ Fig. 13.5, ▶ Fig. 13.6, and ▶ Fig. 13.7.

### Pearls and Pitfalls

- Cortical branches of the ACA are named depending on the cortical territory they supply and are highly variable in their origin from the distal ACA.
- The ACA communicates, via its distal pericallosal branch, with both cortical and choroidal branches of the posterior cerebral artery, and is in hemodynamic balance with the MCA over the convexity.

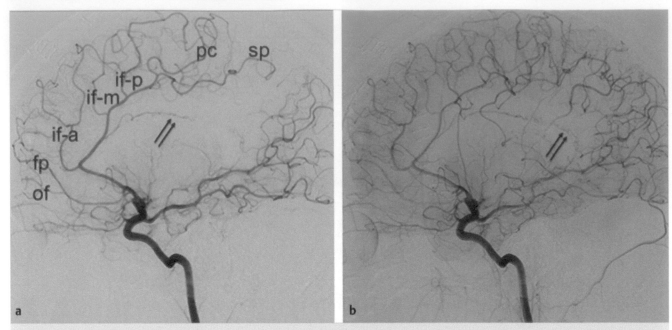

**Fig. 13.4** ACA anatomy; lateral views in early (a) and late (b) arterial phases. In this patient with an acute middle cerebral artery occlusion, the branches of the ACA can be well appreciated. Note also in the late arterial phase the anastomoses between the choroidal artery of the ACA with the posterior medial choroidal artery of the posterior cerebral artery (*arrows*). The cortical branches of the ACA are, in order of appearance, the orbitofrontal (of), frontopolar (fp), internal frontal (if) (anterior [a], middle [m], and posterior [p]), paracentral (pc), and superior parietal (sp) arteries. The inferior parietal artery is the least consistent branch of the ACA.

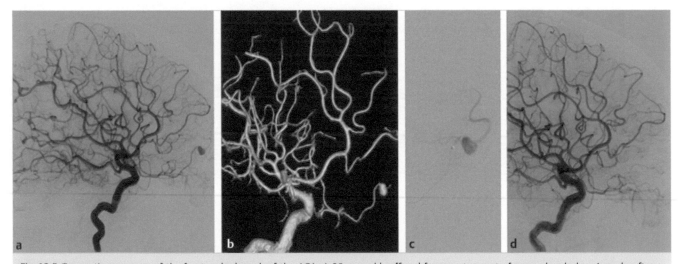

**Fig. 13.5** Traumatic aneurysm of the frontopolar branch of the ACA. A 39-year-old suffered from acute onset of severe headaches 4 weeks after a traumatic head injury. Imaging revealed a small cortical based hemorrhage and an underlying aneurysm of the distal frontopolar branch of the ACA (right internal carotid artery injection lateral view [a], and 3D rotational angiography [b]). Although the pathomechanism of delayed rupture of traumatic aneurysms is more common in the pediatric age group, the distal location and the clinical history made us consider a traumatic aneurysm; therefore, parent vessel occlusion with glue was performed after distal catheterization of the frontopolar branch (c). The control angiography (d) revealed occlusion of the vessel.

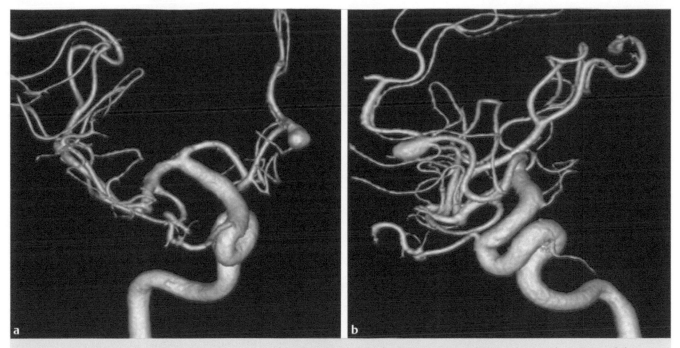

**Fig. 13.6** 3D rotational angiography in anteroposterior and lateral views (a,b) of a distal ACA aneurysm that originates at the junction of the pericallosal artery with the anterior internal frontal artery. The aneurysm has a broad communication with the parent vessel and the cortical branch.

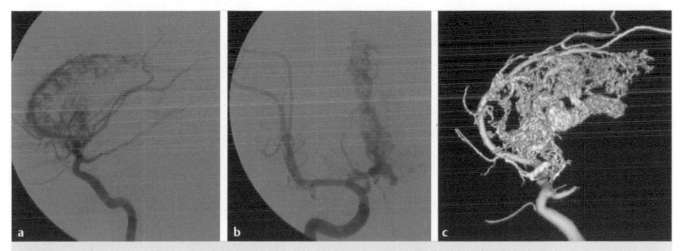

**Fig. 13.7** AVM of the corpus callosum that demonstrates enlargement of the multiple small callosal branches that arise in an "en passage" manner from the pericallosal artery to penetrate the corpus callosum (right internal carotid artery injection, lateral [a], posterior-anterior [b], and 3D rotational [c] angiography).

# Further Reading

[1] Gomes FB, Dujovny M, Umansky F et al. Microanatomy of the anterior cerebral artery. Surg Neurol 1986; 26: 129–141

[2] Morris P. Practical Neuroangiography. 3rd ed. Philadelphia: Lippincott Williams & Wilkins; 2013

[3] Perlmutter D, Rhoton AL, Jr. Microsurgical anatomy of the distal anterior cerebral artery. J Neurosurg 1978; 49: 204–228

[4] Türe U, Yaşargil MG, Krisht AF. The arteries of the corpus callosum: a microsurgical anatomic study. Neurosurgery 1996; 39: 1075–1084, discussion 1084–1085

# 14 The Middle Cerebral Artery Trunk

## 14.1 Case Description

### 14.1.1 Clinical Presentation

A 65-year-old patient with a long-standing history of high blood pressure presented with a stroke in the watershed territory between the lenticulostriate perforators and the penetrating leptomeningeal arteries. Outside magnetic resonance angiography described a filiforme middle cerebral artery (MCA) stenosis, and the patient was scheduled for intracranial percutaneous transluminal angioplasty and stenting

### 14.1.2 Radiologic Studies

See ▶ Fig. 14.1, ▶ Fig. 14.2.

### 14.1.3 Diagnosis

Occlusion of the M1 main trunk in the setting of a fenestrated MCA.

## 14.2 Embryology

The anterior cerebral artery (ACA) is the first and phylogenetically oldest telencephalic vessel and can be considered the terminal branch of the internal carotid artery (ICA). During the first weeks of fetal life, when the embryo is 7 to 12 mm long, lateral striate arteries arise from its wall and provide blood supply for embryonic structures of the telencephalic vesicle that will eventually become the MCA territory. Around the ninth week, after the maturation of the vertebrobasilar system, the MCA develops from the fusion of several ACA perforators of the lateral striate group. This developmental pattern matches that of the recurrent artery of Heubner (RAH). Because both the MCA and the RAH therefore share the same phylogenetic origin, their territories and anatomical variations are related to each other.

Both vessels give rise to perforating centripetal corticostriatal branches supplying, among other territories, the medial putamen, the caudate, and part of the anterior limb of the internal capsule, as is further discussed in Case 15.

Anatomical variations of the MCA have to be recognized when planning interventions to avoid damage or occlusion of perforating vessels that arise from the MCA and to assess their contribution to the perfusion of the deep MCA territory.

These variations are encountered less frequently than variants of other intracranial arteries and include the fenestrated MCA and the presence of a duplicated or accessory MCA (AMCA). Both types of variations are related to a persistence of

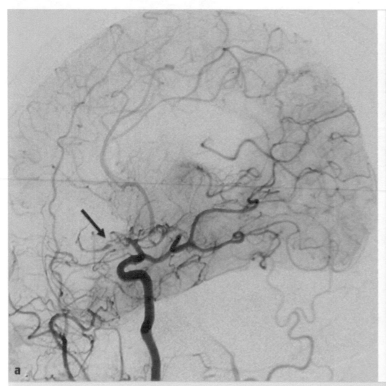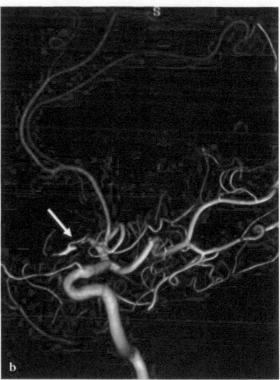

**Fig. 14.1** Right ICA angiogram in lateral view (a) and 3D reconstruction (b) shows a short-segmented occlusion of the right proximal MCA. The distal MCA is filled through a small vessel that arises from the proximal MCA and that enters the M1 distal to the segmental occlusion (*arrows*). There is very slow and incomplete filling of the distal MCA branches. The small-caliber upper limb of this proximal M1 fenestration acts as a natural (but insufficient) bypass. As percutaneous transluminal angioplasty of this small-caliber vessel would have resulted in rupture of the fenestration, the patient underwent extracranial to intracranial bypass surgery to revascularize the distal MCA territory. Case is continued in ▶ Fig. 14.2.

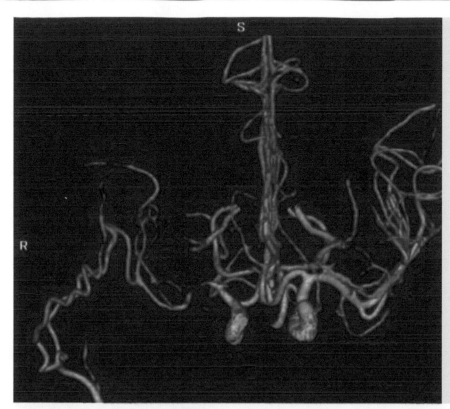

**Fig. 14.2** 3D CTA demonstrates patency of the extracranial to intracranial bypass, reconstituting the distal right MCA branches.

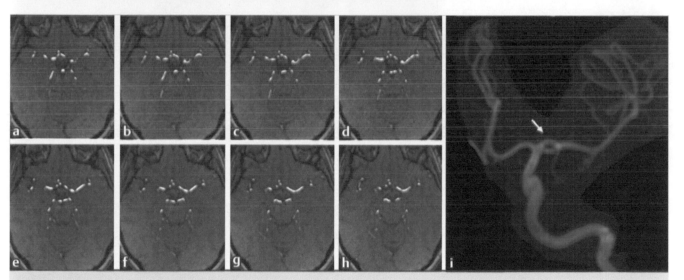

**Fig. 14.3** MRI time-of-flight source images (a–h) from cranial to caudal and 3D reconstruction (i) demonstrate a left-side fenestrated MCA (*arrow*), which fuses to become the M1 segment. This anatomical disposition should not be confused with pathology of the M1 segment (such as dissections or intraluminal thrombus). Note the early temporopolar branch arising from the inferior limb of the fenestrated MCA.

transient embryological vessels with a variant pattern of pruning the definitive vessel tree.

## 14.2.1 Fenestration

A fenestrated MCA arises as a single vessel from the ICA and feeds the MCA territory, but it diverges and reconverges along its course. It is a rare finding, with an incidence of less than 0.5% in angiographic series but as high as 1% in some anatomical series. This variant is usually located in the M1 segment and is often unilateral. A fenestration should not be confused with an early branching of the MCA, with a dissection with a patent pseudolumen, or with a superimposed vessel. The mechanism leading to MCA fenestration remains unclear. In their series of five MCA fenestrations, Gailloud et al. reported an early temporopolar branch arising from the inferior limb of the fenestrated MCA in all cases, suggesting this vessel could play a role in the absent fusion of the early perforating arteries. Perforating branches arise from the upper limb. Although this is a clinically silent anomaly, it is an area of hemodynamic stress and, thus, a site for aneurysmal development, similar to an unfused basilar artery (▶ Fig. 14.3). See also Case 20.

## 14.2.2 Duplicated MCA and AMCA

These two anomalies have usually been described separately, but they probably simply represent the two extremes of the spectrum of anomalies in the coalescence of the ACA embryonic perforating arteries toward the MCA. These branches can feed variable territories. Usually, one vessel supplies the perforators and the other one is purely cortical. There are, however, cases in which both MCAs supply perforators.

Several classifications have been proposed: Teal differentiates the AMCA from the duplicated MCA by the artery from which they arise. The duplicated MCA has its origin in the ICA, whereas the AMCA arises from the ACA. Manelfe classified the AMCA into three types. Type 1 is an anomalous vessel that arises from the internal carotid artery at a point proximal to its bifurcation (the duplicated MCA in Teal's classification), type 2 originates from the proximal portion of the ACA, and type 3 originates from the distal portion of the A1 segment of the ACA near the anterior communicating artery.

Lasjaunias et al. postulated that there is a proximal type AMCA (that comprises Manelfe's type 1 and type 2) and a distal type (Manelfe type 3). In the proximal type, the AMCA (i.e., the more cranial vessel) feeds the medial and lateral striate territories, whereas the MCA (proximal) is purely cortical (▶ Fig. 14.4). In the distal-type AMCA, there is in fact an enlarged RAH arising from the ACA or close to the AComA (▶ Fig. 14.5). In these cases, the MCA will not always be purely cortical but may also give rise to lateral perforators.

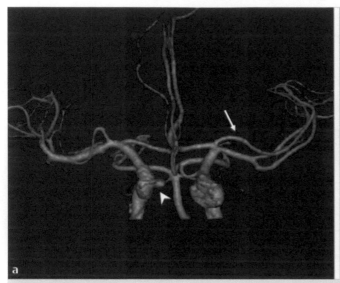
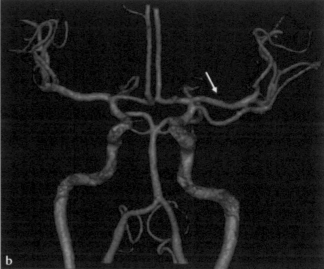

**Fig. 14.4** 3D CTA in AP views in two different cases (a,b) demonstrates left-sided proximal accessory MCAs in both cases (*arrows*). The perforators will typically arise from the more cranial vessel in these instances, whereas the more inferior vessel is typically only supplying the cortex. There is also a right carotid cave aneurysm in the first case (*arrowhead*).

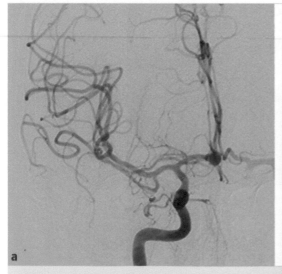
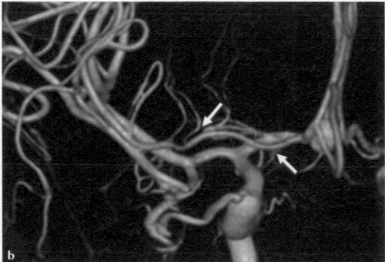

**Fig. 14.5** In this patient with an anterior communicating artery aneurysm, right ICA angiograms in AP view (a) and 3D rotation reconstruction (b) demonstrate the course of the RAH (*arrows*) traveling along the main MCA trunk to give rise to all frontobasal perforators.

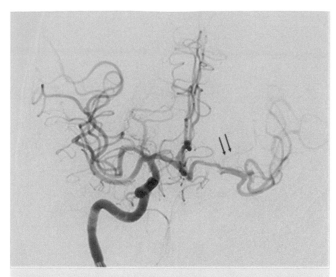

Fig. 14.6 A 55-year-old man with recurrent metastatic squamous cell carcinoma of the neck with left carotid blow out. Right ICA angiogram in AP view under balloon occlusion test of the left ICA demonstrates an incidental finding of a proximal type of right MCA duplication. Note that the more caudal branch is mainly supplying the cortex, whereas the lenticulostriate arteries (*arrows*) arise from the cranial branch.

In all of these scenarios, the true RAH may still be present, which will add complexity to the evaluation of the supply of the perforators and may even lead to the clinical picture of a "triplicated" MCA.

## 14.3 Clinical Impact

In cases with variant MCA trunk anatomy, it is important to identify which artery gives rise to the perforators and which one is purely cortical, or if they both feed the deep and superficial territories. It is quite evident that the planning of an endovascular procedure involving the ICA, ACA, or MCA (i.e., stenting and/or percutaneous transluminal angioplasty to treat an intracranial stenosis, as in our case) should include a thorough assessment of the presence of anatomical variants and their territories, as well as assessment of supply to the perforators, which (as we have seen) can arise from any of the aforementioned vessels with great variability. Without a complete evaluation of these structures, there is a risk that the intervention may interrupt the functional balance or cause occlusion of the perforating arteries.

An association between the duplicated MCA or the AMCA and cerebral aneurysms has been well documented.

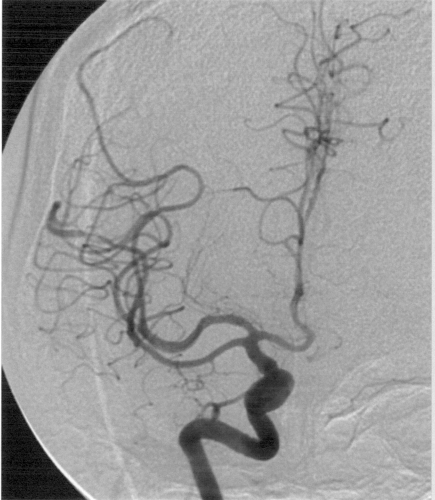

Fig. 14.7 Left ICA angiogram in AP view demonstrates similar findings to those in ► Fig. 14.4 of a proximal duplicated MCA, with the lenticulostriate arteries originating from the cranial branch.

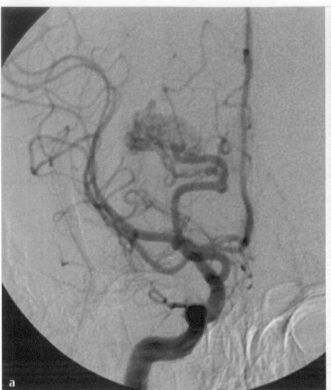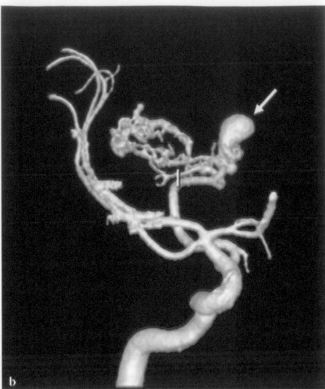

**Fig. 14.8** Right ICA angiogram in AP view (a) and 3D reconstruction (b) reveal an AVM supplied by branches of the right PCA through the right posterior communicating artery, with an intranidal aneurysm (*arrow*). Incidental findings of a proximal type right MCA duplication and fenestration of the A1 segment of the right ACA are also noted.

---

### Pearls and Pitfalls

- In cases of AMCAs, the perforators arise typically from the cranial segment, especially if the AMCA arises proximally from the ICA.
- A fenestrated M1 segment has to be differentiated from a dissection, a stenosis, or an intraluminal thrombus.

## 14.4 Additional Information and Cases

See ▶ Fig. 14.6, ▶ Fig. 14.7, and ▶ Fig. 14.8.

## Further Reading

[1] Dimmick SJ, Faulder KC. Normal variants of the cerebral circulation at multi-detector CT angiography. Radiographics 2009; 29: 1027–1043

[2] Feekes JA, Cassell MD. The vascular supply of the functional compartments of the human striatum. Brain 2006; 129: 2189–2201

[3] Gailloud P, Albayram S, Fasel JH, Beauchamp NJ, Murphy KJ. Angiographic and embryologic considerations in five cases of middle cerebral artery fenestration. AJNR Am J Neuroradiol 2002; 23: 585–587

[4] Kang HS, Han MH, Kwon BJ, Kwon OK, Kim SH, Chang KH. Evaluation of the lenticulostriate arteries with rotational angiography and 3D reconstruction. AJNR Am J Neuroradiol 2005; 26: 306–312

[5] Komiyama M, Nakajima H, Nishikawa M, Yasui T. Middle cerebral artery variations: duplicated and accessory arteries. AJNR Am J Neuroradiol 1998; 19: 45–49

[6] LaBorde DV, Mason AM, Riley J, Dion JE, Barrow DL. Aneurysm of a duplicate middle cerebral artery. World Neurosurg 2012; 77: e1–e4

[7] Lasjaunias P, Berenstein A, ter Brugge KG. Surgical Neuroangiography. Vol. 1. 2nd ed. Berlin: Springer; 2006

[8] Manelfe C, David J, Caussanel JP. L'artère cérébrale moyenne accessoire. Colloque d'anatomie radiologique de la tête, Montpellier. 1972

[9] Lasjaunias P, Berenstein A, ter Brugge KG. Surgical Neuroangiography. Vol 3: Clinical and Interventional Aspects in Children. 2nd ed. Berlin: Springer; 2006

# 15 The Lenticulostriate Arteries and the Recurrent Artery of Heubner

## 15.1 Case Descriptions

### 15.1.1 Clinical Presentation

A 44-year-old male patient presented with acute subarachnoid hemorrhage.

### 15.1.2 Radiologic Studies

See ► Fig. 15.1, ► Fig. 15.2.

### 15.1.3 Diagnosis

Anterior communicating artery aneurysm in the setting of congenital hypoplasia of the left internal carotid artery (ICA) and reconstitution of the left middle cerebral artery (MCA) through two enlarged lenticulostriate arteries.

## 15.2 Embryology and Anatomy

The lenticulostriate arteries are a group of small perforating vessels arising from the proximal segments of the anterior cerebral artery (ACA) and the MCA to supply primarily, but not only, the striatum.

Embryologically, they develop from the lateral striate arteries, a system that arises from the rostral division of the internal cerebral artery, to meet the growing needs of the expanding telencephalic vesicles. This group of arteries will give rise to the lenticulostriate arteries, including the recurrent artery of Heubner (RAH), but will also form the adult MCA. Thus, from an embryological point of view, the MCA represents an enlarged perforator branch of the ACA. See also Case 14.

As discussed in the previous case, there is a broad range of variations related to the perforators as a result of differing coalescences during embryonic life for the different perforator groups; therefore, they may arise as multiple single small vessels from the parent artery or from a common larger trunk or take over each other's territory. From medial to lateral, the following groups can be identified: the RAH, the medial lenticulostriate arteries from the ACA, the medial lenticulostriate arteries from the MCA, and the lateral lenticulostriate artery group. These groups can be interconnected with each other and form a rete (the most prominent example of which is the fenestration of the M1 or A1, as discussed in Case 14).

The RAH originates from the A1/A2 junction or in the first few millimeters of the A2 segment in 90% of cases. In only 10% of cases will it arise from the distal A1. The RAH supplies the anterior inferior striatum, anterior limb of the internal capsule, olfactory region, and anterior hypothalamus and is in a hemodynamic balance with the medial lenticulostriate arterial groups. Occasionally, the RAH can be duplicated or missing. The artery has a recurrent path turning laterally, coursing over the A1 (~60%), anterior to the A1 (~35%), and rarely, posterior to the A1 (3%). The territory supplied by the RAH is variable, as it is in balance with the medial lenticulostriate arteries (► Fig. 15.3; ► Fig. 15.4).

The perforators of the medial lenticulostriate arterial group, which originate from the proximal half of the A1 segment, vary highly in diameter and number, with a mean of eight (range, 2–15). Approximately half of the medial lenticulostriate arterial

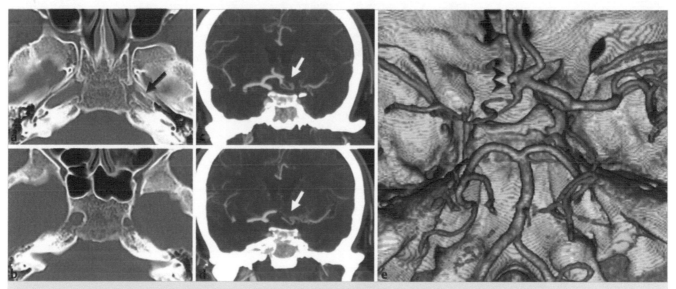

**Fig. 15.1** CT in the bone window (a,b), CTA in coronal view (c,d), and 3D reconstruction (e) demonstrate hypoplasia of the left foramen lacerum and the carotid canal (*black arrow*), indicating congenital ICA hypoplasia. CTA confirms absence of intradural filling of the left ICA and provides evidence for reconstitution of the left MCA via two separate arteries arising from the anterior communicating complex (*white arrows*). As the source of hemorrhage, a small, broad-based anterior communicating artery aneurysm (*black arrowheads*) was found. Case is continued in ► Fig. 15.2.

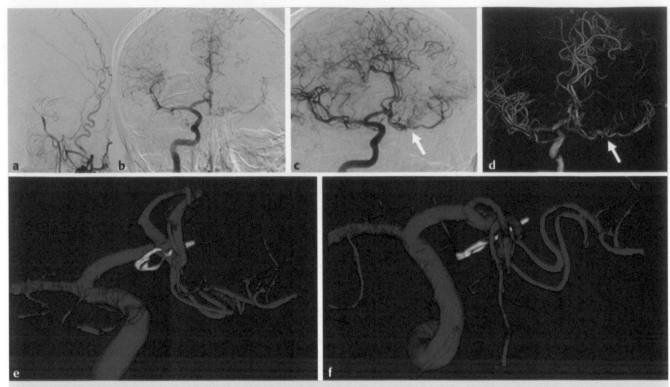

**Fig. 15.2** After clip exclusion of the aneurysm, left common carotid artery angiogram in anteroposterior (AP) view (a) confirms ICA hypoplasia. Right ICA angiogram in AP (b), oblique (c), and 3D reconstruction (d,e,f) demonstrates reconstitution of the MCA via two arteries of the anterior communicating complex that run in parallel and from which the perforating lenticulostriate vessels (*arrows*) arise.

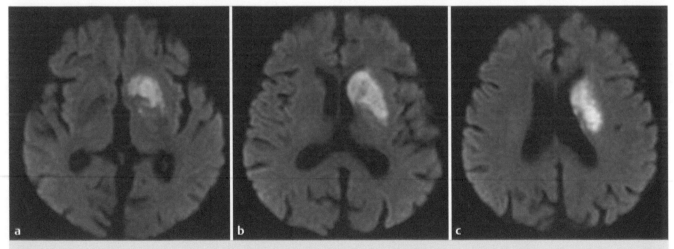

**Fig. 15.3** Diffusion-weighted MRI (a,b,c) in a patient with an extensive left Heubner territory infarction demonstrates abnormal signal intensity within the head of the caudate nucleus and the anterior basal ganglia.

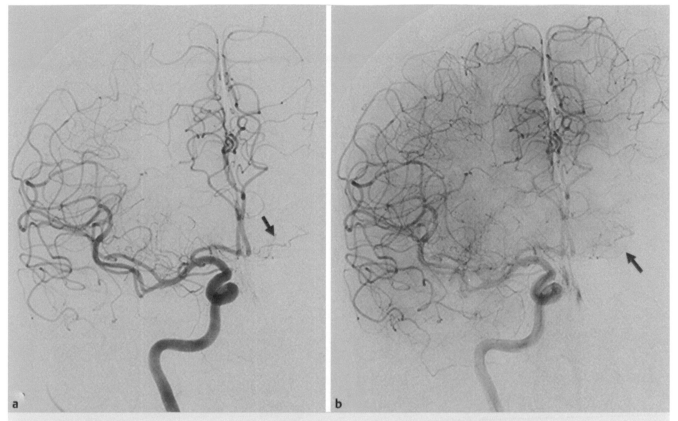

Fig. 15.4 Right ICA angiogram in AP view in arterial (a) and capillary (b) phases demonstrates the course and supply (capillary blush in b) of the left RAH (*arrows*).

groups enter the anterior perforating substance and provide flow to the basal ganglia, septum pellucidum, and anterior limb of the internal capsule. The other half will supply the local structures, including the hypothalamus and the optic chiasm.

The lenticulostriate arteries arising from the MCA can be divided into a smaller medial group and a larger lateral group, even though a clear separation between the two groups is only possible in approximately 40% of cases. They are in balance with the lenticulostriate arteries arising from the ACA, creating an equilibrium that mainly involves the medial group.

There are usually between six and 20 lenticulostriate branches per hemisphere. They may arise from a single vessel or a major trunk (so-called candelabra arteries) in 50% of cases, and subsequently divide into individual small arteries. Most commonly, they arise from the posterosuperior aspect of the M1 segment, but in approximately 20% of cases, they can originate from either the superior or inferior divisions of the MCA or, less commonly, from an early cortical branch of the MCA.

From their site of origin, the medial lenticulostriate arteries ascend through the anterior perforated substance, heading straight to the lenticular nucleus, to supply, together with the medial lenticulostriate arteries from the ACA and the RAH, the anteroinferior portion of the head of the caudate nucleus, the anterior third of the putamen, the anterior limb of the internal capsule, the anterolateral edge of the globus pallidus, the medial aspect of the anterior commissure, and the anterior part of the hypothalamus.

The lateral group describes a sharp posterior and medial recurrent curve in the cisternal segment before entering the lateral two-thirds of the anterior perforated substance. They initially ascend, coursing around and through the lenticular nucleus, and then turn medially through the superior half of the internal capsule, heading toward the caudate nucleus. They will be responsible for the vascularization of the upper portion of the head and the body of the caudate nucleus, the putamen, the lateral segment of the globus pallidus, the lateral half of the anterior commissure, and the superior segments of both limbs of the internal capsule. The blood supply to the structures lateral to the putamen, including the claustrum and the external capsule, is derived from other perforators arising from the insular branches of the MCA (▶ Fig. 15.5).

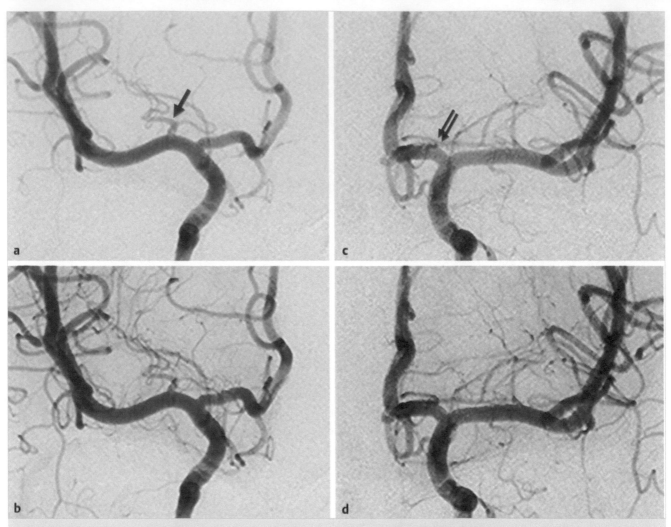

**Fig. 15.5** Variations in the origin of the lenticulostriate arteries: Right ICA angiogram in AP view in early (a) and late (b) arterial phases demonstrates a common trunk for the medial and lateral lenticulostriate group of perforators (*arrow*), whereas the contralateral left ICA angiogram in early (c) and late (d) arterial phases shows a dominant RAH (*thin double arrows*) that gives rise to all perforators on its way laterally, where it anastomoses distally with the main MCA trunk.

## 15.3 Clinical Impact, Additional Information and Cases

In the following, a selection of cases is presented that highlight the anatomical importance of the lenticulostriate artery and the RAH in different clinical scenarios (▸ Fig. 15.6; ▸ Fig. 15.7; ▸ Fig. 15.8; ▸ Fig. 15.9; ▸ Fig. 15.10; ▸ Fig. 15.11; ▸ Fig. 15.12; ▸ Fig. 15.13).

### Pearls and Pitfalls

- Embryologically, the anterior perforators arise from the lateral striate arteries from the ACA. Although, classically, three major groups are present (RAH, medial, and lateral lenticulostriate groups), significant variations with common trunks or multiple separate origins from the proximal A2 to the proximal M2 exist.
- The relation between the perforator origins, their territory, and intracranial stenotic lesions is important in estimating the risk of an intervention in the MCA.

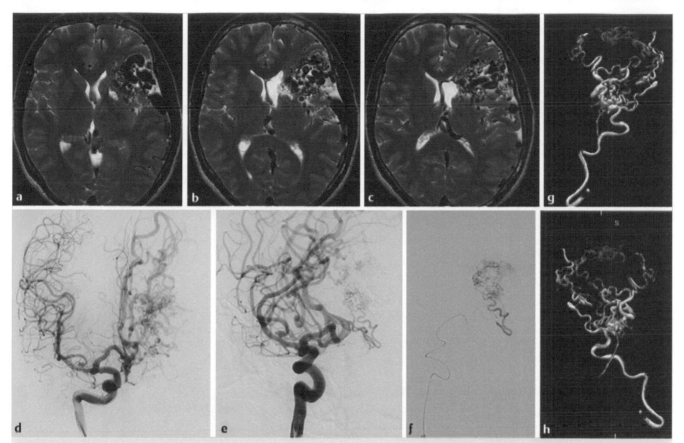

**Fig. 15.6** This 45-year-old male patient with a left frontal arteriovenous malformation (AVM) presented with an intracerebral hemorrhage within the caudate head seen on axial T2-weighted MRI (a,b,c). Given the localized hemorrhage, superselective evaluation of the Heubner artery territory was performed to exclude the possibility of an intranidal aneurysm that would have been regarded as a potential target for embolization. Right ICA angiogram in AP (d) and semioblique (e) views, as well as superselective catheterizations (f) and 3D rotational reconstruction (g,h), demonstrate left Heubner's artery and its territory, as well as its secondarily induced supply to the more cranially located shunt. Superselective injections fail to show any focal angioarchitectural weak spots. As there was no target for embolization therapy identified, the procedure was aborted.

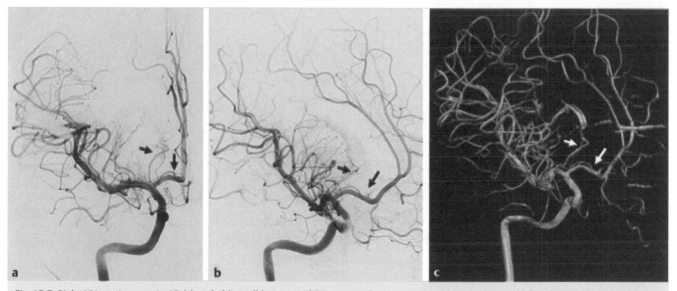

**Fig. 15.7** Right ICA angiograms in AP (a) and oblique (b) views and 3D rotational reconstruction (c) in a 16-year-old female patient demonstrate a micro-AVM, fed by Heubner's artery (*arrows*).

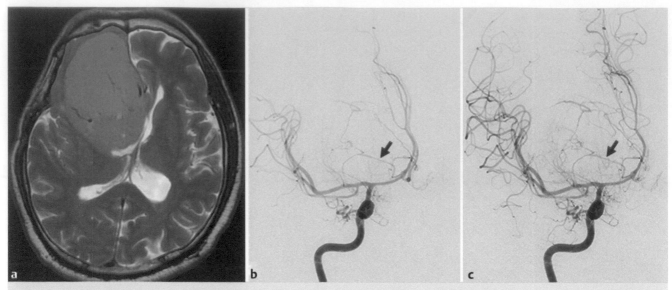

**Fig. 15.8** A 60-year-old man with a large right frontal meningioma, seen on axial T2-weighted MRI (a), was investigated for potential embolization. Right ICA angiogram in AP view in early (b) and late (c) arterial phases demonstrates pial supply to the tumor coming from the right ACA through Heubner's artery (*arrow*). Note that an accessory middle meningeal artery arises from the right ophthalmic artery.

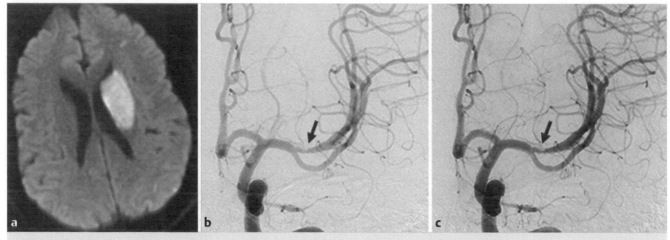

**Fig. 15.9** MRI diffusion-weighted imaging (a) and left ICA angiogram in AP view in early (b) and late (c) arterial phases demonstrate a medial lenticulostriate artery infarction resulting from a thrombus lodging directly at the origin of the artery supplying the infarcted territory (*arrows*).

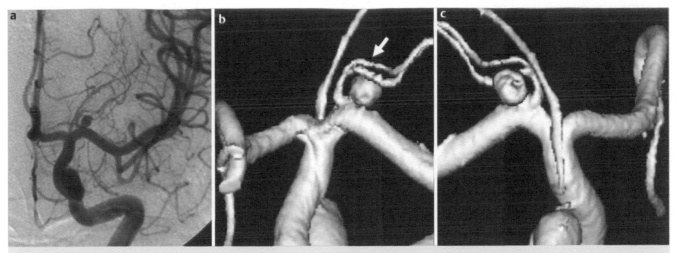

**Fig. 15.10** Left ICA angiograms in AP view (a) and postcoiling 3D rotational reconstruction (b,c) demonstrate a proximal M1 aneurysm at the origin of the medial lenticulostriate perforators (*arrow*).

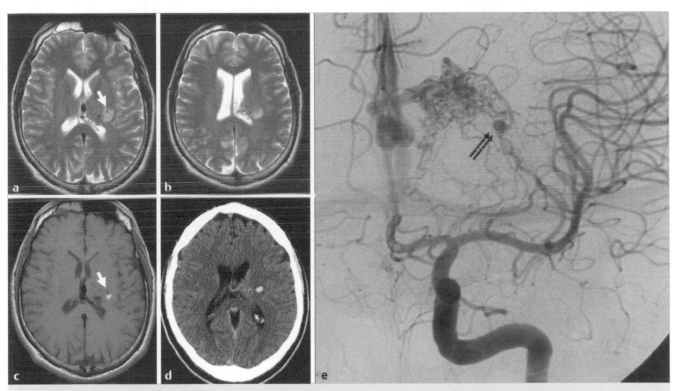

**Fig. 15.11** MRI axial T2-weighted (a,b) and T1-weighted (c) images and unenhanced CT (d) demonstrate a ruptured brain AVM. A round flow-void structure (*white arrows*) adjacent to the hematoma on MRI was confirmed to be a focal aneurysmal outpouching (*double black arrows*), arising from a left lateral lenticulostriate perforator vessel on the left ICA angiogram in AP view (e).

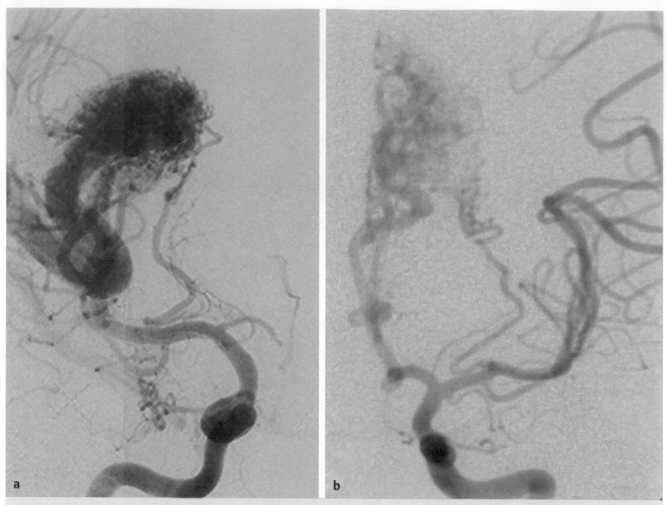

**Fig. 15.12** Right ICA (a) and left ICA (b) angiograms in AP view in two different patients demonstrate secondarily recruited supply from the lenticulostriate perforators in an insular (a) and cingulate (b) AVM. This deep supply to brain AVMs represents a potential target for presurgical embolization.

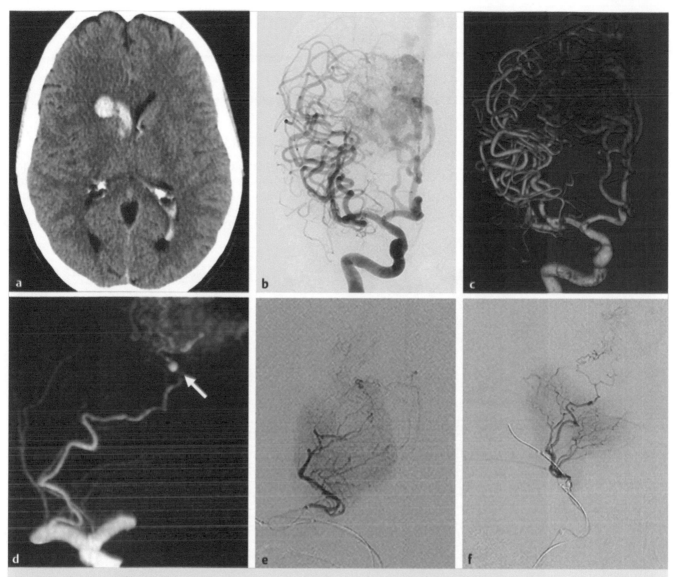

**Fig. 15.13** This 48-year-old patient presented with a right caudate head hemorrhage with intraventricular extension seen on unenhanced axial CT (a). Right ICA angiograms in AP view (b) and 3D rotational reconstruction (c,d) performed on admission showed a small prenidal aneurysm (*arrow*) on the most distal aspect of the secondarily recruited right lateral lenticulostriate artery. After discussion with the vascular neurosurgical team, a decision was made to attempt targeted embolization, which was performed 4 days after the initial angiography. As we were not able to navigate the catheter into the target vessel, a balloon was advanced into the M1, immediately past the origin of the target artery. With balloon inflation, which provided extra support, we were able to navigate the microcatheter into the lateral lenticulostriate artery. Microcatheter injections (e,f) showed that the previously seen pseudoaneurysm was no longer present, presumably because of spontaneous thrombosis. The injections also revealed that the supply to the medial and lateral lenticulostriate territory arose from this single vessel.

# Further Reading

[1] Komiyama M, Nakajima H, Nishikawa M, Yasui T. Middle cerebral artery variations: duplicated and accessory arteries. AJNR Am J Neuroradiol 1998; 19: 45–49

[2] Lasjaunias P, Berenstein A, ter Brugge KG. Surgical Neuroangiography. Vol. 1. 2nd ed. Berlin: Springer; 2006

[3] Newton TH, Potts DG. Radiology of the Skull and Brain. Angiography. Vol. 3, Book 2. St. Louis, MO: Mosby; 1974

[4] Takahashi S, Goto K, Fukasawa H, Kawata Y, Uemura K, Suzuki K. Computed tomography of cerebral infarction along the distribution of the basal perforating arteries. Part I: Striate arterial group. Radiology 1985; 155: 107–118

# 16 The Cortical Branches of the Middle Cerebral Artery

## 16.1 Case Description

### 16.1.1 Clinical Presentation

A 30-year-old woman was investigated with magnetic resonance (MR) in screening for familial aneurysms, and an incidental left-sided broad-based 8-mm middle cerebral artery (MCA) aneurysm was found. The patient was referred to neurosurgery.

### 16.1.2 Radiologic Studies

See ▶ Fig. 16.1, ▶ Fig. 16.2, and ▶ Fig. 16.3.

### 16.1.3 Diagnosis

Acute MCA occlusion with subsequent thrombectomy

## 16.2 Embryology and Anatomy

Distal to the MCA trunk, the MCA typically splits into two divisions—the superior and the inferior trunk—which are in hemodynamic balance and show considerable variations regarding dominance of one trunk over the other (with concomitant annexed territories). The superior division will supply the frontal

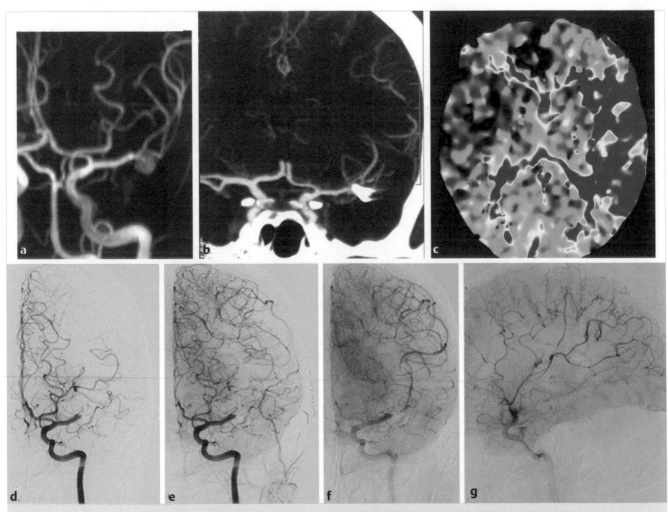

**Fig. 16.1** Immediately after clipping of an incidental left-sided MCA aneurysm (MR angiography in a), this 30-year-old patient presented with a complete right-sided hemiparesis and aphasia. CTA (b) failed to demonstrate a normal MCA bifurcation, whereas CT perfusion (Time to Peak [TTP] Map in c) showed significant hypoperfusion of her left hemisphere. The patient was immediately reoperated, and the clip was repositioned. On surgical inspection, however, the operator noted that thrombus was present within the MCA bifurcation, and emergency thrombectomy was requested. Injection into the left internal carotid artery (ICA) in early (d) and late (e) arterial and capillary (f,g) phases revealed occlusion of the distal M1 with good filling of the lenticulostriate arteries and excellent collaterals from the ACA territory reconstituting the dominant superior division of the MCA. Case continued in ▶ Fig. 16.1.

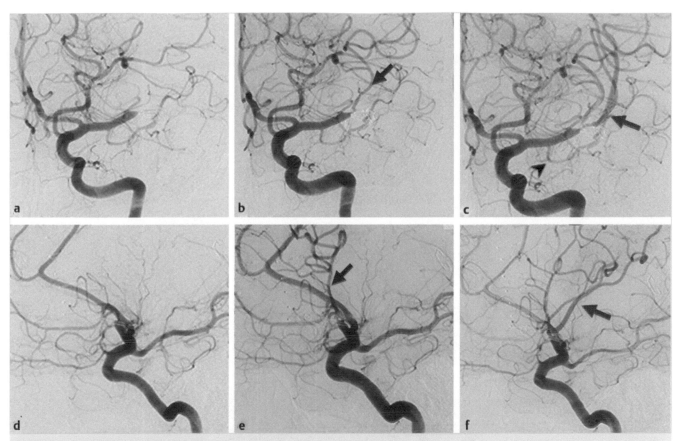

Fig. 16.2 (a,d) Initial angiographic runs; (b,e) runs after the first pass; (c,f) runs after the second pass. After the first pass, the prefrontal or opercular branch was opened (*arrow* in b,e), which supplies the Broca territory. With the second pass, the dominant superior division, including the Rolandic artery, was opened (*arrow* in c,f). Note the early anterior temporal branch of the MCA trunk (*arrowhead* in c). Case continued in ▶ Fig. 16.3.

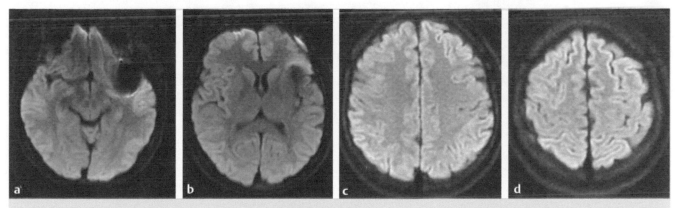

Fig. 16.3 Axial diffusion-weighted imaging at various levels (a–d) 24 hours after the intervention did not show any areas of ischemia, and the patient had no neurological deficit.

convexity, whereas the inferior trunk will supply the temporal lobe. The parietal lobe can be supplied by either trunk (typically the one that is dominant) or by its own division of the MCA; in these cases, a MCA trifurcation is present. An anterior temporal branch can arise proximally from the MCA trunk. Over the frontal and parietal convexity, the distal MCA branches are in hemodynamic balance with the ACA branches (the ACA–MCA watershed), whereas over the temporal lobe, the MCA is in bal-

ance with the PCA (see also Case 17). In addition to their cortical supply, the distal MCA branches also give rise to leptomeningeal perforating arteries that will supply the peripheral white matter and will constitute the hemodynamic watershed with the lenticulostriate arteries of the MCA trunk. The M3 and M4 branches show a certain degree of variability, which is why the nomenclature of these branches varies. In most practices, vessels are named, irrespective of their origin, on the basis of

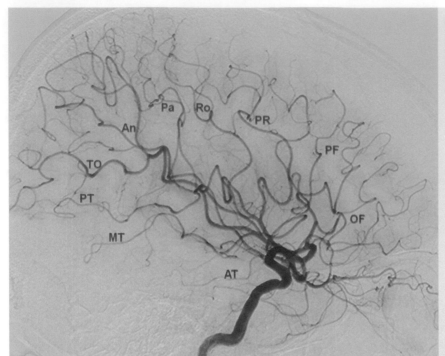

**Fig. 16.4** The MCA branches can be best appreciated on the lateral view in this patient with a hypoplastic A1 segment. OF, orbitofrontal; PF, prefrontal; PR, pre-Rolandic; Ro, Rolandic; Pa, parietal; An, angular; TO, temporooccipital, PT, posterior temporal; MT, middle temporal; AT, anterior temporal.

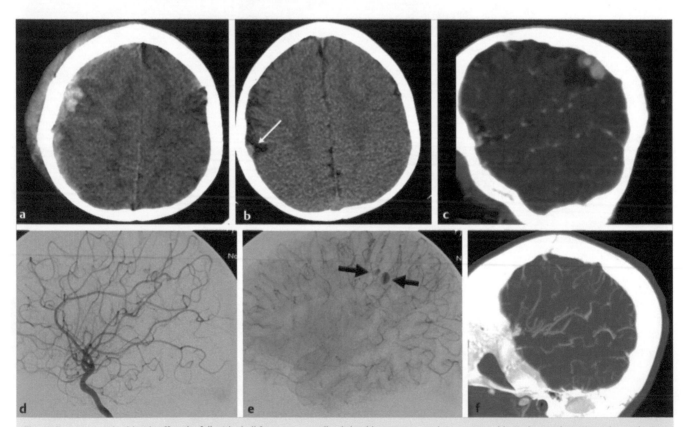

**Fig. 16.5** A 15-month-old girl suffered a fall with skull fracture, a small subdural hematoma, and a contusional brain hemorrhage (unenhanced CT in a). The patient made an excellent recovery with no residual motor deficit. On follow-up imaging 3 months later, an encephalomalacic defect is seen. In the region of the previous fracture, a small extra-axial soft tissue density is seen (*arrow in b*), prompting further evaluation with CTA and, subsequently, digital subtraction angiography. CTA (c), sagittal reconstruction through the area of interest, demonstrates two adjacent aneurysmal outpouchings that were confirmed by digital subtraction angiography to originate from the distal Rolandic artery (right ICA injection lateral view in arterial [d] and capillary [e] phases). Contrast stagnation was seen in the aneurysms in the capillary phase (*arrows in e*). Given the eloquence of the affected vessel and the beginning thrombosis of the aneurysm, conservative management was selected. A follow-up CTA (f) demonstrated complete obliteration of the aneurysm.

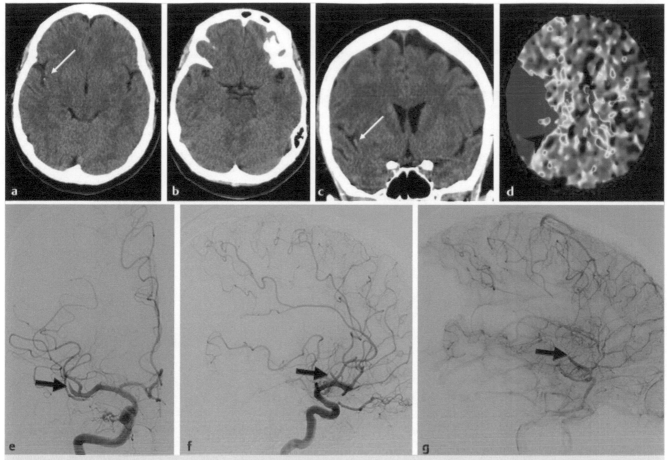

**Fig. 16.6** Unenhanced CT in a 56-year-old female patient who presented with left-sided neglect, mild left upper limb weakness, and dysarthria demonstrates a hyperdense "dot" sign (arrows in a,c) in the right sylvian fissure as a sign of a distal MCA branch (M2) occlusion that was confirmed by CTA (not shown) and CT perfusion (TTP Map, d). Angiography of the right ICA in anteroposterior (e) and lateral (f,g) views demonstrates the sudden cutoff of the dominant inferior division of the right MCA trifurcation (*arrows*) with insufficient collateral flow to the distal MCA territory (belated phase on the lateral view injection). Case continues in ▶ Fig. 16.7.

the cortical territory they supply, which will lead to the following MCA "branches": orbitofrontal, prefrontal, pre-Rolandic, Rolandic, parietal, angular, temporooccipital, posterior temporal, and middle and anterior temporal. These branches are best appreciated on the lateral view (▶ Fig. 16.4).

## 16.3 Clinical Impact, Additional Information and Cases

See ▶ Fig. 16.5, ▶ Fig. 16.6, ▶ Fig. 16.7, ▶ Fig. 16.8, ▶ Fig. 16.9, and ▶ Fig. 16.10.

---

**Pearls and Pitfalls**

- Cortical branches of the MCA are named depending on the cortical territory they supply and are therefore best evaluated from distal to proximal on the lateral view.
- The MCA bifurcates into an inferior and a superior division that are in hemodynamic equilibrium with each other and that supply, respectively, the temporal and the frontal lobes and share the supply to the parietal lobe.

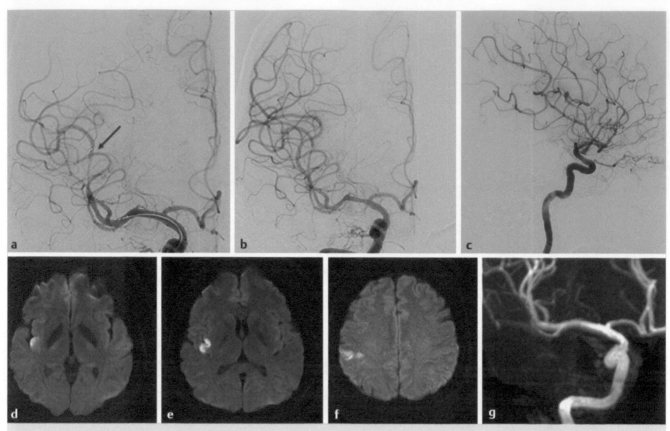

**Fig. 16.7** A stent retriever was placed in the dominant inferior trunk, as verified by the angiographic run during retriever expansion (a; the small arrow points to the distal end). Follow-up angiography after a single pass demonstrated complete reopening of the vessel (b,c). On follow-up MR (axial diffusion-weighted imaging; d–f), a small area of (clinically silent) ischemia and persistent opening of the MCA branches on MR angiography (g) is seen.

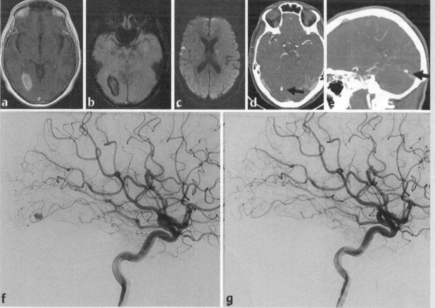

**Fig. 16.8** A patient with endocarditis and vegetations on his mitral valve presented with a right occipital hemorrhage (MR imaging with T1 [a] and susceptibility weighting [b]) and embolic hits (diffusion-weighted imaging in c). CTA in axial (d) and sagittal (e) cuts demonstrates a distal aneurysm as the source of the hemorrhage (*arrows*). As the patient was scheduled for urgent cardiac valve replacement surgery, embolization of the presumed mycotic aneurysm was requested. Right ICA injection in lateral view before embolization (f) demonstrated the peripheral MCA aneurysm that arises from the temporooccipital branch of the MCA that was subsequently catheterized. The aneurysm was occluded with glue embolization (immediate postembolization result [g]).

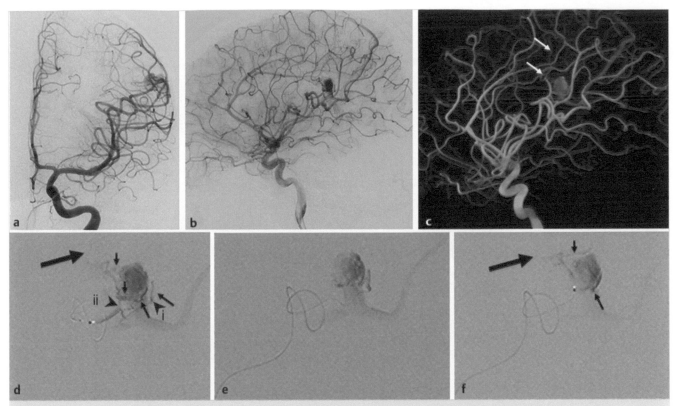

**Fig. 16.9** A 14-year-old boy presented with seizures. On investigation, a brain arteriovenous malformation (AVM) was found that was subsequently evaluated by conventional angiography for potential embolization. Left ICA injections in anteroposterior (a) and lateral view (b) and 3D rotational angiography in a semioblique view (c) demonstrate that the AVM was fed by the Rolandic artery and that, distal to the AVM nidus, the feeding vessel to the precentral gyrus continued (*arrows* in c). Microcatheter injections into the proximal Rolandic artery (d) demonstrate four feeding arteries (*small black arrows*) into the shunt. The Rolandic artery continues distally (*large arrow*) to feed the primary motor cortex. Subsequently, injections were performed at the positions denoted by the arrowheads (I and II). (e) The microcatheter injection in position (i). This is a safe vessel to embolize, as it is of the terminal type, with a sufficient security margin to the feeding artery. However, glue will likely enter the venous pouch and occlude the vein, which is the only venous outlet of the AVM. If additional arterial input is still present, bleeding of the AVM is likely to happen. Microcatheter injection in position (ii) (f) demonstrates two small vessels entering the AVM (*arrows*) that arise "en passage" from the Rolandic artery. The faint distal continuation to the ICA is again seen. Given these anatomical and angio-architectonic considerations, no embolization was performed.

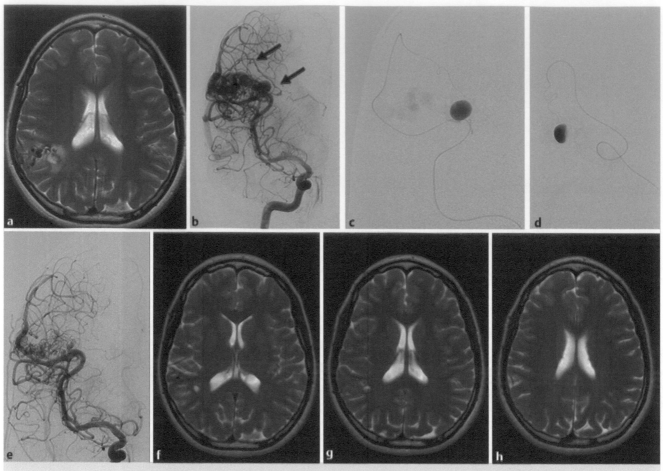

**Fig. 16.10** MR imaging in T2 weighting (a) demonstrates a right parietal AVM in a young patient with unspecific symptoms. There is peripheral edema surrounding a focal deep-seated outpouching of the AVM. Right ICA injection (b) demonstrates an enlarged leptomeningeal penetrating artery that feeds the medial (deep) portions of the AVM in which MR had demonstrated the outpouching (*arrow* in b). This feeder was subsequently catheterized and revealed a large intranidal aneurysm (c,d) that was subsequently embolized (immediate postembolization result seen in e). The patient underwent subsequent gamma knife radiosurgery, and 2-year follow-up axial T2 W MR sequences (f,g,h), show that the AVM was obliterated in a neurologically intact individual.

# Further Reading

[1] Gibo II, Carver CC, Rhoton AL, Jr, Lenkey C, Mitchell RJ. Microsurgical anatomy of the middle cerebral artery. J Neurosurg 1981; 54: 151–169

[2] Morris P. Practical Neuroangiography. 3rd ed. Philadelphia: Lippincott, Williams & Wilkins; 2013

[3] Umansky F, Gomes FB, Dujovny M et al. The perforating branches of the middle cerebral artery. A microanatomical study. J Neurosurg 1985; 62: 261–268

[4] van der Zwan A, Hillen B, Tulleken CAF, Dujovny M, Dragovic L. Variability of the territories of the major cerebral arteries. J Neurosurg 1992; 77: 927–940

[5] van der Zwan A, Hillen B, Tulleken CAF, Dujovny M. A quantitative investigation of the variability of the major cerebral arterial territories. Stroke 1993; 24: 1951–1959

# 17 The Leptomeningeal Anastomoses

## 17.1 Case Description

### 17.1.1 Clinical Presentation

A 30-year-old man with history of prosthetic mitral valve replacement associated with rheumatic disease was poorly compliant with his anticoagulation therapy regimen. He presented to the emergency department with aphasia and left-sided hemiplegia, with the arm more pronounced then the leg. Because he had an absolute contraindication to the use of intravenous recombinant tissue plasminogen activator, he was brought to the angio-suite for mechanical thrombectomy.

### 17.1.2 Radiologic Studies

See ▶ Fig. 17.1, ▶ Fig. 17.2.

### 17.1.3 Diagnosis

Acute stroke resulting from embolic occlusion of the superior division of the middle cerebral artery (MCA) with excellent leptomeningeal collateral circulation.

## 17.2 Anatomy

Leptomeningeal anastomoses (LMAs), or leptomeningeal collaterals, are small arteriolar connections (~50–400 μm) between two cerebral arteries supplying two different but adjacent cortical territories. They were initially described by Sir Thomas Willis in 1684, but the first well-documented work demonstrating their presence was done by Heubner in 1874. These vessels form an extensive network that provides a potential route for collateral perfusion, together with the large arterial communications and the circle of Willis.

In LMAs, blood can flow in both directions, depending on the hemodynamic and metabolic needs, thus allowing retrograde perfusion of adjacent territories. Their presence, number, size, and location have a high degree of variability between individuals as well as between hemispheres in the same person. They tend to be more extensive along the convexity, connecting the MCA with the anterior cerebral artery (ACA) and posterior cerebral artery (PCA) territories, but there are also LMAs connecting the ACA and PCA territories (precuneus and splenium of the corpus callosum), as well as both ACA territories (through callosal arteries) and between distal branches of the MCA, PCA, and ACA (▶ Table 17.1).

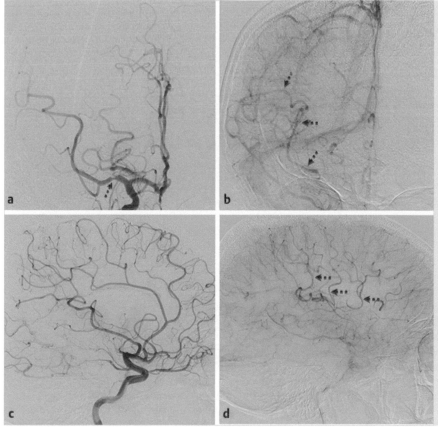

**Fig. 17.1** Right internal carotid artery (ICA) angiogram in anteroposterior (AP) (a,b) and lateral (c,d) views in arterial (a,c) and late capillary (b,d) phase. There is occlusion of the superior division of the middle cerebral artery (MCA), with a focal extrinsic filling defect in the M1 trunk (arrow). The late-capillary-phase angiograms show retrograde filling of the superior division of the MCA via LMAs from the ACA (thin arrows in b,d). Case continued in ▶ Fig. 17.2.

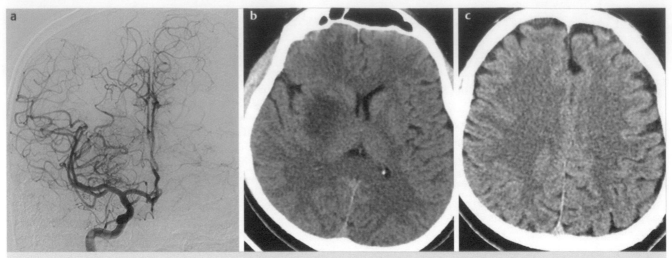

**Fig. 17.2** Right ICA angiogram in AP view after thrombectomy (a) demonstrates complete recanalization of the superior division of the MCA with good antegrade flow and no distal filling defects. Control unenhanced axial computed tomography 24 hours after thrombectomy (b,c) shows an infarct in the right striatum but no cortical infarct in the territory of the superior division of the MCA, as the cortex received collateral supply during MCA trunk occlusion, whereas the perforators did not.

**Table 17.1** Territories, arteries involved, and location of the most common leptomeningeal anastomoses: Orbito-frontal (MCA) with fronto orbital and fronto-polar (ACA).

| Territory | Anastomosing Arteries | Location of the Anastomosis |
|---|---|---|
| MCA and ACA | Orbito-frontal (MCA) with fronto-orbital and fronto-polar (ACA) | Inferior and middle frontal gyrus |
|  | Pre-frontal artery (MCA) with anterior/middle internal frontal artery (ACA) | Superior frontal sulcus |
|  | Pre-central artery (MCA) with posterior internal frontal artery (ACA) | Pre-central sulcus |
|  | Central artery (MCA) with paracentral artery (ACA) | Central sulcus |
|  | Parietal artery (MCA) with superior parietal (ACA) | Post-central sulcus or intraparietal sulcus |
| MCA and PCA | Angular or posterior temporal artery (MCA) with parieto-occipital artery (PCA) | Parieto-occipital or intraparietal sulcus |
|  | Temporal arteries (MCA) with inferior temporal trunk branches (PCA) | Middle temporal sulcus |
| ACA and PCA | Superior parietal or pericallosal arteries (ACA) with parieto-occipital artery (PCA) | Parieto-occipital sulcus |
|  | Pericallosal artery (ACA) with splenial artery (PCA) | Splenium of the corpus callosum |

ACA = anterior cerebral artery; MCA = middle cerebral artery; PCA = posterior cerebral artery

The ability of LMAs to compensate for a vascular occlusion depends on four main factors: presence and number of LMAs, systemic blood pressure, onset of the occlusion, and age of the patient. As stated earlier, the number and diameter of the LMAs vary significantly among different individuals, but the pressure gradient magnitude between the unaffected and affected vascular territory, and thus the flow rate, is influenced by the systemic blood pressure. Nevertheless, it has been seen that patients with chronic systolic hypertension will have less-functional LMAs because of impairment of the cerebral blood flow autoregulation. Patients with a gradual onset of a vascular occlusion (moyamoya syndrome or intracranial or extracranial stenosis) develop a more extensive LMA network that allows for better compensatory collateral flow changes than does an abrupt arterial occlusion. The functional compensatory capacity of LMAs also diminishes with age. This is probably mediated by a decrease in the number of LMAs, as well as "stiffening" of these vessels mediated by atherosclerosis, decreasing their ability to dilate properly in response to flow or metabolic demands.

## 17.3 Clinical Impact

At this time, there is a general consensus that the ability of LMAs to compensate for a vascular occlusion is one of the main determinants of outcome in patients with acute stroke and is, therefore, critical in patient selection for intra-arterial endovascular stroke treatments. Good collateral flow via the LMAs is assumed to be independently associated with a favorable outcome because of the capacity to maintain the ischemic penumbra until reperfusion occurs. Computed tomographic angiography gives a rough estimation of the collateral flow, specifically

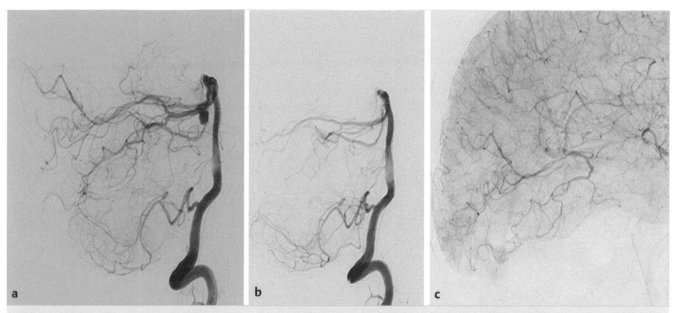

**Fig. 17.3** A 66-year-old man presenting with an acute subarachnoid hemorrhage. Right vertebral artery angiogram in lateral view before (a) and after (b) coil occlusion of the distal P1 segment for treatment of a right PCA dissecting aneurysm located in the P1/P2 segment junction. Right ICA angiogram in lateral view immediately after the procedure (c) shows retrograde filling of the distal PCA branches via LMAs, with contrast filling seen up to the P3 segment of the PCA.

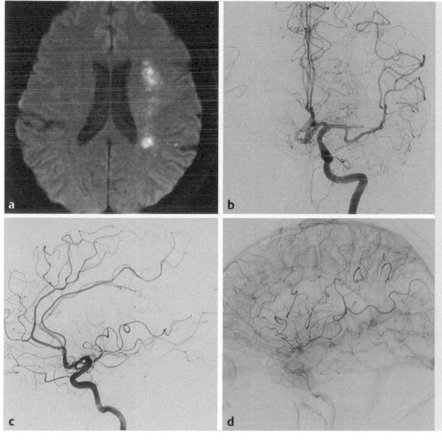

**Fig. 17.4** A 57-year-old woman with acute onset of focal neurological deficits. Diffusion-weighted MRI (a) shows acute ischemic lesions in the ACA/MCA watershed territory. Left ICA angiogram in AP view (b) shows an occlusion in the superior division of the left MCA. Left ICA angiogram in lateral view in arterial (c) and late (d) capillary phase shows significantly decreased antegrade flow through the superior division of the MCA, with retrograde filling of the distal cortical branches through LMAs from the ACA.

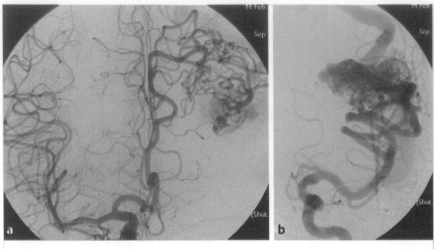

**Fig. 17.5** LMAs are often recruited in high-flow AVMs because of the "sump" effect. This can be explained by the low resistance of the high-flow shunt, as there is no intervening capillary bed at the level of the shunt, with subsequently increased flow from neighboring territories. The high-flow nature of the AVM may also lead to relative perinidal hypoxemia with secondarily enlarged leptomeningeal collaterals. Both factors will lead to a "shift of the watershed" (i.e., an apparent supply from neighboring branches to the AVM) as indicated in this example. Right (a) and left (b) ICA angiograms in AP view demonstrate that the ACA branches do not feed the AVM proper but are only secondarily recruited to anastomose via the leptomeningeal vessels to the MCA branches that supply the AVM. Caution must be taken not to include the secondarily recruited vessels in the treatment plan.

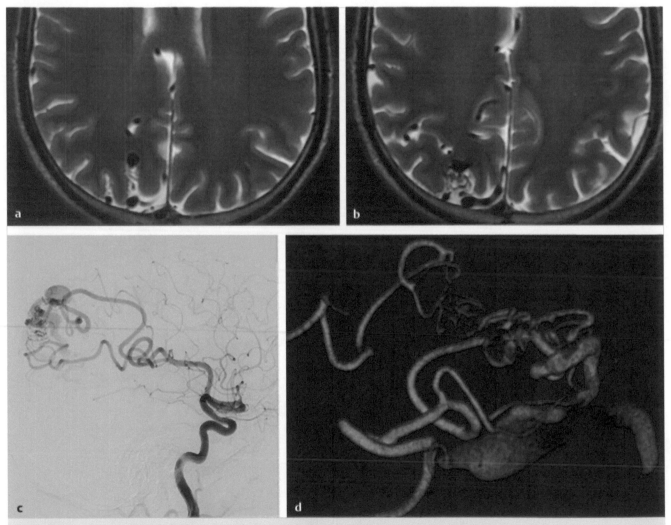

**Fig. 17.6** Although in its most dramatic form the shift of the watershed resulting from leptomeningeal collaterals is visible from one large vessel territory into the other (ACA to MCA or vice versa), it may also be present between neighboring distal pial branches, as visualized in this case with a fistulous high parietal AVM, where high-resolution T2-weighted MRI (a,b) demonstrate dilated transgyral vessels and right ICA angiograms in lateral view (c) and 3D rotational reconstruction (d) demonstrates that the angular artery (via dilated leptomeningeal branches) secondarily contributes to the supply of the posterior parietal branch that is the sole feeding vessel of the AVM.

on delayed angiographic images, but the optimal imaging modality to quantify and properly classify the grade of collateral flow remains controversial. Not only the imaging technique but also timing of imaging is important, as changes in the flow are a dynamic process. The ability to compensate for an acute occlusion is also relevant in cases in which an intracranial parent vessel occlusion is needed for treatment of aneurysms. It is important to keep in mind that LMAs may be sufficient to supply the distal arterial territories but may not provide enough flow to retrogradely fill the perforator artery territory.

LMAs are also important in the assessment and treatment planning of brain arteriovenous malformations (AVMs). Patients with AVMs with a significant fistulous component will show a shift of the watershed territory seen on angiograms, which is a process mediated by the LMA. LMAs can be secondarily recruited by an AVM because of an increase in flow demand. When recruited, they provide blood supply to normal brain parenchyma and should be preserved regardless of the treatment modality. This is of special relevance for treatment planning in AVM radiosurgical candidates. LMAs are also involved in arterial steal, when blood flow from an adjacent part of the brain cortex is "sumped" into the AVM nidus via this network of vessels, leading to focal neurological deficits or chronic hypoperfusion (resulting in gliosis and atrophy). In treated AVMs, LMAs will be an important route to fill the AVM nidus in those cases with incomplete resection or when the liquid embolic material did not reach the venous side of the AVM, leading to continued demand from indirect sources (LMA). "Ligation"-type embolizations (i.e., purely arterial occlusion without penetration into the first

segment of the vein) will therefore lead to reconstitution of the AVM over time through the LMA. In contrast, a liquid embolic agent with a propensity to penetrate deep into adjacent vessels or a wedge-type embolization can open these collaterals, which can cause perinidal ischemia.

## 17.4 Additional Information and Cases

See ▶ Fig. 17.3, ▶ Fig. 17.4, ▶ Fig. 17.5, ▶ Fig. 17.6, and ▶ Fig. 17.7.

---

### Pearls and Pitfalls

- The number and diameter of LMAs vary significantly from patient to patient, and even between the hemispheres of the same individual.
- The capacity of LMAs to compensate for an arterial occlusion is a significant factor in stroke outcome. Efforts are underway to standardize the classification of the magnitude of collateral to improve patient selection for stroke therapy.
- LMAs are involved in AVM recurrence/persistence and in cases of arterial steal in AVMs with high fistulous components. When present, they supply normal brain en route to the AVM; therefore, they should be preserved, regardless of the treatment modality.

---

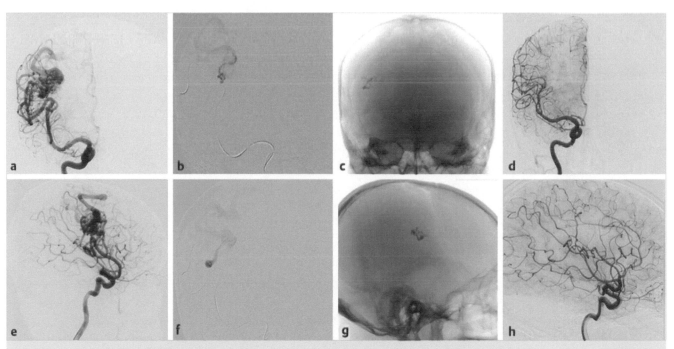

**Fig. 17.7** The clinical relevance of the leptomeningeal recruitment surrounding a fistulous AVM is demonstrated in this example of a 63-year-old patient with an AVM, seen on right ICA angiogram in AP (a) and lateral (b) views, which has led to significant leptomeningeal collateral supply. After embolization of two fistulous components in this AVM (c,d) with a rather small glue cast on the plain radiography (e,f), the secondarily recruited leptomeningeal collaterals regress, as there is no further "sump effect" toward the AVM once occlusion of the distal artery and the proximal vein draining the fistula is achieved. Complete obliteration of the AVM can thus be achieved, as seen on the follow-up right ICA angiograms (g,h). If AVM treatment leads to ligation of the artery without reaching the vein, these leptomeningeal collaterals will secondarily reopen the AVM, further highlighting the importance of recognizing the proper anatomy to target the embolization.

# Further Reading

[1] Brozici M, van der Zwan A, Hillen B. Anatomy and functionality of leptomeningeal anastomoses: a review. Stroke 2003; 34: 2750–2762

[2] Kim DJ, Krings T. Whole-brain perfusion CT patterns of brain arteriovenous malformations: a pilot study in 18 patients. AJNR Am J Neuroradiol 2011; 32: 2061–2066

[3] Liebeskind DS. Collateral circulation. Stroke 2003; 34: 2279–2284

[4] Liebeskind DS. Collaterals in acute stroke: beyond the clot. Neuroimaging Clin N Am 2005; 15: 553–573, xx

[5] McVerry F, Liebeskind DS, Muir KW. Systematic review of methods for assessing leptomeningeal collateral flow. AJNR Am J Neuroradiol 2012; 33: 576–582

[6] Nambiar V, Sohn SI, Almekhlafi MA, et al. CTA collateral status and response to recanalization in patients with acute ischemic stroke. AJNR Am J Neuroradiol 2014; 35: 884–890

[7] Shuaib A, Butcher K, Mohammad AA, Saqqur M, Liebeskind DS. Collateral blood vessels in acute ischaemic stroke: a potential therapeutic target. Lancet Neurol 2011; 10: 909–921

[8] Tan IY, Demchuk AM, Hopyan J et al. CT angiography clot burden score and collateral score: correlation with clinical and radiologic outcomes in acute middle cerebral artery infarct. AJNR Am J Neuroradiol 2009; 30: 525–531

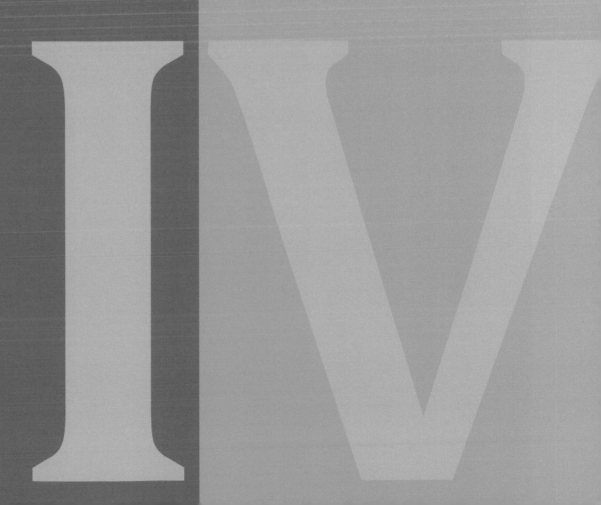

# Section IV

## Posterior Circulation

# 18 Variations of the Origin of the PICA

## 18.1 Case Description

### 18.1.1 Clinical Presentation

A 59-year-old man presented with a perimesencephalic subarachnoid hemorrhage. Computed tomography angiogram was negative for aneurysm, and digital subtraction angiography was obtained.

### 18.1.2 Radiologic Studies

See ▶ Fig. 18.1.

### 18.1.3 Diagnosis

Posterior inferior cerebellar artery (PICA) origin of a trigeminal artery. No cause for the hemorrhage was found.

## 18.2 Embryology and Anatomy

The PICA is the cerebellar artery with the most variations, which may range from unilateral or bilateral absence to being duplicated with different possible origins. The proximal PICA is the equivalent of a radiculopial artery that enlarged because of its annexed cerebellar territory via the primitive choroidal plexus of the fourth ventricle. The variations of the PICA origin follow the metameric arrangement also seen at the spinal cord level. Possible variations include the C3 origin from the vertebral artery (VA) or the ascending cervical artery; the C2 and C1 origins from the occipital artery via the embryonic proatlantal arteries (occipito-cerebellar variant); the ascending pharyngeal artery via the embryonic hypoglossal artery (pharyngo-cerebellar variant); and origin from various meningeal branches through the artery of the falx cerebelli. In exceedingly rare cases, there have also been reports of the PICA originating from the trigeminal artery.

The PICA is divided into five segments: the anterior medullary segment along the front of the medulla; the lateral medullary segment, which courses beside the medulla and extends to the origin of the glossopharyngeal, vagal, and accessory nerves; the tonsillomedullary segment, which courses around the caudal half of the cerebellar tonsil; the telovelotonsillar segment, which courses in the cleft between the tela choroidea and the inferior medullary velum rostrally and the superior pole of the cerebellar tonsil caudally; and finally, its cortical segment, with its course over the cerebellar surface.

Perforator supply to the lateral medulla is present from the PICA in approximately 50% of the population. By applying the same analogy as at the spinal cord level, it can be deduced that the more ventral (or medial) the origin of the PICA, as in cases of the pharyngo-cerebellar variant, the greater the chances of the PICA having medullary perforators, similar to that of a ventral pial artery of the spinal cord. The same rules hold true for the possibility of the spinal cord supply originating from the PICA. Therefore, PICAs that have an extradural origin are extremely unlikely to give any supply to the spinal cord. Origins from the proximal VA and occipito-cerebellar variants would produce a dorsoradiculopial pattern and are thus less likely to supply any eloquent territories of the brainstem.

## 18.3 Clinical Impact

Because of the potential supply to the lateral medulla, occlusion of the PICA can result in lateral medullary syndrome, which includes ipsilateral hemifacial numbness (injury to the spinal tract of the trigeminal nerve) and contralateral hemiparesthesia (spino-thalamic tract). Other symptoms of PICA infarction are

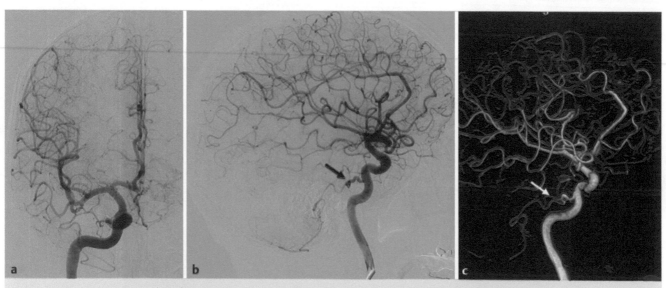

**Fig. 18.1** Right ICA angiogram in lateral view in early (a) and late (b) arterial phases and 3D reconstruction (c) reveal a persistent trigeminal artery on the right side supplying the right PICA (*arrows*). The remainder of the intracranial arteries is unremarkable.

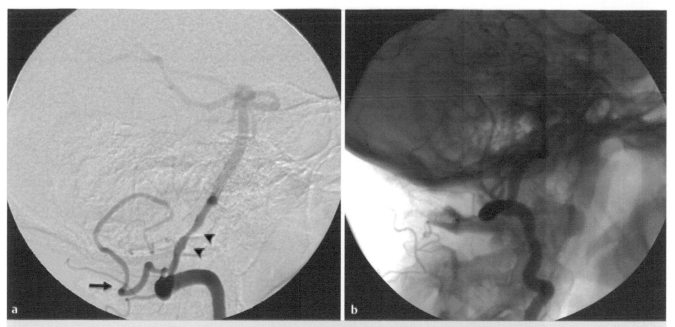

**Fig. 18.2** Left VA angiograms in oblique (a) and lateral unsubtracted (b) views demonstrate an extradural origin of the left PICA (*arrow*). Note the irregularity of the intradural left VA distal to the PICA origin up to the basilar origin (*arrowheads*), resulting from dissection. In this case, the right VA was patent; therefore, the dissected portion could be sacrificed without any complications.

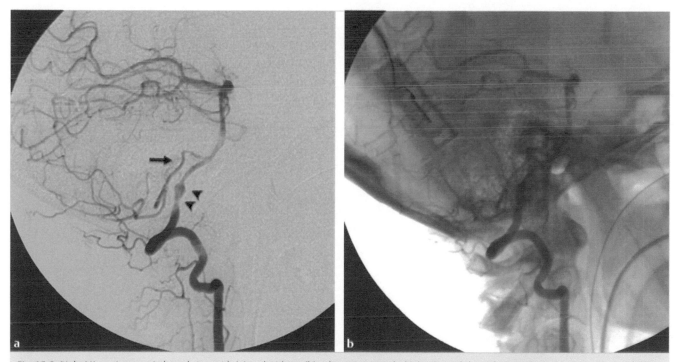

**Fig. 18.3** Right VA angiograms in lateral view with (a) and without (b) subtraction reveal a high origin of the right PICA (*arrow*), originating just before the basilar origin. There is a fusiform outpouching at the intradural right VA, proximal to the PICA (*arrowheads*), with narrowing proximal and distal to the lesion, representing a dissecting aneurysm. Because the origin of the PICA is not involved, if there is sufficient collateral from the left VA, the dissecting aneurysm may also be treated by parent vessel sacrifice.

dysphagia, dysarthria, and hoarseness (involvement of the nucleus ambiguus); ataxia, dizziness, vertigo, nystagmus, and homolateral cerebellar signs (damage to the vestibular nuclei and cerebellar tracts); an ipsilateral Horner's syndrome (disruption of the oculosympathetic fibers in the lateral medullary reticular substance); and vomiting (involvement of the nucleus and tractus solitarius).

In cases with intracranial vertebral artery dissection, the origin of the PICA will determine the feasibility of endovascular treatment. If the origin of the PICA is not involved, when the patient presents with a subarachnoid hemorrhage and the patient has good collaterals from the contralateral vertebral artery or posterior communicating arteries, sacrifice of the dissected vertebral artery segment is the preferred treatment. However, if the PICA origin is included within the involved segment and/or there are no collaterals, other treatment options (i.e., the use of flow-diverting stents or bypass surgery) may have to be considered.

## 18.4 Additional Information and Cases

See ▶ Fig. 18.2, ▶ Fig. 18.3, ▶ Fig. 18.4, and ▶ Fig. 18.5.

### Pearls and Pitfalls

- The origin of the PICA is extremely variable and follows the metameric arrangement seen at the spinal cord level.
- The more medial (or ventral) the origin of the PICA, the more likely for it to have perforators to the medulla.
- Cases with extradural origin of the PICA are extremely unlikely to give any supply to the spinal cord or the brainstem.
- Proximal PICA aneurysms are often dissecting in nature.

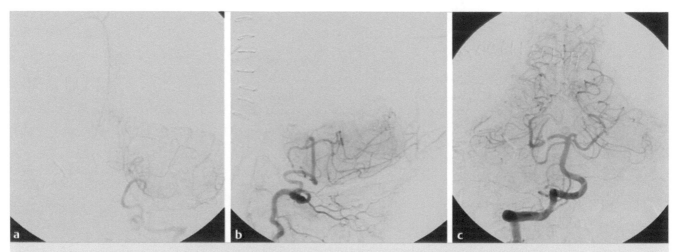

**Fig. 18.4** Left VA angiogram in anteroposterior (a) and lateral (b) views and right VA angiogram in anteroposterior view (c) reveal termination of the left VA at the left PICA.

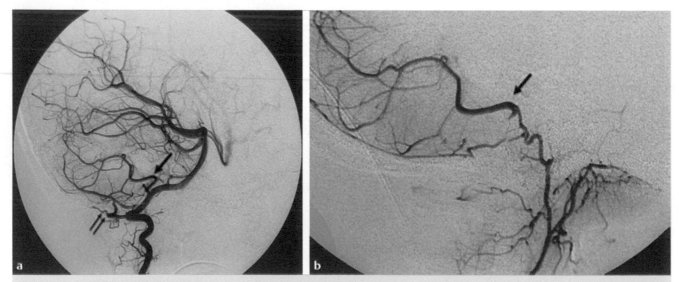

**Fig. 18.5** Right VA (a) and right ascending pharyngeal artery (b) angiograms in lateral view reveal an anastomosis between the neuromeningeal trunk and the right PICA (*arrows*). Note the occipital artery originates from a hypertrophied musculospinal branch of the atlantal loop (*thin double arrows*).

# Further Reading

[1] Lasjaunias P, Berenstein A, ter Brugge KG. Surgical Neuroangiography. Vol. 1. 2nd ed. Berlin: Springer; 2006

[2] Lister JR, Rhoton AL, Jr, Matsushima T, Peace DA. Microsurgical anatomy of the posterior inferior cerebellar artery. Neurosurgery 1982; 10: 170–199

[3] Peluso JP, van Rooij WJ, Sluzewski M, Beute GN, Majoie CB. Posterior inferior cerebellar artery aneurysms: incidence, clinical presentation, and outcome of endovascular treatment. AJNR Am J Neuroradiol 2008; 29: 86–90

[4] Uchino A, Suzuki C. Posterior inferior cerebellar artery supplied by the jugular branch of the ascending pharyngeal artery diagnosed by MR angiography: report of two cases. Cerebellum 2011; 10: 204–207

# 19 The Cerebellar Arteries

## 19.1 Case Description

### 19.1.1 Clinical Presentation

This 49-year-old man presented to medical attention with a large subarachnoid hemorrhage. CTA failed to demonstrate a source for the subarachnoid hemorrhage, and the patient was referred for diagnostic catheter angiography. This initially also failed to demonstrate a definitive source for the subarachnoid hemorrhage. Given the large quantity of subarachnoid blood, repeat vascular imaging was recommended in short course.

### 19.1.2 Radiologic Studies

See ▶ Fig. 19.1, ▶ Fig. 19.2.

### 19.1.3 Diagnosis

Dissecting aneurysm of the distal medial division of the superior cerebellar artery (SCA).

## 19.2 Embryology and Anatomy

The cerebellum is essentially supplied by three pairs of arteries that are in balance with each other; namely, the SCA, the anterior inferior cerebellar artery (AICA), and the posterior inferior cerebellar artery (PICA). However, these arteries have distinctly different embryological origins: the SCA belongs to the anterior circulation, as it originates from the caudal ramus of the carotid artery, distal to the trigeminal artery; the AICA develops from the longitudinal neural system, a forerunner of the basilar artery; and the PICA, the latest acquisition to the cerebellar supply, can be regarded as a radiculopial artery that annexed a

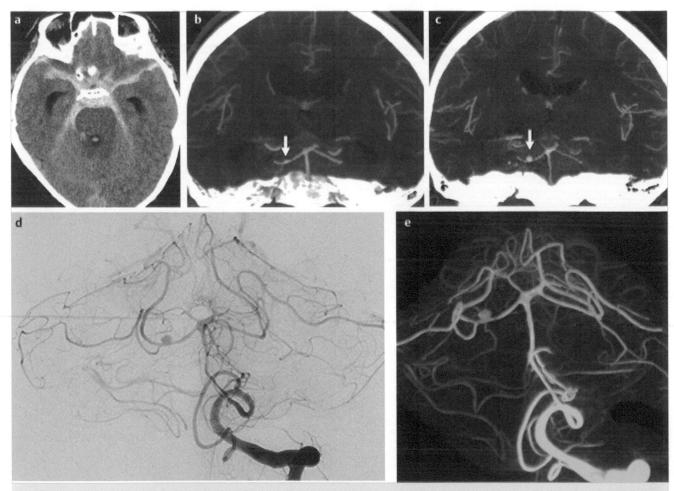

**Fig. 19.1** Unenhanced axial CT (a) shows diffuse subarachnoid hemorrhage. Initial CTA in coronal view (b) was read as normal, although in retrospect and in light of the second CTA (c), a focal irregularity in the distal SCA could be appreciated that after 1 week had become more apparent and enlarged (*arrows*) to a fusiform outpouching. Left VA angiogram in anteroposterior (AP) view (d) and three-dimensional rotational reconstruction (e) demonstrate the fusiform aneurysm with adjacent proximal narrowing and which was therefore presumed to be of the dissecting type. Case continued in ▶ Fig. 19.2.

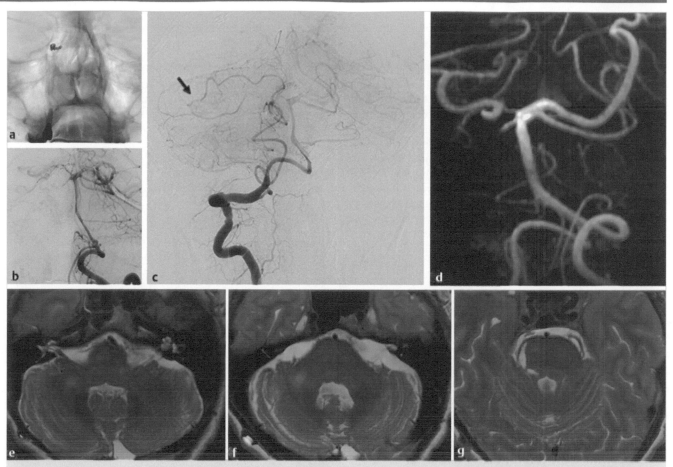

Fig. 19.2 Occlusion of the aneurysm and the parent vessel was performed (a,b), given the nature of the disease. On the control right VA angiography (c), there is collateralization from the vermian branch of the PICA to the medial vermian branch of the SCA (arrow). Follow-up time-of-flight MRA (d) demonstrated complete obliteration of the aneurysm. T2-weighted MRIs (e,f,g) demonstrate some small areas of ischemia in the brachium pontis, the superior cerebellar peduncle, and the dorsal tegmentum.

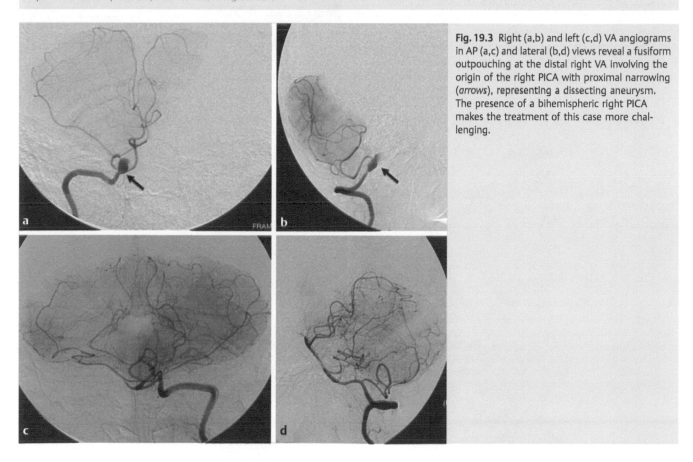

Fig. 19.3 Right (a,b) and left (c,d) VA angiograms in AP (a,c) and lateral (b,d) views reveal a fusiform outpouching at the distal right VA involving the origin of the right PICA with proximal narrowing (arrows), representing a dissecting aneurysm. The presence of a bihemispheric right PICA makes the treatment of this case more challenging.

cerebellar territory when the cerebellum rolled over the myelencephalon.

The PICA is highly variable in both its origin (see Case 18) and territorial supply. Common variations include unilateral agenesis/hypoplasia, double or duplicated origin, and extracranial or epidural origin. The territorial supply of the PICA varies with its origin and branching arrangement. It can be absent in up to 26% of patients, and if so, its territory is typically annexed by a dominant AICA through the lateral medullary anastomotic network in the pontomedullary sulcus. An alternative supply of the PICA territory is the contralateral PICA, which can then lead to a bihemispheric supply. This is less common than an AICA–PICA complex, as the vascular territory has to be annexed by an artery that has to cross the midline. Intradural arteries can cross the midline via a commissure (e.g., bihemispheric supply by a single pericallosal artery) or a midline structure, such as the vermis, which permits the formation of a vessel that is not constrained to a single lateralized territory.

Most commonly, the PICA arises from the vertebral artery (VA) near the inferior olive and then courses posteriorly around the medulla and, at its posterior margin, ascends behind the posterior medullary velum, describing a cranial loop above or across the cerebellar tonsil. Multiple small arterial branches emerge from this proximal section of the PICA to supply the posterolateral aspect of the medulla. The apex of the cranial loop (where the PICA also sends some branches to the choroid plexus of the fourth ventricle) is described as the "choroidal point," the distal limit for perforator arteries to arise from the PICA trunk. The PICA then turns downward in the retrotonsillar fissure and terminates a short distance distal to the cranial loop by dividing into the tonsillohemispheric (lateral) and vermian (medial) branches. The vermian branches supply the inferior vermis and anastomose with the superior vermian branches of the SCA. The lateral branch further divides into tonsillar branches that supply the tonsils, as well as into hemispheric branches that vascularize the posteroinferior aspect of the cerebellar hemisphere and anastomose with the AICA and SCA. The PICA can also give rise to meningeal branches, with the major branch being the artery of the falx cerebelli, also known as the

posterior meningeal artery. Other origins of this branch are directly from the VA and occasionally from the ascending pharyngeal or occipital arteries from the external carotid system. Although it is typically a midline branch with a dorsal territorial supply — hence its name — several smaller branches can supply the dural covers more laterally. It is in hemodynamic equilibrium with other meningeal branches from the middle meningeal artery, the stylomastoid artery, and various branches from the ICA. See also Case 31.

The AICA is considered part of the arterial labyrinthine system, as it consistently gives off the internal auditory artery. The AICA itself is a heterogeneous conduit that supplies several

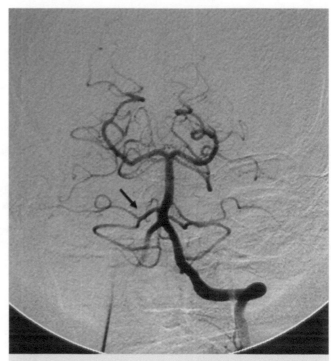

**Fig. 19.4** Left VA angiogram in AP view demonstrates a right AICA–PICA complex (*arrow*).

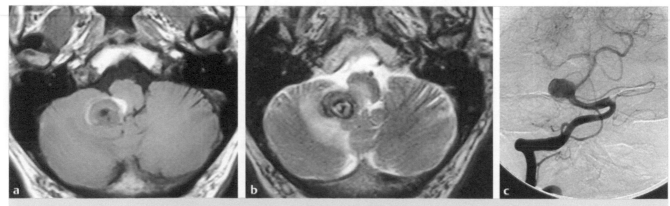

**Fig. 19.5** Giant partially thrombosed or chronic dissecting aneurysms with recurrent intramural hemorrhage that appear bright on T1-weighted scans indicating recent progression of the dissection. The patient had acute symptoms with significant headaches that were followed by a dorsolateral medulla oblongata syndrome. T1-weighted (a) and T2-weighted (b) MRI revealed not only the recent intramural hematoma but also an acute infarction in the dorsolateral medulla oblongata, a structure that is typically perfused by arteries that arise from the proximal PICA. Right VA angiogram in AP view (c) demonstrates the intraluminal compartment of the giant aneurysm. Given the nature of the disease, it was presumed that a perforator got occluded because of the recurrent intramural hematoma with expansion of the aneurysmal wall.

territories that include the trigeminal and acoustic nerves, as well as the cerebellum. In 99% of the cases, the AICA originates from the basilar artery, most commonly as a single trunk. In rare instances in which the trigeminal persistence is incomplete, the AICA, the SCA, or even the PICA may arise from the ICA. From its basilar artery origin, the AICA runs posterior, lateral, and inferiorly toward the cerebellopontine angle cistern, where, after giving rise to the internal auditory artery, it divides into two major branches. The lateral branch courses laterally toward the superior and inferior semilunar lobules, forming a loop around the flocculus, to anastomose with branches of the SCA and PICA. The medial branch courses downward toward the biventral lobule to anastomose with branches of the PICA. The AICA also gives rise to small perforating branches to the lateral aspect of the pons and superolateral aspect of the medulla, choroidal branches to the lateral recess of the fourth ventricle, and a dural branch, the subarcuate artery, that runs in the petromastoid or subarcuate canal and anastomoses with the middle meningeal artery at the cerebellopontine angle and with the stylomastoid artery branches in the petrous bone.

The SCA is the most constant artery to supply the cerebellum. It arises bilaterally just before the basilar artery bifurcation or, less commonly, from the P1 segment of the posterior cerebral artery. Most SCAs arise as a single trunk, although they may

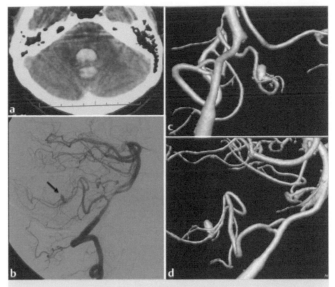

**Fig. 19.6** Unenhanced axial CT (a) shows hemorrhage in the cerebellar vermis with intraventricular hemorrhage. Right vertebral angiograms in lateral view (b) and 3D reconstruction (c,d) demonstrate the dissecting distal AICA aneurysm (*arrow*) that caused the hemorrhage.

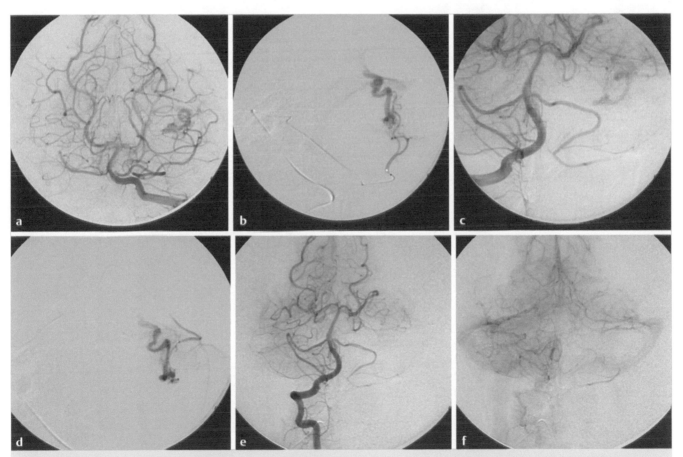

**Fig. 19.7** AVM fed by a left-sided AICA–PICA and a superior cerebellar artery branch. This 11-year-old patient had a left hemispheric cerebellar hemorrhage, and left VA angiogram in AP view (a) revealed an AVM that was fed by both the hemispheric branch of the AICA–PICA and the SCA, indicating that all cerebellar arteries are in equilibrium with each other. Selective catheterization of the AICA–PICA was done with glue embolization (b), and control angiogram (c) demonstrated the residual part of the AVM supplied by the SCA branches, which was subsequently catheterized and embolized (d). Left VA angiogram in arterial (e) and venous (f) phases after the procedure confirmed the complete occlusion of the AVM.

also have a duplicate or even a triplicate origin. The more caudal the fusion of the basilar artery, the higher the probability of a P1 origin of the SCA and the greater the likelihood of a duplicate origin of the SCA. Duplicated origin of the SCA corresponds to separated origins of its medial and lateral divisions, and the triplicated origin represents additional separation of the medial and lateral branches of the medial division (see following). After its origin, the proximal trunk of the SCA courses posterolaterally below the oculomotor nerve, encircling the brainstem near the pontomesencephalic junction and providing small perforators that contribute to the vascular supply of this region. The SCA usually bifurcates at the lateral pontomesencephalic level into a lateral and a medial division, which then courses in the cerebellomesencephalic fissure. The lateral division is responsible for the blood supply to the deep nuclei of the cerebellum and extends posterolaterally in the region of the horizontal fissure (as the marginal artery), supplying the superolateral aspect of the cerebellar hemisphere and anastomosing with the AICA and PICA. The medial division further divides into a medial branch that contributes to the tectal anastomotic network that covers the colliculi and to the vascularization of the superior cerebellar peduncle, as well as into a lateral branch that supplies the superomedial surface of the cerebellar hemisphere and the superior vermis through superior vermian branches.

## 19.3 Clinical Impact

Because of the different variations of the AICA and PICA, injection of both VAs is necessary during a diagnostic work-up of posterior fossa arteriovenous malformations (AVMs) or vascular tumors. In cases of bihemispheric PICAs, treatment of an aneurysm located at its origin or VA dissections must be done with extreme caution to avoid the potential bilateral posterior fossa infarction.

Symptoms of PICA occlusion are discussed in detail in Case 18.

Occlusion of the AICA results in several symptoms, including palsies of the facial and vestibulocochlear nerves; vertigo, nausea, vomiting, and nystagmus caused by involvement of the vestibular and vagal nuclei; ipsilateral hemifacial numbness and corneal hypesthesia; Horner's syndrome; cerebellar ataxia; and contralateral hemiparesthesia.

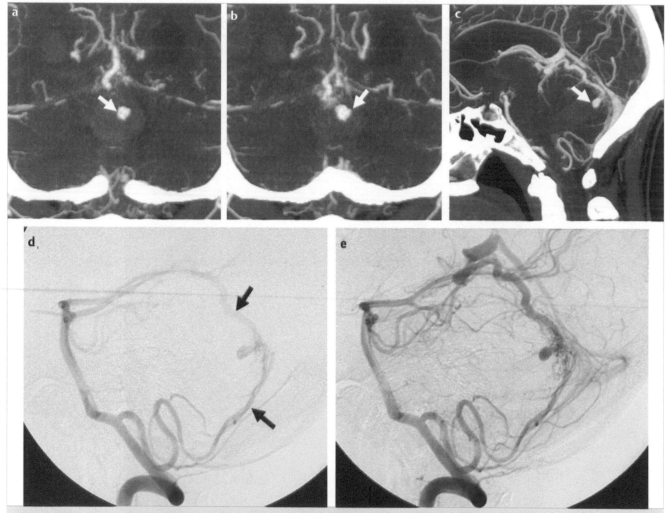

**Fig. 19.8** CTA in coronal (a,b) and sagittal (c) views in a patient with a recently bled cerebellar AVM demonstrates a focal outpouching pointing into the hemorrhagic cavity as the source of hemorrhage (*arrows*). Angiography in lateral view (d,e) in early and late arterial phases demonstrates the AVM fed by the vermian midline anastomosis between the superior and posterior inferior cerebellar arteries, which are in hemodynamic balance over the midline vermis.

## Pearls and Pitfalls

- The AICA is considered part of the arterial labyrinthine system because of its major branch, the internal auditory artery.
- It classically originates from the basilar artery; however, variations with an AICA–PICA complex are common.
- In rare cases with incomplete trigeminal persistence, the AICA or SCA may originate from the cavernous ICA.
- In cases with bihemispheric PICAs, extreme caution must be used to avoid potential bilateral posterior fossa infarctions during endovascular procedures.
- The SCA supplies, with its lateral branch, the deep cerebellar nuclei.

Total occlusion of the SCA may cause vertigo, an ipsilateral Horner's syndrome, limb and gait ataxia, intention tremor, dysarthria, contralateral spinothalamic sensory loss, contralateral upper motor neuron-type facial palsy, and occasionally, a contralateral fourth nerve palsy.

## 19.4 Additional Information and Cases

See ► Fig. 19.3, ► Fig. 19.4, ► Fig. 19.5, ► Fig. 19.6, ► Fig. 19.7, and ► Fig. 19.8.

# Further Reading

[1] Cullen SP, Ozanne A, Alvarez H, Lasjaunias P. The bihemispheric posterior inferior cerebellar artery. Neuroradiology 2005; 47: 809–812

[2] Lasjaunias P, Berenstein A, ter Brugge KG. Surgical Neuroangiography. Vol. 1. 2nd ed. Berlin: Springer; 2006

[3] Lasjaunias P, Vallee B, Person H, Ter Brugge K, Chiu M. The lateral spinal artery of the upper cervical spinal cord. Anatomy, normal variations, and angiographic aspects. J Neurosurg 1985; 63: 235–241

[4] Naidich TP, Kricheff II, II, George AE, Lin JP. The normal anterior inferior cerebellar artery. Anatomic-radiographic correlation with emphasis on the lateral projection. Radiology 1976; 119: 355–373

[5] Newton TH, Potts DG. Radiology of the Skull and Brain. St. Louis: Mosby; 1974

[6] Reinacher P, Krings T, Buergel U, Hans FJ. Posterior inferior cerebellar artery (PICA) aneurysm arising from a bihemispheric PICA. Clin Neuroradiol. 2006; 16: 190–191

[7] Rodríguez-Hernández A, Rhoton AL, Jr, Lawton MT. Segmental anatomy of cerebellar arteries: a proposed nomenclature. Laboratory investigation. J Neurosurg 2011; 115: 387–397

[8] Takahashi M, Wilson G, Hanafee W. The anterior inferior cerebellar artery, Its radiographic anatomy and significance in the diagnosis of extraaxial tumors of the posterior fossa. Radiology 1968; 90: 281–287

# 20 The Basilar Artery Trunk

## 20.1 Case Description

### 20.1.1 Clinical Presentation

A 39-year-old man collapsed at work and was brought to the emergency department. CT demonstrated a diffuse subarachnoid hemorrhage and associated hydrocephalus. CTA demonstrated an aneurysm at the proximal portion of the basilar artery just distal to its origin from the vertebral arteries. For further evaluation and treatment, the patient underwent conventional angiography.

### 20.1.2 Radiologic Studies

See ▶ Fig. 20.1.

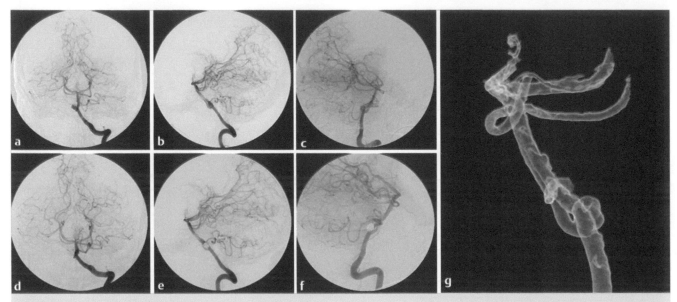

**Fig. 20.1** Left vertebral artery (VA) angiogram in anteroposterior (AP) (a,d), lateral (b,e), and oblique (c,f) views with 3D reconstruction (g) before (a,b, c,g) and after (d,e,f) embolization of a saccular basilar trunk aneurysm. 3D rotational angiography revealed its origin to be at the caudal portion of a focal unfused ("fenestrated") basilar artery pointing cranially. Unassisted coil embolization was performed and resulted in complete obliteration of the aneurysm.

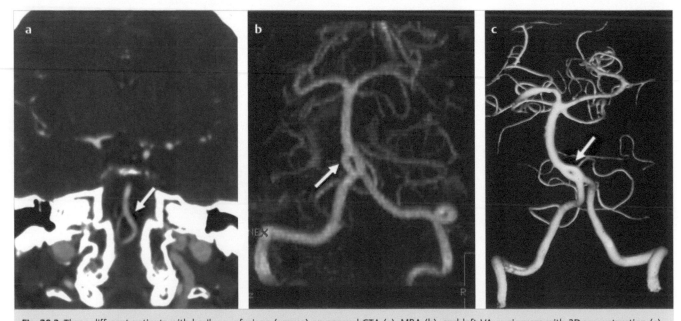

**Fig. 20.2** Three different patients with basilar nonfusions (*arrows*) on coronal CTA (a), MRA (b), and left VA angiogram with 3D reconstruction (c). These anatomic variations are typically present in the inferior third of the basilar artery and result from incomplete fusion of the paired longitudinal neural arteries.

### 20.1.3 Diagnosis

Ruptured mid-basilar aneurysm in the setting of a proximal focal unfused segment of the basilar artery.

## 20.2 Embryology and Anatomy

The basilar artery is a result of two simultaneous fusion phenomena that concur with the regression of the primitive trigeminal arteries. When the embryo is about 4 mm long, the primitive posterior circulation is constituted caudally by the paired ventral longitudinal neural arteries that are connected laterally at multiple locations with the primitive hindbrain plexus, and cranially by the caudal divisions of the internal carotid arteries. Cranially, at the pontomesencephalic sulcus, these caudal divisions of the internal carotid arteries fuse to form the basilar tip, whereas caudally, the paired longitudinal neural arteries fuse to form a single basilar artery. The fusion process is typically completed when the embryo is 9 mm long (i.e., around the fifth fetal week). Failure of fusion of the neural arteries and regression of the bridging vessels between longitudinal arteries will lead to varying degrees of nonfusion, from duplicated basilar arteries (as the extreme form of an incomplete fusion process) to focal nonfused segments. The lateral walls of the unfused artery have a normal intrinsic architecture; however, at the base of the medial wall, the media layer is absent. In addition, there is discontinuity of elastin, the subendothelium is thinned, and the muscular layer of the basilar artery can be absent. This

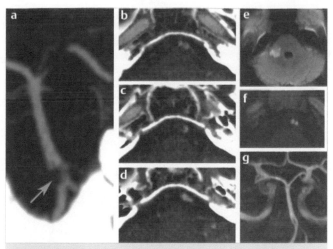

**Fig. 20.3** An 84-year-old man presented with acute brainstem symptoms. CTA coronal (a) and axial 0.5-mm images (b,c,d, from top to bottom) show a clot, seen as a filling defect, in the right inferior basilar artery (*arrow*). Follow-up diffusion-weighted MRI (e), axial T1-weighted image with fat suppression (f), and 3D time-of-flight MRA (g) after autolysis of the clot demonstrate that the thrombus had actually lodged in the right limb of an unfused basilar artery. The diffusion-weighted image shows the corresponding area of ischemia, indicating that perforators arise from both limbs of the unfused segment. It is important to recognize this variation prospectively when contemplating mechanical thrombectomy, for example with a stent-retriever.

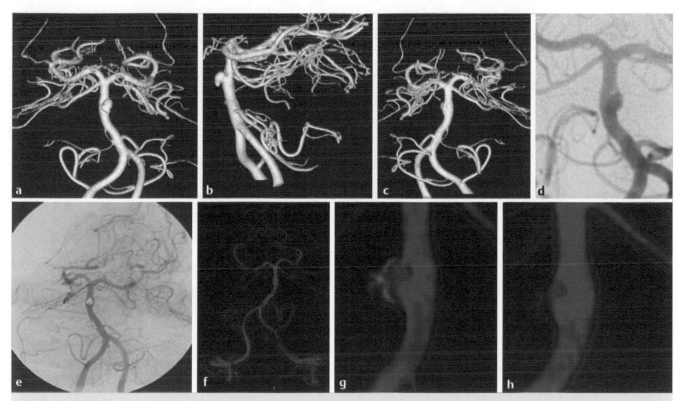

**Fig. 20.4** Left VA angiogram and 3D reconstruction, before (a–d) and after (e–h) embolization of a saccular basilar trunk aneurysm in the context of a very small unfused segment that is best apparent after coiling. Failure to recognize these very small unfused segments may lead to catastrophic outcomes if a balloon remodeling technique is used, as it may rupture the basilar artery if the balloon is inflated in the smaller channel.

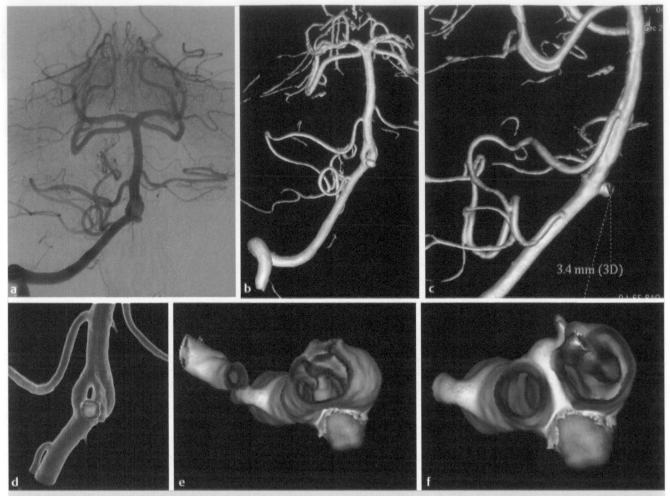

**Fig. 20.5** Right VA angiograms in AP view (a) and 3D reconstruction (b–f), before (a,b,c) and after (d,e,f) embolization of a saccular basilar trunk aneurysm in the context of an unfused segment in the caudal portion of the basilar artery. Note that this patient also harbors a tiny "mirror" aneurysm at the level of the nonfusion pointing posteriorly. These types of "kissing" or mirror aneurysms are present in up to 10% of patients with aneurysms at nonfusion sites. The in-vessel view of the 3D reconstructions demonstrates that between the two channels, a solid septation is present.

structural weakness may lead to the formation of aneurysms at nonfused segments, as the wall architecture resembles those of arterial bifurcations. In addition, one may presume that an incomplete fusion points to an incomplete maturation process of the arterial wall. The lack of cell selection that such pattern, imply may preserve "weaker" (i.e., less matured) endothelial cells, which will later reveal arterial aneurysms when secondary, revealing, triggers, such as hemodynamic stress, are present.

## 20.3 Clinical Impact

Given the location at the midline, anterior to the brainstem, aneurysms that are associated with a focal unfused basilar artery are best treated with coil embolization.

Because of their embryological development, both limbs of the unfused basilar artery carry brainstem-perforating arteries to their respective sides. Vessel sacrifice of one limb of the fenestration may therefore result in unilateral brain stem stroke resulting from occlusion of perforators and should not be performed.

Failure to recognize a small nonfusion may lead to catastrophic events if the balloon remodeling technique is performed and the balloon is overinflated, which may lead to rupture at the level of the nonfusion site.

## 20.4 Additional Information and Cases

Four differential diagnoses of a "double lumen of a single artery" have to be discussed that are often mistakenly grouped together under the name "fenestration."

Given the above-mentioned embryology, a lack of fusion of embryologically paired vessels leads to segmentally unfused arteries. This condition can only exist where two embryological arteries fuse during development; therefore, the basilar artery, as described here, or the anterior spinal artery can harbor unfused segments.

Second, duplications can be present. Here, the "double lumen" is a result of persistence of two embryologically different vessels, of which one normally regresses during development. If both vessels persist, the vessel is duplicated. Duplications can be encountered in the internal carotid artery (ICA; segmental agenesis of the first ICA segment with reconstitution of the distal ICA via different arteries from the ascending pharyngeal artery system) (see Case 3's ▸ Fig. 3.3 ), the anterior cerebral artery (ACA; duplicated ACA with persistent infraorbital origin of the ACA) (see Case 10's ▸ Fig. 10.4 ), or at the vertebrobasilar junction. Here, the duplication recruits two separate vessels (the lateral spinal artery and vertebral artery), one of which enters the spinal canal while the other remains in the vertebral canal.

Third, extracerebral anastomoses between perforators can lead to the aspect of a double lumen of a single artery (see Case 14's ▸ Fig. 14.3). This condition can be encountered close to both the anterior and posterior perforating substance and is established from the embryologically present rete of perforators.

Finally, a true fenestration is defined as a single artery with two luminal channels. This fenestration can, for example, be a result of a nerve or other anatomical structure "piercing" the artery and is typically encountered in the vertebral artery or the ICA at the neck and can rarely be seen in the A1 segment (▸ Fig. 20.2; ▸ Fig. 20.3; ▸ Fig. 20.4; ▸ Fig. 20.5; ▸ Fig. 20.6; ▸ Fig. 20.7; ▸ Fig. 20.8; ▸ Fig. 20.9; ▸ Fig. 20.10). See also Cases 11 and 14.

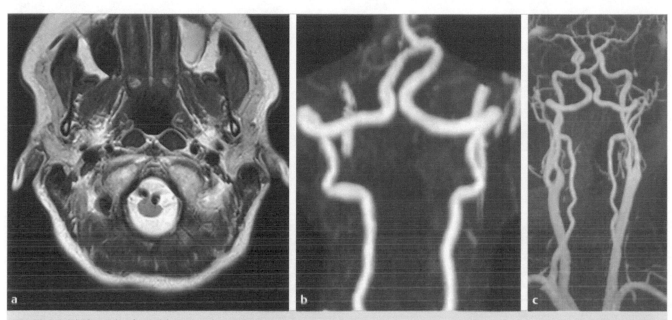

Fig. 20.6 Axial T2-weighted MRI (a), MRA without (b) and with (c) contrast enhancement reveal "kissing" of the vertebral arteries at the level of the foramen magnum.

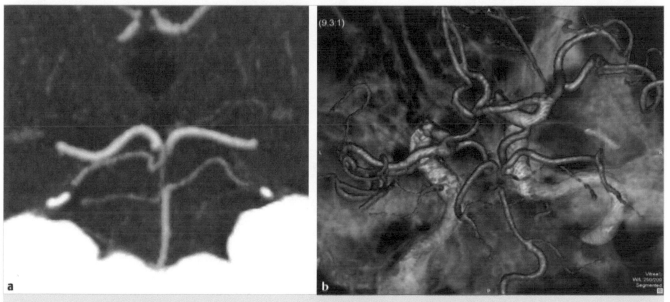

Fig. 20.7 Coronal CTA (a) and 3D reconstruction (b) in oblique view demonstrate absence of the distal basilar artery.

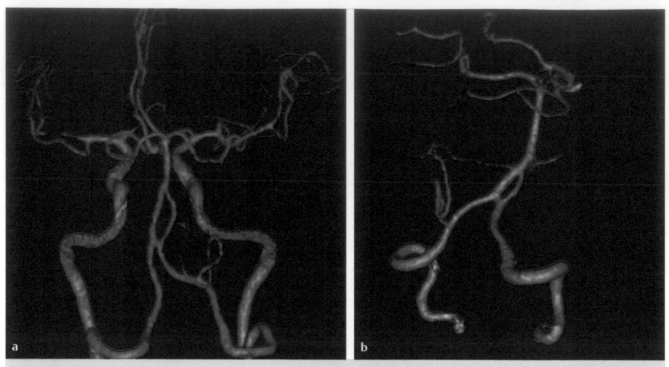

**Fig. 20.8** 3D CTA reconstructions in posterior-anterior (a) and oblique (b) views in two different cases demonstrate nonfusion of the basilar artery. This variation should not be confused with dissections or thrombus within the basilar artery.

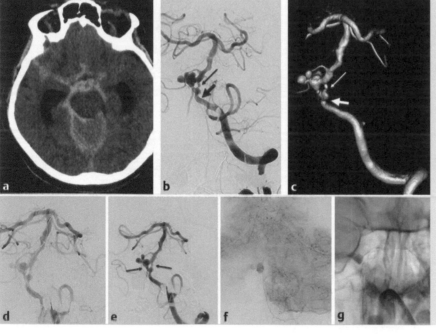

**Fig. 20.9** Acute subarachnoid hemorrhage (non-enhanced CT in a) related to a dissecting aneurysm that commenced (*arrow* in b,c) just proximal to a local unfused basilar artery segment (*small arrows* in b,c) and that extended over the right lateral limb of the nonfused segment ([b] left VA injection in AP projection; [c] 3D rotational angiography). As the dissection started proximal to the nonfused segment, parent vessel sacrifice was not contemplated, and instead, a flow diverter was inserted through the right lateral limb (d), keeping both limbs open (*arrows* in e) and leading to significant stagnation in the aneurysmal outpouching (f,g).

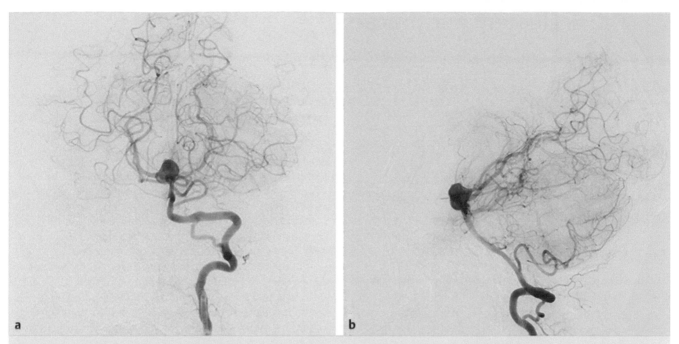

**Fig. 20.10** Left VA angiograms in AP (a) and lateral (b) views in a patient with a basilar tip aneurysm demonstrate an incidental finding of a distal VA duplication resulting from persistence of the lateral spinal artery channel at C2 level.

## Pearls and Pitfalls

- Midbasilar saccular aneurysms are extremely rare, and if present, a focal nonfusion has to be specifically looked for (including 3D rotational angiographies).
- Kissing aneurysms (i.e., mirror-type aneurysms) occur in up to 10% of patients with an aneurysm at a basilar artery nonfusion site and have to be searched for by 3D rotational angiography.
- If the flow is antegrade, aneurysms at local nonfusions nearly always occur at the proximal limb of the nonfusion.
- Basilar artery nonfusions do not predispose to the formation of aneurysms; the occurrence rate is similar to those at other bifurcations of the circle of Willis.

## Further Reading

[1] Black SP, Ansbacher LE. Saccular aneurysm associated with segmental duplication of the basilar artery. A morphological study. J Neurosurg 1984; 61: 1005–1008

[2] Islak C, Kocer N, Kantarci F, Saatci I, Uzma O, Canbaz B. Endovascular management of basilar artery aneurysms associated with fenestrations. AJNR Am J Neuroradiol 2002; 23: 958–964

[3] Krings T, Baccin CE, Alvarez H, Ozanne A, Stracke P, Lasjaunias PL. Segmental unfused basilar artery with kissing aneurysms: report of three cases and literature review. Acta Neurochir (Wien) 2007; 149: 567–574, discussion 574

[4] Padget DH. The development of the cranial arteries in the human embryo. Contrib Embryol 1948; 32: 205–261

[5] Sanders WP, Sorek PA, Mehta BA. Fenestration of intracranial arteries with special attention to associated aneurysms and other anomalies. AJNR Am J Neuroradiol 1993; 14: 675–680

# 21 The Brainstem Perforators

## 21.1 Case Description

### 21.1.1 Clinical Presentation

An 80-year-old man presented with progressive symptoms of dizziness, ataxia, multiple episodes of loss of consciousness, double vision, and skew deviation. His symptoms progressed despite best medical treatment.

### 21.1.2 Radiologic Studies

See ▶ Fig. 21.1, ▶ Fig. 21.2.

### 21.1.3 Diagnosis

Basilar artery perforator stroke after percutaneous transluminal angioplasty and stenting of a mid-basilar artery stenosis.

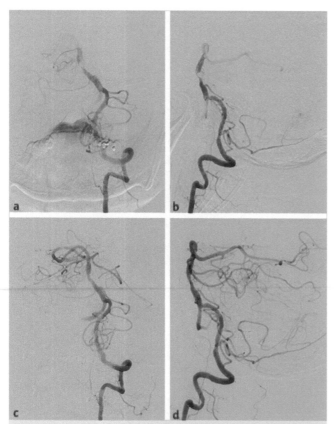

**Fig. 21.1** Left vertebral artery (VA) angiograms in anteroposterior (a,c) and lateral (b–d) views before (a,b) and after (c,d) angioplasty and stenting. There is a tight midbasilar artery stenosis resulting from a posteriorly located plaque, with a slow flow toward the basilar tip (a,b). This was thought to be responsible for the patient's symptoms, and treatment with stent-assisted angioplasty was performed, with good reopening of the basilar artery and brisk filling of the basilar circulation (c,d). Note the improved flow to the posterior circulation after the procedure. The patient woke up from anesthesia with a left facial droop, slurred speech, and mild weakness in the left arm and left leg.

## 21.2 Embryology and Anatomy

The basilar artery gives rise to three different groups of arteries: the cerebellar arteries (anterior inferior cerebellar artery [AICA] and superior cerebellar artery, and in approximately one-quarter of patients, the posterior inferior cerebellar artery as well), the pontine arteries (pontomedullary, superior and inferior long lateral pontine, and posterolateral arteries) and the basilar perforators.

While the pontine arteries are circumferential arteries to supply the lateral (short circumferential) and the dorsolateral (long circumferential branches) parts of the pons in its caudal (pontomedullary arteries), middle (long lateral pontine arteries), and superior (posterolateral artery) portion, the central parts of the pons are supplied by the basilar artery perforators. Three groups of perforators can be distinguished: the caudal, the middle, and the rostral groups. Within each of these groups, 1 to 10 individual perforators can be identified that may originate from a common trunk or, less commonly, individually from the basilar artery.

The caudal perforators originate from the dorsal wall of the basilar artery cranial to the junction of the vertebral arteries and caudal to the origin of the AICA and descend along the basilar sulcus to enter the foramen caecum at the junctional point of the pontomedullary sulcus and the anterior median sulcus. The middle perforators arise typically from the dorsal or dorsolateral wall of the basilar artery between the AICA and the posterolateral artery or along with the basilar artery collateral branches, whereas the rostral perforators originate from the terminal dorsal and superior part of the basilar artery, as well as from the superior cerebellar artery and the posterolateral artery. They enter the most caudal part of the interpeduncular fossa, just caudal to the penetration sites of the mesencephalic perforators of the posterior cerebral artery.

Each perforator group has short and long terminal intrapontine branches that course close to the raphe of the pons. The short arteries supply the medial part of the pyramidal bundles, whereas the long arteries supply the pontine tegmentum close to the raphe and the fourth ventricle, particularly the raphe nuclei, the paramedian reticular formation, the medial longitudinal fasciculus, the medial part of the medial lemniscus, and the abducens nucleus. As the basilar artery is formed by fusion of the paired longitudinal neural arteries, it is extremely uncommon to have a common origin of both the right and the left perforators in the dorsal midline; instead, separate dorsolateral trunks of the perforators are most commonly present.

## 21.3 Clinical Impact

Although this anatomical description of the origin and the type of perforators may sound somewhat abstract, they do have a direct effect on patient treatment in a variety of clinical scenarios: Given the dorsal or dorsolateral location of the perforators, intracranial balloon angioplasty or stenting will be of greater risk if the atherosclerotic plaque to be treated is located on the posterior wall of the basilar artery, as the "snow-plowing" effect of the angioplasty may dislodge debris into the perforators.

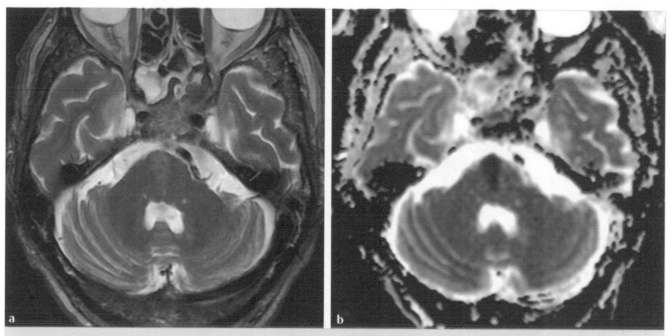

**Fig. 21.2** Axial T2-weighted MRI (a) and apparent diffusion coefficient map (b) after angioplasty and stenting reveal a right medial brainstem perforator infarct.

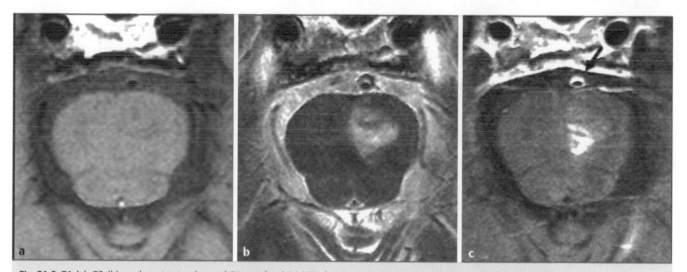

**Fig. 21.3** T1 (a), T2 (b), and contrast-enhanced T1-weighted (c) MRI demonstrate an acute perforator ischemia in a patient with a ventrolateral enhancing plaque (*black arrow*) that incorporates a perforator on its lateral wall. Ischemia is present in the short paramedian midpontine segment.

Plaques that are located on the anterior wall will harbor a smaller risk. Patients who are symptomatic only because of perforator ischemia in the basilar artery territory will not benefit from intracranial stenting, as the perforators will not open because of the stenting of the parent artery and the location of the plaque will be dorsolateral, thereby putting additional perforators at risk. This anatomy of the basilar artery perforators may explain why patients with intracranial stenting and balloon angioplasty did worse if the percutaneous transluminal angioplasty was performed in the posterior circulation.

In giant, "partially thrombosed" fusiform aneurysms, reconstruction of the basilar artery by using flow-diverting stents with additional coil embolization to promote thrombosis in the fusiform aneurysm has been reported to have a very high morbidity and mortality, which, given the above-mentioned considerations, will not come as a surprise, as the reconstruction of the basilar artery will not lead necessarily also to reconstruction of the perforating branches, which in fact may occlude after this particular type of treatment, especially if additional coils are packed between the flow diverter and the vessel wall.

## 21.4 Additional Information and Cases

See ▸ Fig. 21.3, ▸ Fig. 21.4, ▸ Fig. 21.5, ▸ Fig. 21.6, and ▸ Fig. 21.7.

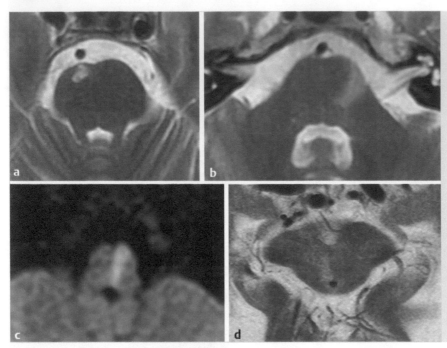

**Fig. 21.4** T2-weighted (a,b,d) and diffusion-weighted (c) MRI in four different patients with perforator ischemia involving the short circumferential vessels (a), the long circumferential vessels (b), the long paramedian territory (c), or the short paramedian territory (d).

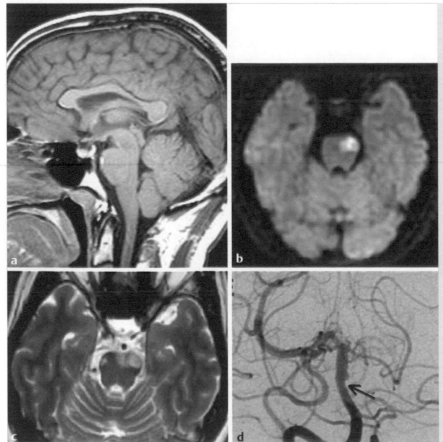

**Fig. 21.5** A 48-year-old woman developed sudden onset of dysarthria, right facial droop, and decreased coordination on her right. Sagittal T1-weighted (a), axial diffusion-weighted (b), and T2-weighted (c) MRI show partial pontine infarction caused by basilar dissection that involved the short paramedian and circumferential territories on the left. Right VA angiogram in anteroposterior view (d) confirms the dissection (*arrow*), seen as focal narrowing with a small distal outpouching, at the midbasilar artery.

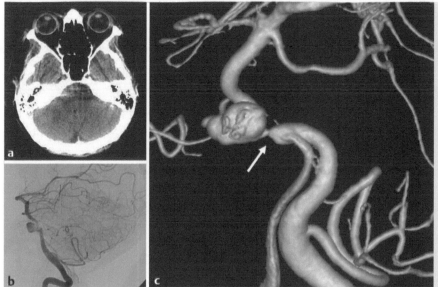

**Fig. 21.6** Unenhanced axial CT (a), left VA angiograms in lateral view (b), and 3D rotation reconstruction (c) demonstrate a hemorrhagic dissecting midbasilar artery aneurysm with the characteristic preaneurysmal narrowing (*arrow*) as the origin of the dissection. Depending on the location along the basilar artery and its circumferential position, a variable number of perforators will be involved in the dissection or are at risk in case of parent vessel occlusion.

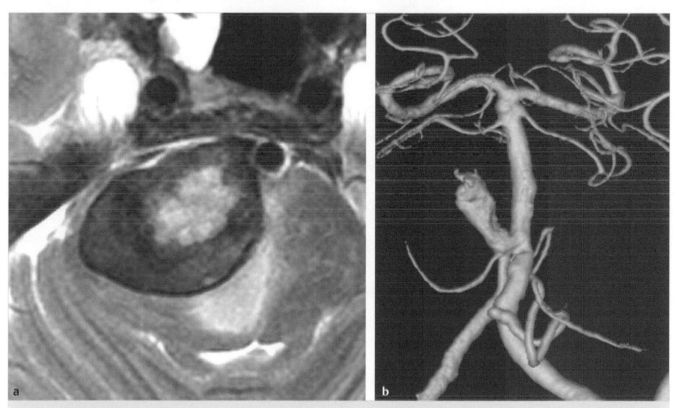

**Fig. 21.7** Chronic dissecting midbasilar aneurysm with recent symptoms. T2-weighted MRI (a) demonstrates both infarction of a paramedian perforator, presumably resulting from chronic dissection, which is seen on the 3D rotational reconstruction of the VA angiogram (b), as well as involvement of the origin of the perforator in the dissection.

Pearls and Pitfalls

- Plaque on the anterior wall of the basilar artery is less likely to involve perforators compared with plaque on the posterior and lateral walls.
- Three groups of perforators and pontine circumferential vessels can be differentiated: the caudal, middle, and superior ones. Areas that are rich in perforators will be localized to the area of the foramen caecum for the inferior group, at the level of the interpeduncular fossa for the superior group, and cranial to the AICA origin for the middle group. The basilar artery just inferior to the AICA is therefore often not as rich in perforators as other regions.
- The paramedian perforators resemble the sulcocommissural arteries of the spine and will therefore commonly supply the brainstem nuclei, whereas the circumferential pontine arteries are linked to the vasocorona system of the spine and therefore supply the white matter tracts.

# Further Reading

[1] Kulcsár Z, Ernemann U, Wetzel SG et al. High-profile flow diverter (silk) implantation in the basilar artery: efficacy in the treatment of aneurysms and the role of the perforators. Stroke 2010; 41: 1690–1696

[2] Kumral E, Bayulkem G, Akyol A, Yunten N, Sirin H, Sagduyu A. Mesencephalic and associated posterior circulation infarcts. Stroke 2002; 33: 2224–2231

[3] Marinković SV, Gibo H. The surgical anatomy of the perforating branches of the basilar artery. Neurosurgery 1993; 33: 80–87

# 22 The Basilar Tip

## 22.1 Case Description

### 22.1.1 Clinical Presentation

Forty-eight hours after subarachnoid bleed, a 44-year-old female patient was transferred to our institution. Unenhanced CTA demonstrated a blood clot in the interpeduncular cistern. On CTA, a basilar tip aneurysm was seen and the patient underwent catheter angiography.

### 22.1.2 Radiologic Studies

See ▸ Fig. 22.1, ▸ Fig. 22.2.

### 22.1.3 Diagnosis

Saccular aneurysm in the presence of an asymmetric fusion of the basilar tip.

## 22.2 Embryology and Anatomy

The termination of the basilar artery can be subdivided into three distinct types, depending on the time when the caudal portions of the distal internal carotid artery (ICA) merge with the paired ventral longitudinal neural arteries: a cranial symmetric fusion type, a caudal symmetric fusion type, or an asymmetric fusion type. As pointed out in the previous case, formation of the basilar artery occurs via a bidirectional fusion

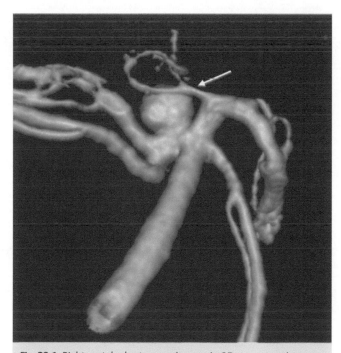

**Fig. 22.1** Right vertebral artery angiogram in 3D reconstruction demonstrates a broad-based basilar tip aneurysm that is arising from the caudal P1 in the setting of asymmetric fusion of the basilar tip. Note that a single bithalamic perforator (*arrow*) to the thalamus (so-called artery of Percheron) is present, arising from the cranial P1.

process. The fusion process cranial to the trigeminal point incorporates merging of both caudal divisions of the embryonic ICAs with the anterior longitudinal neural arteries. If the fusion occurs early, it will be completed from its most cranial point onward and will lead to fusion of both the right and the left caudal division of the ICA to the level of the pontomesencephalic sulcus, leading to an adult T-shape of the basilar tip (▸ Fig. 22.3). This fusion type constitutes the most "mature" or complete fusion and is referred to as a "cranial" fusion type. If the fusion of both limbs occurs later, it will be below the pontomesencephalic sulcus, and a V-shape of the basilar tip will ensue; this is referred to as a "caudal" fusion type. The third type of fusion is when merging is asymmetrical, with one caudal division merging with the anterior longitudinal neural arteries earlier (more cranially) than the other caudal division of the ICA. This disposition is called an asymmetric fusion.

## 22.3 Clinical Impact, Additional Information and Cases

The presented anatomical variations have two potential effects on treatment of basilar tip aneurysms: one being its relation to the anatomy of the thalamic perforators of the P1 and the basilar tip, and the other being the occurrence rates of aneurysm in relation to each of the different types of fusion.

The recognition of the specific basilar tip anatomy will enable prediction of the origin and size of the supplied territory of the basilar tip perforators arising in proximity to the basilar artery aneurysm. When the fusion is symmetrical, independent of whether it is a caudal (late) or cranial (early) fusion, the origins of the perforating arteries of the interpeduncular fossa are more or less equally distributed; however, when merging is asymmetric, the great majority of the perforating diencephalic and mesencephalic arteries stem from the P1 segment on the side that merged earlier (i.e., the cranial limb). Patients with a caudal variant (V-type) will have a smaller vascular territory being supplied from the proximal P1 segment, whereas in cranial fusion types, the supplied territory can be larger. In asymmetric dispositions, the cranial limb will classically harbor the major supply to the thalamus and a unilateral supply type, the so-called Percheron artery (see also Case 23), can be present (▸ Fig. 22.4; ▸ Fig. 22.5).

Regarding occurrence rates, it has been shown that basilar tip aneurysms arise preferentially on an asymmetric basilar artery fusion (with the neck of the aneurysm commonly located in the caudal P1 segment), followed by symmetric caudal fusion. Aneurysms in the most mature form of basilar tip configurations (i.e., the symmetrical cranial fusion) occur significantly less often. This observation gains additional weight by the fact that these two fusion types (asymmetric and caudal) are far less common than the cranial symmetric fusion types (1:5), thereby indicating that specific anatomical dispositions are more prone than others to aneurysm occurrence.

When evaluating their patients with multiple aneurysms, the Bicêtre group found in 280 aneurysms in 113 consecutive patients that aneurysms occurred more frequently in caudal or

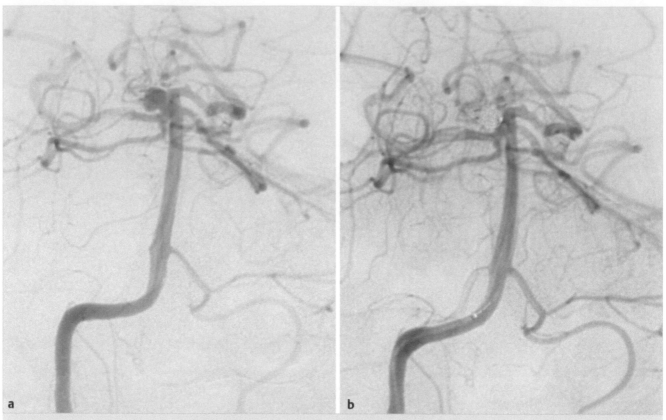

**Fig. 22.2** Right vertebral artery angiograms in the working projection before (a) and after (b) coiling. In this scenario, the caudal P1 is at higher risk of occlusion, given its broad communication with the aneurysm. A working projection should, however, also ensure that the origin of the Percheron artery is well visualized.

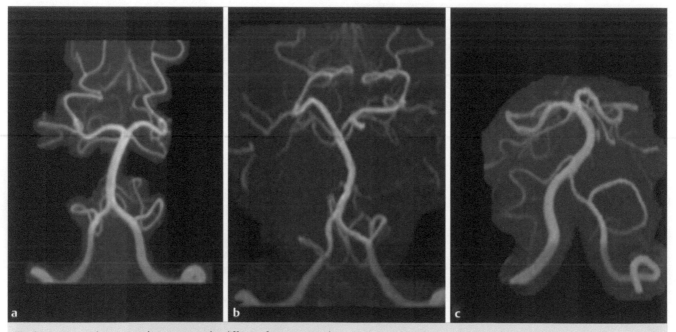

**Fig. 22.3** MRA in three cases demonstrates the different fusion types: the cranial symmetric fusion (a), the caudal symmetric fusion (b), and the asymmetric fusion (c).

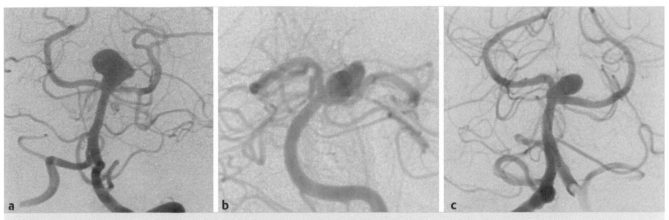

**Fig. 22.4** Vertebral artery angiograms in anteroposterior view demonstrate basilar tip aneurysms in three different fusion types: the cranial symmetric fusion (a), the caudal symmetric fusion (b), and the asymmetric fusion (c).

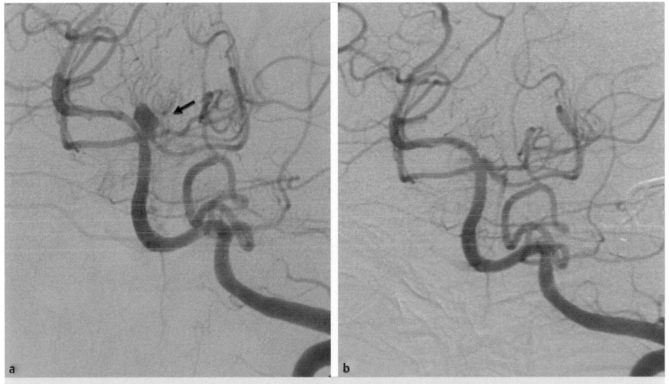

**Fig. 22.5** Left vertebral artery angiograms in anteroposterior view before (a) and after (b) coiling of a basilar tip aneurysm. In very rare circumstances, the thalamoperforators arise in an asymmetric fusion from the caudal P1 limb (*arrow*), as in this case. These are potentially dangerous cases, as the aneurysm neck has classically a wide communication with the inferior P1 limb.

delayed fusion types of the basilar artery, embryonic arterial persistence, nonfused segments, and an incomplete anterior communicating artery complex. They related these findings to the relative immaturity of the vasculature and its vulnerability to secondary events. However, this observation can also be interpreted in terms of the hemodynamic stress that is secondarily caused by the variation. It is known that degenerative changes of the elastic lamina and media caused by hemody-namic stress close to branching structures are the initial lesions existing before aneurysm formation. As variations in inflow conditions related to anatomic variations of the basilar artery tip result in changes of the average wall shear stress magnitude for the vessel wall, hemodynamic stress may be higher in certain basilar tip fusion types, and therefore explain the higher proportion of aneurysms encountered.

## Pearls and Pitfalls

- Certain basilar tip configurations are more commonly associated with aneurysms than others.
- In asymmetric basilar tip configurations, the aneurysm neck is typically located on the caudal segment.
- In asymmetrical dispositions, the cranial limb will classically harbor the major supply to the thalamus, and a unilateral supply type, the so-called Percheron artery, can be present.
- The most "mature" type of basilar tip configuration is the symmetric cranial fusion.

# Further Reading

[1] Brassier G, Morandi X, Fournier D, Velut S, Mercier P. Origin of the perforating arteries of the interpeduncular fossa in relation to the termination of the basilar artery. Interv Neuroradiol 1998; 4: 109–120

[2] Campos C, Churojana A, Rodesch G, Alvarez H, Lasjaunias P. Basilar tip aneurysms and basilar tip anatomy. Interv Neuroradiol 1998; 4: 121–125

[3] Songsaeng D, Geibprasert S, Willinsky R, Tymianski M, TerBrugge KG, Krings T. Impact of anatomical variations of the circle of Willis on the incidence of aneurysms and their recurrence rate following endovascular treatment. Clin Radiol 2010; 65: 895–901

# 23 The Thalamoperforating Arteries

## 23.1 Case Description

### 23.1.1 Clinical Presentation

A 48-year-old patient presented with acute onset of confusion and ataxia to the emergency room.

### 23.1.2 Radiologic Studies

See ▶ Fig. 23.1, ▶ Fig. 23.2.

### 23.1.3 Diagnosis

Thalamic micro-arteriovenous malformation (AVM) fed by the principal group of the inferolateral thalamoperforators.

## 23.2 Anatomy

There are three major thalamoperforating artery (ThPA) groups that supply the different thalamic vascular territories. The nomenclature varies, but for this chapter they are referred to as the tuberothalamic, paramedian, and inferolateral arteries. These groups have also been referred to as the anterior ThPA, posterior ThPA, and thalamogeniculate arteries. There is high individual variability in the number, origin, and arterial territory supplied by each group. The small size of the perforator branches makes them often difficult to visualize, but they can be seen on lateral angiograms.

The tuberothalamic arteries arise from the middle third of the posterior communicating artery (PcomA) and supply the ventral section of the thalamus, which includes the reticular nucleus, the ventral anterior nucleus, the rostral section of the ventrolateral nucleus, the ventral pole of the medial dorsal nucleus, the mamillothalamic tract, the ventral amygdalofugal pathway, the ventral section of the internal medullary lamina, and the anterior thalamic nuclei. They can be divided into interpeduncular, hypothalamic, and thalamic segments. The interpe-

duncular segment loops posterior to the optic tract. It is extremely short and sometimes nonexistent. The hypothalamic segment enters the hypothalamus in close relationship to the lateral wall of the third ventricle. The thalamic segment appears as a characteristic cluster of vessels that supplies the nuclei mentioned earlier. The tuberothalamic group can be absent in ~30% (up to 60%, according to some series) of the normal population. In these cases, the tuberothalamic arterial territory is taken over by the paramedian group.

The paramedian arteries are usually two arteries that arise from the P1 segment of the posterior cerebral artery (PCA), but their number can range between one and five. They supply the dorsomedial nucleus, internal medullary lamina, and intralaminar nuclei and are presumed to represent the most cranial group of paramedian arteries of the basilar artery. They can be divided into interpeduncular, mesencephalic, and thalamic segments. The interpeduncular segment has a characteristic short but very sinuous course. The mesencephalic segment, in contrast, has a characteristically straight course as it traverses the midbrain, allowing the differentiation between the segments. The thalamic segment appears as a cluster of vessels, similar to the one from the tuberothalamic arteries. The paramedian arteries can arise as a pair from each P1, but also as a common trunk, thus supplying the thalamus bilaterally (artery of Percheron) (▶ Fig. 23.3). When the tuberothalamic arteries are absent, the paramedian arteries take over their territory.

The inferolateral arteries are between 5 and 10 arteries that arise from the P2 segment of the PCA. They are subdivided into three groups: medial geniculate, principal inferolateral, and inferolateral pulvinar. The medial group supplies the external half of the medial geniculate nucleus. The principal inferolateral group penetrates between the geniculate bodies, ascends in the lateral medullary lamina, and supplies the major part of the ventral posterior nuclei and parts of the ventrolateral nucleus. The inferolateral pulvinar group supplies the rostral and lateral parts of the pulvinar and the lateral dorsal nucleus.

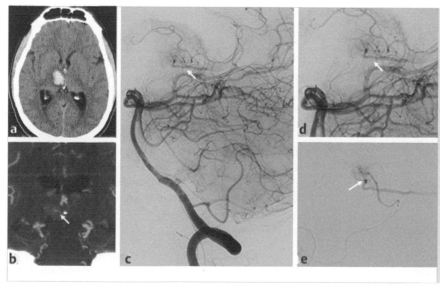

**Fig. 23.1** Unenhanced CT (a) demonstrated a right thalamic hemorrhage. As there was no evidence for microangiopathy on the CT and no history regarding cardiovascular risk factors, CTA (b) and, subsequently, digital subtraction angiography were performed. In retrospect, the CTA demonstrated a tiny asymmetry in the vascularity of the thalamus showing a vessel coursing through the area of hemorrhage (arrow). Vertebral artery injection (b,c) (lateral view with magnification of the area of interest in d) demonstrated a microshunt that was only visible because of early venous shunting (arrows in b,c, d). Superselective catheterization of the principal group of the inferolateral thalamoperforators arising from the P2 segment of the PCA (e) demonstrated the shunt (arrow). After more distal catheterization, the shunt was treated with liquid embolic agent embolization. Case continued in ▶ Fig. 23.2.

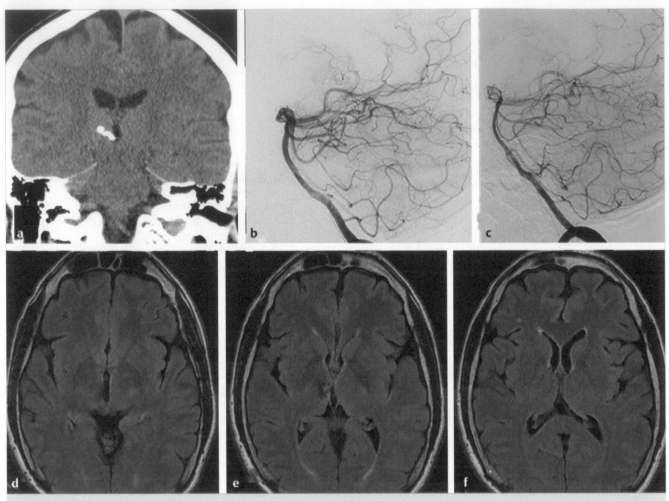

**Fig. 23.2** After the procedure, the patient awoke without new neurological deficits. Coronal unenhanced CT (a) demonstrates the glue cast and angiographic controls immediately after the procedure (vertebral artery lateral view) (b) and, after 1 year (c), demonstrated complete obliteration of the shunt. Axial fluid-attenuated inversion recovery weighted scans (d,e,f) in adjacent cuts after embolization demonstrate the sequelae of the hemorrhage and no focal ischemia.

## 23.3 Clinical Impact

### 23.3.1 PcomA and Tuberothalamic Arteries

There is no consistent relationship between the size of the PcomA and the thalamic territory it supplies. For this reason, surgical or endovascular occlusion of a hypoplastic PcomA during treatment of an aneurysm based on the assumption that it will have a small or no arterial thalamic territory is erroneous. In fact, a hypoplastic PcomA may even increase the chance of a tuberothalamic infarct, as there is less possibility of recruiting supply from P1.

### 23.3.2 Caudal Fusion of the Basilar Artery and ThPA Origin

The more caudal the P1 fusion, the smaller the chance of finding a bilateral common trunk for the perforators. This is an important feature, as in cases of asymmetric caudal fusion (see Case 22), the paramedian arterial group is likely to arise from the most cranial limb. Because of this, catheterization and excessive maneuvering in the higher limb of an asymmetric caudal fusion should be avoided when possible.

### 23.3.3 Artery of Percheron

Percheron described three variations involving the paramedian thalamic-mesencephalic arterial supply: small branches arising from both P1 segments, a common trunk arising from one P1 segment (i.e., artery of Percheron), and an arterial arcade arising from a bridging artery between the two P1 segments. The artery of Percheron is a well-known but relatively uncommon anatomic variant and represents bilateral supply to the medial thalami from a single dominant trunk. There can be variable contributions to the rostral midbrain. Occlusion results in a characteristic imaging pattern of ischemia involving the paramedian thalami with or without midbrain involvement. Clinically, it will present with the classic triad of altered mental status, vertical gaze palsy, and memory impairment.

In cases of basilar tip aneurysms in proximity to an artery of Percheron, special care must be taken in preserving the patency

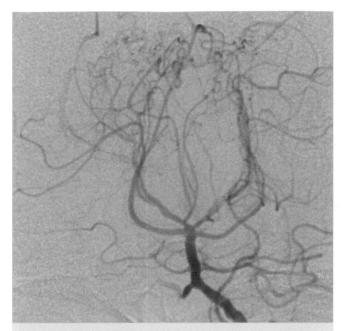

**Fig. 23.3** A 52-year-old man was evaluated for moyamoya disease. Anteroposterior (AP) left vertebral artery angiogram revealed a single right arterial trunk supplying the paramedian thalami bilaterally, in keeping with an artery of Percheron. The patient showed an unusually straight course of the interpeduncular segment.

of the P1 segment. In addition, in cases of balloon remodeling, the balloon must be inflated for short periods of time, as there is no other potential supply to that thalamic territory.

### 23.3.4 Subependymal versus Trans-mesencephalic AVM Supply

In choroidal or third ventricular AVMs, it is important to differentiate a subependymal course of a recruited ThPA from the trans-mesencephalic supply. The former can be used for embolization if a distal position is reached, whereas the latter is considered to be dangerous. The differentiation between both can be done in the lateral angiogram, as the ThPA subependymal course will be longer and will follow the wall of the third ventricle before joining the nidus or one of the choroidal arteries. In contrast, the trans-mesencephalic arteries will be shorter and more direct, connecting directly to the nidus rather than to another vessel.

## 23.4 Additional Information and Cases

See ▶ Fig. 23.4, ▶ Fig. 23.5, ▶ Fig. 23.6, ▶ Fig. 23.7, ▶ Fig. 23.8, and ▶ Fig. 23.9.

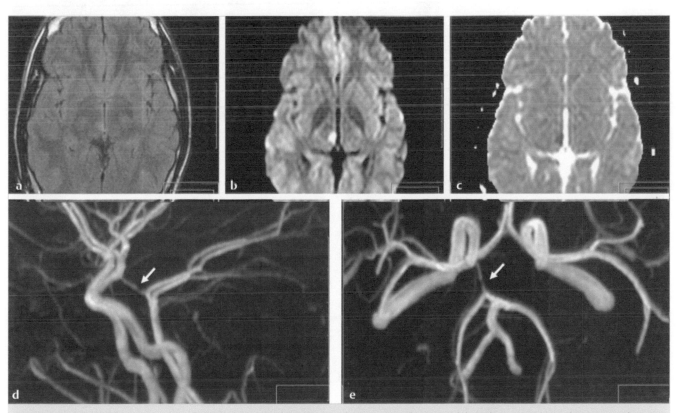

**Fig. 23.4** A 16-year-old patient presented to the emergency department with acute onset of hypo- and dysesthesia. He admitted to using a "designer drug." Drug screening was positive for amphetamines. Fluid-attenuated inversion recovery, diffusion-weighted imaging, and apparent diffusion coefficient scans (a,b,c) demonstrate a focal area of restricted infarction in the right paramedian thalamus (ventral pole of the dorsomedial thalamic nuclei). This territory is classically supplied by the thalamotuberal arteries that arise from the PcomA artery segment. On high-resolution time-of-flight MRA, there is a focal narrowing of this segment (*arrows* in d,e) that was believed to be related to either drug-induced vasculitis or drug-induced vasospasm.

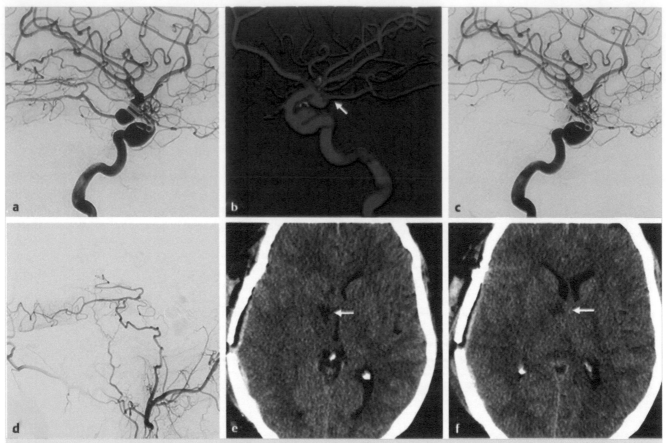

**Fig. 23.5** A 54-year-old woman presented with a past history of subarachnoid hemorrhage secondary to a ruptured right PcomA aneurysm that was clipped 18 years earlier, which now showed a large local recurrence. A right fetal PCA originated from the medial aspect of the aneurysm sac. After multidisciplinary discussion, we decided to treat this patient with a superior temporal artery/PCA bypass followed by endovascular coiling, sacrificing the origin of the right fetal PCA. (a) Lateral and (b) 3D angiography of the right internal carotid artery show a recurrent PcomA aneurysm with a fetal PCA arising from the medial wall of the aneurysm sac (*arrow* in b). (c) Postcoiling lateral ICA angiogram shows complete occlusion of the aneurysm and no filling of the fetal PCA. (d) Right external carotid artery angiogram shows a widely patent extracranial–PCA bypass, with good opacification of the distal PCA branches but no retrograde filling of the proximal P2 segment or PcomA. After the procedure, the patient presented with left upper extremity weakness with no personality changes or memory impairment. (e,f) Nonenhanced CT 24 hours later reveals a recent thalamic infarct in the tuberothalamic artery territory (*arrow* in e,f).

## Pearls and Pitfalls

- The ThPAs are divided into three groups that arise from the PcomA, P1 segment, and P2 segment.
- The tuberothalamic group can be absent in ~30% of cases. In such patients, the paramedian group takes over that arterial territory.
- There is no consistent relationship between PcomA size and arterial supply (i.e., presence of tuberothalamic arteries), so sacrificing a hypoplastic PcomA should be avoided.
- The artery of Percheron is a well-known but unusual variant in which a single trunk supplies both paramedian thalamic territories plus a variable extent of the midbrain.
- In choroidal AVM treatment, it is important to differentiate the subependymal course of a recruited ThPA from trans-mescencephalic supply, as the former can be potentially used for embolization.

## Further Reading

[1] Endo H, Sato K, Kondo R, Matsumoto Y, Takahashi A, Tominaga T. Tuberotha-lamic artery infarctions following coil embolization of ruptured posterior communicating artery aneurysms with posterior communicating artery sac-rifice. AJNR Am J Neuroradiol 2012; 33: 500–506

[2] George AE, Raybaud C, Salamon G, Kricheff II. Anatomy of the thalamoperfo-rating arteries with special emphasis on arteriography of the third ventricle: Part I. Am J Roentgenol Radium Ther Nucl Med 1975; 124: 220–230

[3] Lazzaro NA, Wright B, Castillo M et al. Artery of percheron infarction: imag-ing patterns and clinical spectrum. AJNR Am J Neuroradiol 2010; 31: 1283–1289

[4] Rangel-Castilla L, Gasco J, Thompson B, Salinas P. Bilateral paramedian thala-mic and mesencephalic infarcts after basilar tip aneurysm coiling: role of the artery of Percheron. Neurocirugia (Astur) 2009; 20: 288–293

[5] Schmahmann JD. Vascular syndromes of the thalamus. Stroke 2003; 34: 2264–2278

[6] Uz A. Variations in the origin of the thalamoperforating arteries. J Clin Neuro-sci 2007; 14: 134–137

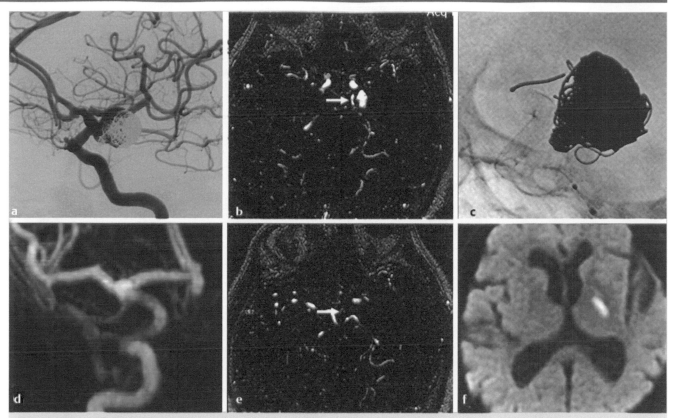

**Fig. 23.6** A 72-year-old woman presented 6 years ago with intracranial bleeding from a large left PcomA aneurysm that was coiled at the time. She made good clinical recovery; however, follow-up imaging demonstrated aneurysm recanalization, and she was retreated with coil embolization. The aneurysm recurred again (a), despite dense packing, and flow-diverter treatment was therefore performed. Note the patency of the PcomA on the time-of-flight MRA source images (b) before retreatment (*arrow*). After flow-diverter treatment (c), the patient was discharged without neurological deficits on dual antiplatelet medication. After 1 year, clopidogrel was discontinued and the patient experienced right weakness and dysarthria with sudden onset 1 week later. Angiography demonstrated occlusion of the aneurysm (d). On the source images, the PcomA is no longer filling (*arrow* in e). The infarction is in the rostral parts of the ventrolateral nucleus, in the territory of the thalamotuberal arteries (diffusion-weighted MRI in f) that arise from the PcomA.

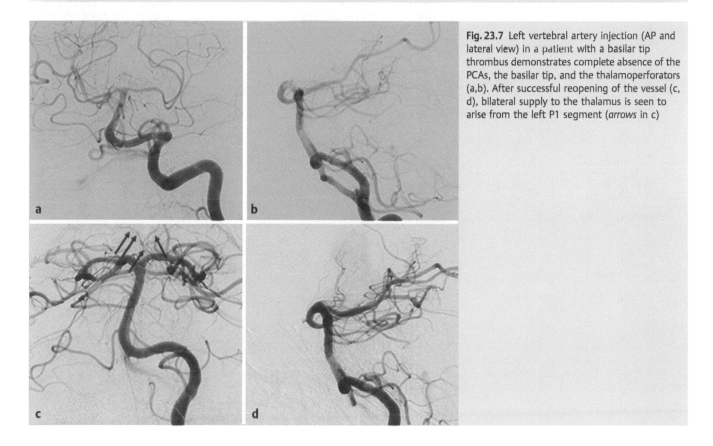

**Fig. 23.7** Left vertebral artery injection (AP and lateral view) in a patient with a basilar tip thrombus demonstrates complete absence of the PCAs, the basilar tip, and the thalamoperforators (a,b). After successful reopening of the vessel (c, d), bilateral supply to the thalamus is seen to arise from the left P1 segment (*arrows* in c)

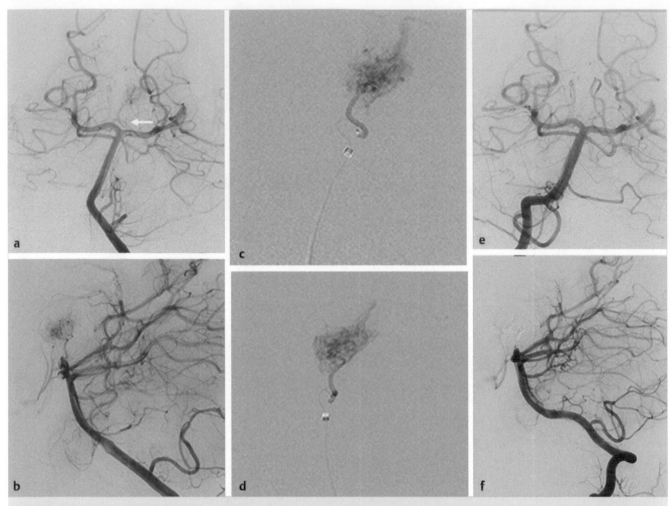

**Fig. 23.8** A 6-year-old boy presented with a left thalamic hematoma secondary to a small thalamic AVM. (a,b) AP and lateral left vertebral artery angiograms show a small nidal-type AVM supplied by a large paramedian perforator arising from the contralateral P1 segment. The angiogram shows the characteristic sinuous course of the interpeduncular segment (*arrow* in a), followed by a straight mesencephalic segment. (c,d) Microcatheter superselective injections (AP and lateral) with the tip placed in the midinterpeduncular segment. (e,f) AP and lateral left vertebral artery angiogram postembolization, showing occlusion of the AVM nidus.

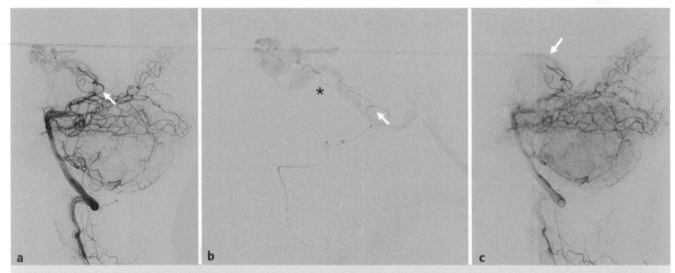

**Fig. 23.9** This patient presented with intraventricular hemorrhage, the cause of which was identified to be a choroidal-type AVM that was fed by the medial choroidal artery from the distal P2 segment (*arrow* in a). This artery follows a recurrent course around the splenium of the corpus callosum (arrow in b) before it reaches the choroid plexus (*asterisk*: tip of the microcatheter). (c) Lateral view after embolization of the AVM demonstrates persistent choroidal blush from the lateral choroidal arteries (*arrow* in c) and complete obliteration of the AVM.

# 24 The Cortical Branches of the Posterior Cerebral Artery

## 24.1 Case Description

### 24.1.1 Clinical Presentation

A 12-year-old boy presented with nausea, vomiting, headaches, and a visual field deficit. An outside CT scan demonstrated a left occipital hemorrhage.

### 24.1.2 Radiologic Studies

See ▶ Fig. 24.1, ▶ Fig. 24.2, and ▶ Fig. 24.3.

### 24.1.3 Diagnosis

Ruptured arteriovenous malformation fed by a medial recurrent branch of the calcarine artery of the distal posterior cerebral artery (PCA).

## 24.2 Embryology and Anatomy

Four major arterial territories are fed by the cortical branches of the PCA: the inferior temporal territory with a hippocampal and an anterior, middle, and posterior temporal subdivision; the calcarine territory; the parieto-occipital territory; and the splenial territory.

The inferior temporal arteries may arise as separate arteries or from a common trunk of the P2 segment. The first branch to arise from the inferior temporal branches is the hippocampal artery, which is in equilibrium with the anterior choroidal artery at the uncus and supplies the hippocampus; the remainder of the inferior temporal branches will be in balance with the middle cerebral artery (MCA) anteriorly and laterally and supply the undersurface of the brain.

The calcarine artery supplies the visual cortex, and its branching of the main PCA trunk is considered the termination of the PCA, with the second continuing branch being the parietooccipital artery. Accessory supply to this territory can arise from the MCA (posterior temporal branch).

The parietooccipital artery supplies the medial surface of the brain in its posterior aspect, including the cuneus and precuneus and the superior parietal lobule, but also the lateral occipital gyrus. It can supply parts of the convexity and is in equilibrium with the anterior and middle cerebral arteries at their respective border zones. An accessory calcarine supply can arise from the parietooccipital artery.

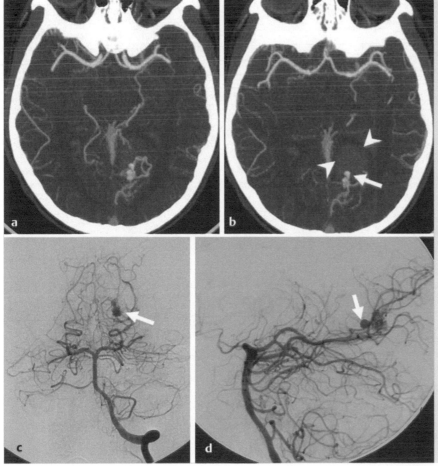

Fig. 24.1 CTA in axial cuts (a,b) demonstrates the left medial occipital hemorrhage (*arrowheads*) and a focal outpouching (*arrow*) arising from the arteriovenous malformation nidus and pointing into the hemorrhagic cavity. Conventional angiography of the left vertebral artery (c,d anteroposterior and lateral view) demonstrates a small left inferior parietal AVM fed by the proximal calcarine artery with a focal outpouching pointing anteriorly (*arrows*).

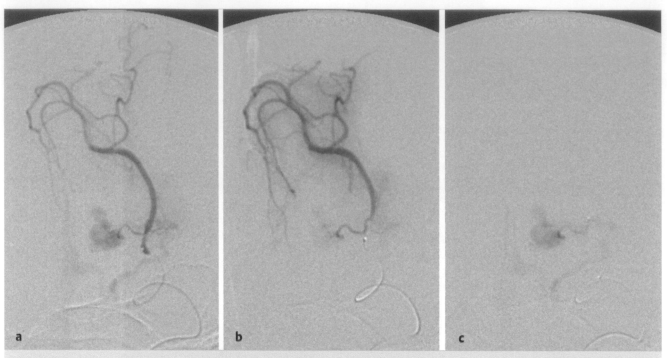

**Fig. 24.2** Distal catheterization of the calcarine artery (a,b) demonstrates the distal territory supplied by this vessel and the AVM arising from a small recurrent medial branch that was subsequently catheterized (c), allowing embolization.

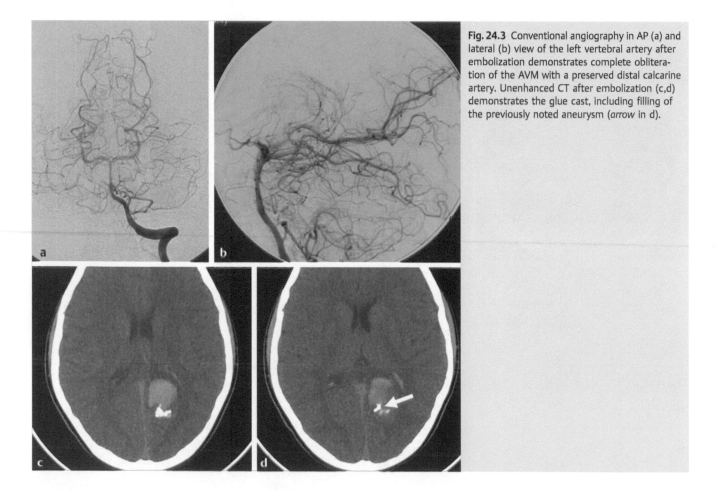

**Fig. 24.3** Conventional angiography in AP (a) and lateral (b) view of the left vertebral artery after embolization demonstrates complete obliteration of the AVM with a preserved distal calcarine artery. Unenhanced CT after embolization (c,d) demonstrates the glue cast, including filling of the previously noted aneurysm (*arrow* in d).

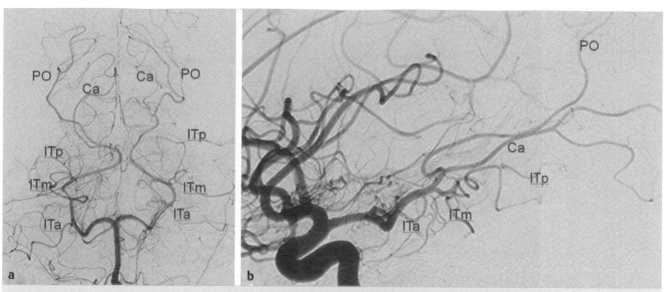

Fig. 24.4 Left vertebral artery injection in AP (a) and left internal carotid artery injection in lateral view (b) in two different patients. The distal cortical branches of the PCA territory are best appreciated on AP views, whereas the proximal temporal branches are best seen on the lateral view. PO, parietooccipital; Ca, calcarine; IT, inferior temporal (a, anterior; m, middle; and p, posterior).

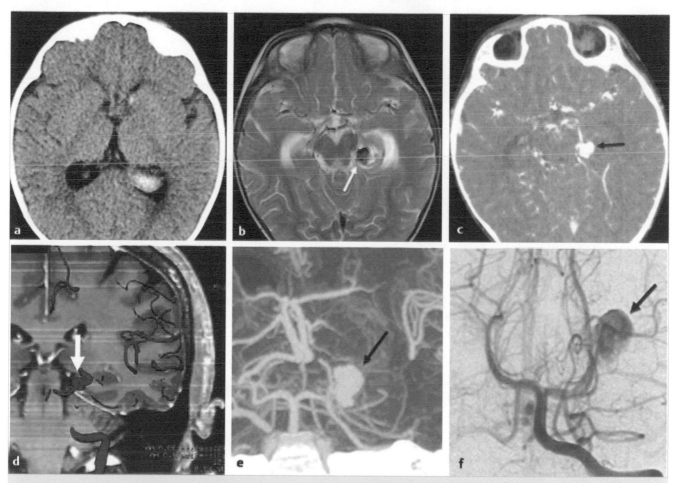

Fig. 24.5 Axial unenhanced CT (a), axial T2-weighted MRI (b), axial CTA (c), coronal fusion image of digital subtraction angiography and MRI (d), coronal CTA (e), and left vertebral artery injection in AP view (f) in a child with intraventricular hemorrhage. As the P2 segment courses through the ambient cistern, it traverses the free margin of the tentorium in its P2/3 segment (*white arrow* in d). It is believed that because of repeated microtrauma, dissecting aneurysms can form at this level (*arrows* in b,c,e,f). These aneurysms may arise from the main PCA stem or from smaller lateral branches. As this is a symptomatic distal dissecting aneurysm, treatment of choice is parent vessel occlusion.

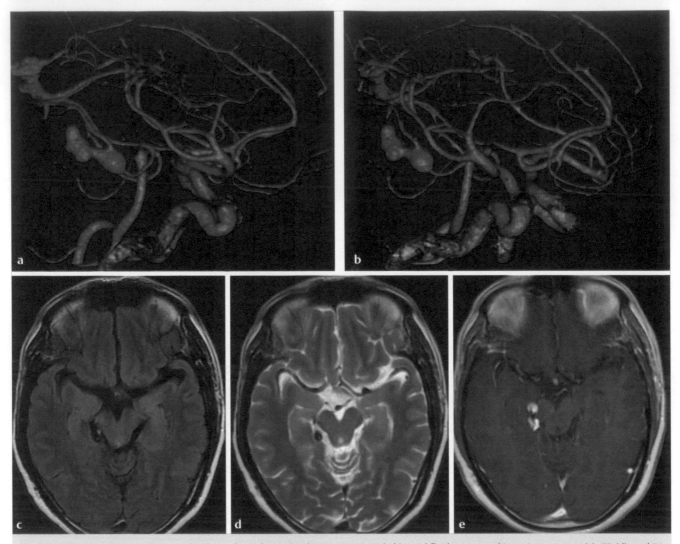

**Fig. 24.6** Companion case to ▸ Fig. 24.5: CTA in three-dimensional reconstructions (a,b), axial fluid-attenuated inversion recovery (c), T2 (d), and T1 postcontrast (e) sequences show a fusiforme aneurysm in the distal ambient cistern in close contact with the free margin of the tentorium. Case continued in ▸ Fig. 24.7.

The splenial artery either arises separately or from the parie-tooccipital branch to supply the posterior corpus callosum. It represents an important collateral pathway to the anterior cere-bral artery. In this regard, it is of interest that in cases of PCA occlusion, this collateral is typically not used and, instead, the cortical branches (especially the posterior temporal branches) will supply the PCA territory (▸ Fig. 24.4).

## 24.3 Clinical Impact, Additional Information and Cases

See ▸ Fig. 24.5, ▸ Fig. 24.6, ▸ Fig. 24.7, and ▸ Fig. 24.8.

### Pearls and Pitfalls

- The main branches of the PCA are the inferior temporal branches and the calcarine, parietooccipital, and splenial arteries.
- Cortical branches of the PCA are in hemodynamic equili-brium with the anterior cerebral artery and MCA, mainly via their cortical branches and via the hippocampal artery, as well as with the anterior choroidal artery.
- If the final division of the PCA into calcarine and parietoocci-pital arteries is proximal on the P2 segment, it will be the parietooccipital artery that will supply the choroidal and thalamus territories.

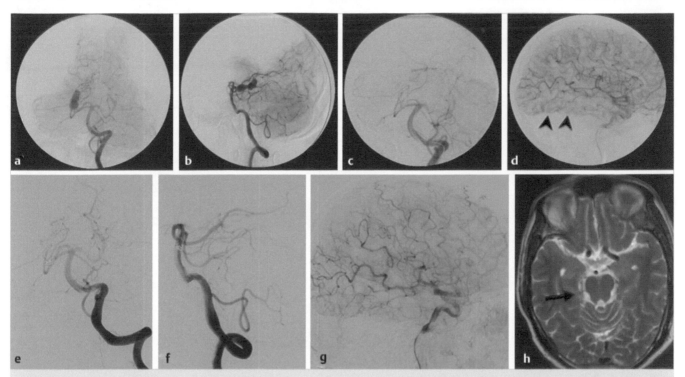

**Fig. 24.7** Angiography of the left vertebral artery in AP (a) and lateral (b) views confirms the diagnosis of a dissecting aneurysm. In the same setting, a balloon test occlusion of the proximal P2 segment was performed (inflated balloon in c), and injection of the left internal carotid artery was done (d), showing excellent filling of the undersurface of the brain (*arrowheads* in d) via leptomeningeal collaterals of a dominant posterior temporal branch from the MCA. Subsequently, the distal PCA was sacrificed with dense coil packing (e,f), and the follow-up digital subtraction angiography demonstrates complete filling of the PCA territory (g). T2-weighted scan after treatment demonstrates that the aneurysm is no longer visible (*arrow*) and no PCA territory infarction is present.

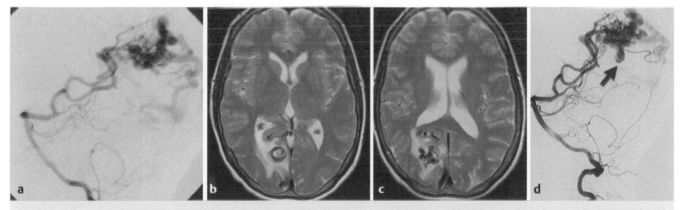

**Fig. 24.8** Eight years before the current presentation, a 47-year-old patient had presented with a single seizure, and a right posterior AVM was found (angiography in lateral view in (a) that was fed by both the parietooccipital and the calcarine branch. The patient had refused treatment. On present hospitalization, resulting from repeated seizures and visual disturbances, axial T2 weighted MRI (b,c) demonstrates perifocal edema surrounding a focal outpouching in the inferior parts of the AVM. Repeat angiography (d) demonstrates a newly developed, intranidal, inferiorly pointing outpouching (*arrow*) that was subsequently targeted with embolization.

# Further Reading

[1] Morris P. Practical Neuroangiography. 3rd ed. Philadelphia, PA: Lippincott Williams & Wilkins; 2013

[2] Párraga RG, Ribas GC, Andrade SE, de Oliveira E. Microsurgical anatomy of the posterior cerebral artery in three-dimensional images. World Neurosurg 2011; 75: 233–257

[3] Zeal AA, Rhoton AL. Microsurgical anatomy of the posterior cerebral artery. J Neurosurg 1978; 48: 534–559

# Section V

## External Carotid Artery

# 25 The "Dangerous" Anastomoses I: Ophthalmic Anastomoses

## 25.1 Introduction

The "dangerous" anastomoses are further subdivided into three separate cases (this case, Case 26, and Case 27), as we believe that a thorough understanding of potential anastomotic routes between the extracranial and the intracranial arteries is of utmost importance for all types of endovascular procedures in the external carotid artery (ECA) territory, including embolization of tumors of the skull base or the face, vascular malformations of the face and the orbit, dural arteriovenous malformations, and epistaxis.

The ECA is closely linked to the internal carotid artery (ICA) through embryology and phylogenetic development. This explains why although many anastomotic channels may not be visualized on routine (i.e., global) catheter angiographies, they are always present and will therefore necessarily open under certain predictable circumstances. As inadvertent embolization through these anastomoses can lead to major complications, such as stroke or cranial nerve palsies, both the circumstances under which the anastomoses may open and their potential localization have to be known by the interventional radiologist.

Anastomoses may open as a) a result of increased pressure on the feeding site of the anastomosis, b) because of increased demand on the receiving site of the anastomosis, or c) as a result of a "sump" effect of flow from the feeding to the receiving end of the anastomosis. Increased pressure in the feeding artery can build up during superselective injections, distal catheterizations, injections in wedged catheter position, or when using an embolizing agent that has the tendency to polymerize slowly and penetrate deep into the vascular bed. An increased demand is present when the proximal receiving artery is occluded or nearly occluded (e.g., a high-degree ICA stenosis may lead to recruitment of the ophthalmic collateral), and finally, high-flow shunts will sump the blood flow toward the shunt and, therefore, keep the anastomotic channels open.

Lasjaunias introduced the concept of functional vascular anatomy by subdividing the arterial anatomy of the head and neck by their territories (i.e., the internal maxillary, linguofacial, pharyngooccipital, thyroidal, cervical, internal carotid, and vertebral territories). He demonstrated that adjacent territories have close vascular and anastomotic interrelationships and will therefore function as potential vascular collaterals. Of these territories, there are three regions that serve as the major extracranial–intracranial anastomotic pathways: the orbital region, where the ophthalmic artery will act as the interface between the internal maxillary and internal carotid territories; the petrocavernous region, where the inferolateral and the meningohypophyseal trunk will be the major route to connect ECA and ICA vessels; and the upper cervical region, where the ascending pharyngeal, the occipital, and the ascending and deep cervical arteries will connect with the vertebral artery. In the following three cases, we discuss these three different regions separately.

## 25.2 Case Description

### 25.2.1 Clinical Presentation

A 72-year-old patient presented with idiopathic epistaxis refractory to nasal packing.

### 25.2.2 Radiologic Studies

See ▶ Fig. 25.1.

### 25.2.3 Diagnosis

Anastomosis between the anterior deep temporal artery from the distal internal maxillary artery (IMA) to the ophthalmic artery through the lacrimal system.

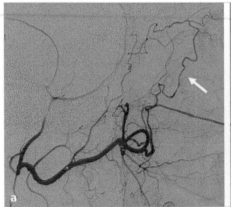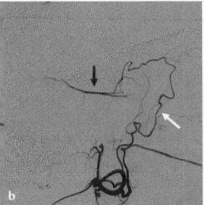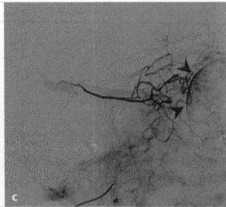

**Fig. 25.1** On injection of the left common carotid artery, occlusion of the ICA was seen (not shown). Right ECA angiogram (a) and selective internal maxillary injection in arterial (b) and capillary (c) phase in lateral views demonstrate the anastomosis between the anterior deep temporal artery (*white arrow*) from the distal IMA to the ophthalmic artery (*black arrow*) through the lacrimal system. Note the choroidal blush (*arrowheads*) in the capillary phase that in patients with a patent ICA is not seen because of antegrade washout. No embolization was performed, and the patient was referred to surgery.

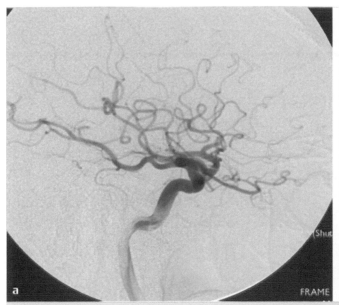
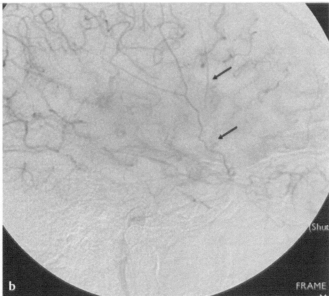

**Fig. 25.2** Right ICA angiogram in lateral view in the arterial (a) and capillary (b) phases demonstrates the MMA originating from the ophthalmic artery (*arrows*). This represents failure of the embryonic stapedial artery annexation by the ventral pharyngeal artery.

## 25.3 Embryology

The ECA develops from the remnants of the branchial arteries (or aortic arches) to supply the metameric territories of the neural crest in the maxillofacial region and from the ventral aorta and ventral pharyngeal artery to supply the floor of the mouth and digestive regions. The stapedial artery, part of the embryonic hyostapedial artery (from the second aortic arch), has two branches: the maxillomandibular artery, which leaves the cranial cavity through the foramen spinosum, and the supraorbital branch (see Case 3), which runs forward and gives off the orbital artery. In the most common variation, by the end of the 40-mm stage, the transsphenoidal part of the orbital artery regresses and the supply to the orbital artery has been taken over by the primitive ophthalmic arteries (see Case 7). The endocranial part of the stapedial artery will form the middle meningeal artery (MMA), and the maxillomandibular artery is later annexed by the ventral pharyngeal system to become part of the ECA. In the most extreme variation, a "meningo-ophthalmic artery" is encountered when the stapedial system, through the MMA and IMA, takes over the entire orbital supply, resulting in the MMA giving rise to the distal ophthalmic artery, including the central retinal artery and ciliary arteries (see Case 8).

On the opposite end, in rare cases in which the stapedial artery fails to be annexed by the ventral pharyngeal system, the MMA may arise directly from the ICA or the ophthalmic artery. Other MMA collaterals to the ophthalmic artery, which also represent remnants of the stapedial artery, are through the superficial recurrent meningeal branch of the lacrimal artery, which anastomoses with the corresponding orbital branches through the superior orbital fissure, and the anterior falcine artery, a meningeal branch arising from the distal ophthalmic artery supplying the anterior falx, anastomosing indirectly with the anterior branch of the MMA through the meninges. The orbital branches can be best seen on the lateral projection,

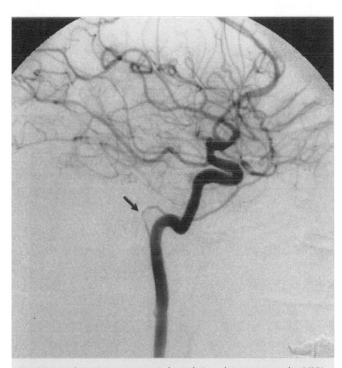

**Fig. 25.3** Right ICA angiogram in lateral view demonstrates the MMA originating from the right ICA through the persistent stapedial artery (*arrow*).

typically just inferior to the sphenoid ridge, similar to the location of the meningo-ophthalmic artery origin.

Other potential collaterals to the orbit include branches of the distal IMA and cutaneous branches of the face. The inferior branch of the lacrimal artery of the ophthalmic artery has anastomoses with the anterior deep temporal artery and the infraorbital artery, both branches of the distal IMA. Another branch of the distal IMA, the sphenopalatine artery, is

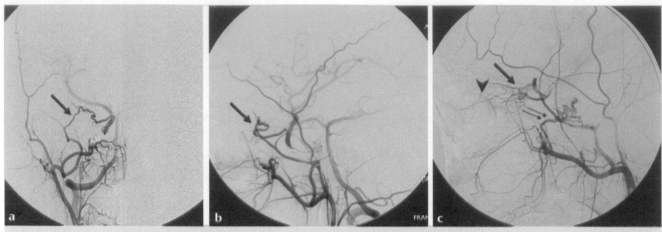

**Fig. 25.4** Right ECA angiogram in anteroposterior (a) and lateral (b) views and left ECA angiogram in lateral view (c) demonstrate the meningolacrimal anastomosis between the MMA and the ophthalmic artery (*arrows*). Note the presence of the choroidal blush (*arrowhead*), which serves as a landmark for the central retinal artery in the second case (c). Anastomosis between the artery of the foramen rotundum (*thin double arrows*) from the distal IMA and the inferolateral trunk is also observed.

connected with the anterior and posterior ethmoidal arteries of the ophthalmic artery through the septal arteries, which are classically enlarged in cases of large juvenile angiofibromas (see Case 29). The cutaneous branches are connected to the distal third portion of the ophthalmic artery, the frontal branch of the superficial temporal artery, through the supraorbital artery, and to the distal end of the facial artery through the dorsal nasal artery at the angular termination.

## 25.4 Clinical Impact

Because of occlusion of the ICA in the index case, the IMA was the sole supply to the ophthalmic artery, and therefore, particle embolization within the IMA carries a high risk of blindness. The treatment alternative for epistaxis that is refractory to nasal packing is direct endoscopic cauterization, which we opted for in this case.

The most important risk when embolizing within the orbital region is occlusion of the central retinal artery, which results in blindness of the patient. Infrequently, embolic stroke may also occur through retrograde filling of the ICA. Because the central retinal artery typically originates with, or close, to the posterior ciliary arteries, the choroidal blush, best seen on the lateral angiographic view in the capillary and early venous phases, is used as a landmark to identify its origin (see also Case 8).

In the presence of a meningo-ophthalmic artery, embolization including proximal occlusion of the MMA carries a high risk of monocular blindness and must be avoided, as this MMA branch represents the sole supply to the distal ophthalmic artery and central retinal artery. The other anastomotic channels from the MMA are typically not visualized on global injections and only open with increased pressure during embolization procedures within the MMA.

The distal IMA and cutaneous collaterals are typically small and connect only distally to the ophthalmic artery; therefore, they carry a smaller risk during endovascular procedures. However, they may enlarge in cases with tumors involving the skull

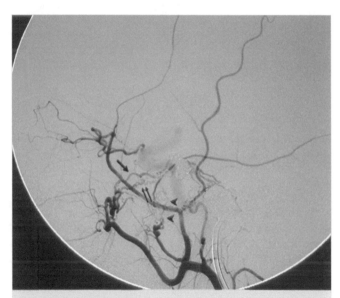

**Fig. 25.5** Right ECA angiogram in lateral view after transvenous coiling of a cavernous sinus dural arteriovenous fistula demonstrates retrograde filling of the ICA through the meningolacrimal anastomosis from the MMA to the ophthalmic artery. Note the enlarged artery of foramen rotundum (*arrow*), vidian artery (*thin double arrows*), artery of foramen ovale (*arrowheads*), and petrous branches of the MMA, previously supplying the dural arteriovenous fistulas at the cavernous sinus and clival regions.

base, such as a large juvenile angiofibroma, but because their diameters rarely exceed 80 μm, it is generally considered safe to embolize within this region, using larger particles.

## 25.5 Additional Information and Cases

See ▸ Fig. 25.2, ▸ Fig. 25.3, ▸ Fig. 25.4, and ▸ Fig. 25.5.

## Pearls and Pitfalls

- The choroidal blush, best seen on the lateral angiographic view in the capillary and early venous phases, is used as a landmark to identify the origin of the central retinal artery at the time of selective internal and external carotid angiography.
- The major MMA–ophthalmic anastomotic channels are located slightly inferior to the sphenoid ridge on lateral angiographic views.
- Identification of a meningo-ophthalmic artery contraindicates embolization of the MMA.

# Further Reading

[1] Berenstein A, Lasjaunias P, Kricheff II. Functional anatomy of the facial vasculature in pathologic conditions and its therapeutic application. AJNR Am J Neuroradiol 1983; 4: 149–153

[2] Countee RW, Vijayanathan T. External carotid artery in internal carotid artery occlusion. Angiographic, therapeutic, and prognostic considerations. Stroke 1979; 10: 450–460

[3] Geibprasert S, Pongpech S, Armstrong D, Krings T. Dangerous extracranial-intracranial anastomoses and supply to the cranial nerves: vessels the neurointerventionalist needs to know. AJNR Am J Neuroradiol 2009; 30: 1459–1468

[4] Hayreh SS. Orbital vascular anatomy. Eye (Lond) 2006; 20: 1130–1144

[5] Lasjaunias P, Berenstein A, ter Brugge KG. Surgical Neuroangiography. Vol. 1. 2nd ed. Berlin: Springer; 2006

[6] Lasjaunias P, Berenstein A, ter Brugge KG. Surgical Neuroangiography. Vol 3: Clinical and Interventional Aspects in Children. 2nd ed. Berlin: Springer; 2006

[7] Liebeskind DS. Collateral circulation. Stroke 2003; 34: 2279–2284

[8] Perrini P, Cardia A, Fraser K, Lanzino G. A microsurgical study of the anatomy and course of the ophthalmic artery and its possibly dangerous anastomoses. J Neurosurg 2007; 106: 142–150

# 26 The "Dangerous" Anastomoses II: Petrous and Cavernous Anastomoses

## 26.1 Case Description

### 26.1.1 Clinical Presentation

A 59-year-old man presented with two right-sided hemodynamic hemispheric ischemic strokes, the last one 10 months before the angiogram. He is a heavy smoker and has a history of peripheral and coronary artery vascular disease. He was being considered for extracranial–intracranial bypass.

### 26.1.2 Radiologic Studies

See ▶ Fig. 26.1, ▶ Fig. 26.2.

### 26.1.3 Diagnosis

Right internal carotid artery (ICA) occlusion with hemodynamic infarctions and secondary opening of petrocavernous extracranial–intracranial anastomoses.

## 26.2 Embryology and Anatomy

There are three major anastomotic areas within the petrocavernous region of the ICA: the petrous, the clivus, and the cavernous sinus. The corresponding branches along the ICA are the mandibular artery (remnant of the dorsal part of the first aortic arch) and the caroticotympanic artery (remnant of the embryologic hyoid artery) for the petrous territory and the meningohypophyseal trunk (remnant of the embryologic primitive maxillary artery) and the inferolateral trunk (ILT) (remnant of the embryologic dorsal ophthalmic artery) for the cavernous region and the clivus. See also Case 5.

The ascending pharyngeal artery divides into two main trunks: the pharyngeal and neuromeningeal trunks (see Case 30). The superior pharyngeal artery branch of the anteriorly located pharyngeal trunk has two major petrocavernous anastomotic routes, including one through the eustachian tube anastomotic circle and one at the foramen lacerum. The former connects with the mandibular artery from the petrous ICA, a branch of the accessory meningeal artery and the pterygovaginal artery from the distal internal maxillary artery (IMA), whereas the latter, a small carotid canal branch, enters the cranium through the foramen lacerum to the cavernous sinus to join the recurrent artery of the foramen lacerum, a branch of the lateral clival artery, and the ILT.

The neuromeningeal trunk branches into two major arteries, the jugular and hypoglossal branches, entering the cranial cavity through the corresponding foramen/canal, with the former giving supply to cranial nerves IX and X and the latter to cranial nerve XII as they traverse the foramen (see Case 28). Both

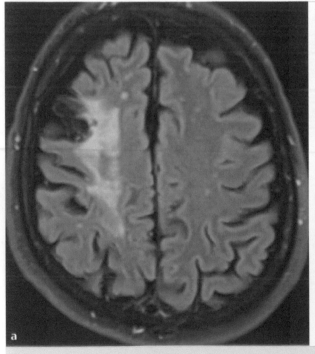
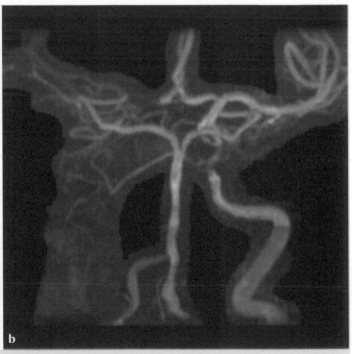

**Fig. 26.1** FLAIR MRI (a) shows infarction in the right frontoparietal lobe with associated volume loss. Small T2 bright spots are observed in the remaining white matter. MRA (b) reveals nonvisualization of the right ICA, likely because of chronic occlusion, and the right A1 segment, which could be related to severe hypoplasia and/or stenosis. The right middle cerebral artery branches are also poorly visualized. Irregularity of the basilar artery and some narrowing of cavernous left ICA are observed, suggesting diffuse underlying atherosclerotic disease. Case is continued in ▶ Fig. 26.2.

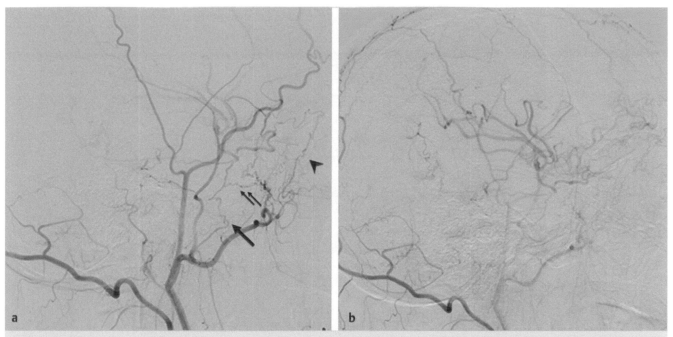

**Fig. 26.2** Cerebral angiography confirmed the right ICA occlusion. There was no A1 segment and minimal leptomeningeal collaterals to the distal middle cerebral artery branches from the PCA branches. Small collaterals through anastomotic channels from the right ECA to the middle cerebral artery were also observed; however, these were insufficient, and there was a delayed venous phase within the middle cerebral artery territory. Right ECA angiogram in lateral view in early (a) and late (b) arterial phases demonstrates collaterals to the ICA from the artery of the foramen ovale (*arrow*) and the vidian artery (*thin double arrows*) via the ILT and the MMA and anterior deep temporal artery (*arrowhead*) via the ophthalmic artery.

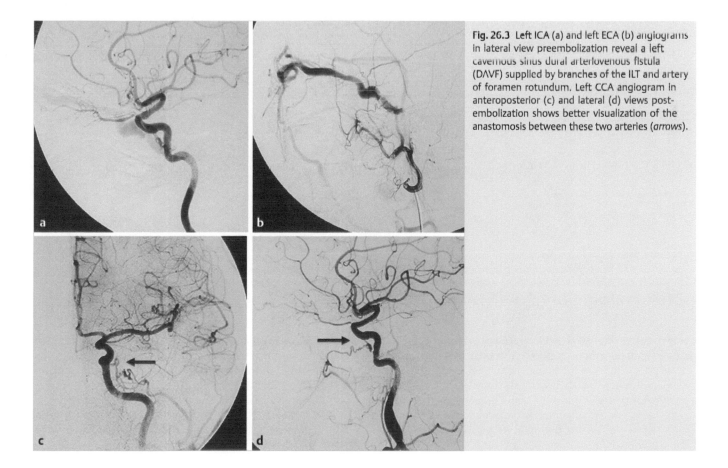

**Fig. 26.3** Left ICA (a) and left ECA (b) angiograms in lateral view preembolization reveal a left cavernous sinus dural arteriovenous fistula (DAVF) supplied by branches of the ILT and artery of foramen rotundum. Left CCA angiogram in anteroposterior (c) and lateral (d) views postembolization shows better visualization of the anastomosis between these two arteries (*arrows*).

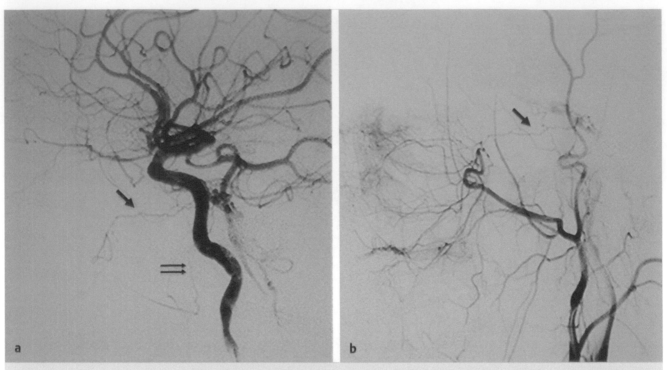

**Fig. 26.4** Right ICA (a) and right ECA (b) angiograms in lateral view demonstrate a DAVF at the posterior cavernous sinus, supplied via the lateral clival artery through anastomoses from the artery of foramen rotundum (*single arrow*) and the small MMA (*thin double arrows*), which is hypoplastic related to prior embolizations.

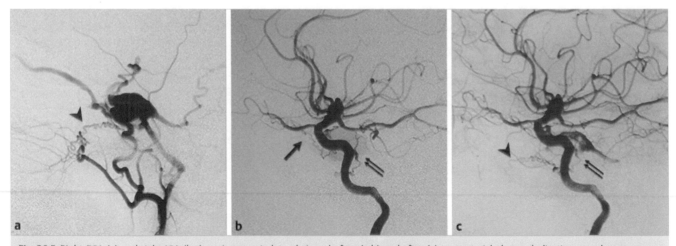

**Fig. 26.5** Right ECA (a) and right ICA (b,c) angiograms in lateral views before (a,b) and after (c) transarterial glue embolization reveal a cavernous DAVF, supplied by the recurrent meningeal artery from the ophthalmic artery (*arrow*), the lateral clival artery (*thin double arrows*), the artery of the foramen rotundum (*arrowheads*), and the artery of the foramen ovale from the accessory meningeal artery. The anastomosis between the artery of the foramen rotundum and the lateral clival artery is better visualized on the postembolization angiogram.

branches give off medial and lateral clival branches immediately after exiting the foramens to join with branches from the lateral clival artery and the meningohypophyseal trunk. The inferior tympanic artery, which may arise from the main ascending pharyngeal artery or one of its major branches, enters the tympanic cavity through the inferior tympanic foramen with Jacobson's nerve and retains the embryologic connection between the artery of the third branchial arch and the hyoid artery (or caroticotympanic artery) from the petrous ICA. Within the middle ear, it also anastomoses with the superior tympanic artery (from the petrous branch of the middle meningeal artery [MMA]), the anterior tympanic artery (from proximal IMA), the stylomastoid artery (from the posterior auricular/occipital artery), and the mandibular branch of the ICA. This arterial network, but in particular the petrous branch of the MMA and stylomastoid artery, forms the facial arcade, which supplies the geniculate ganglion of cranial nerve VII. See also Case 28.

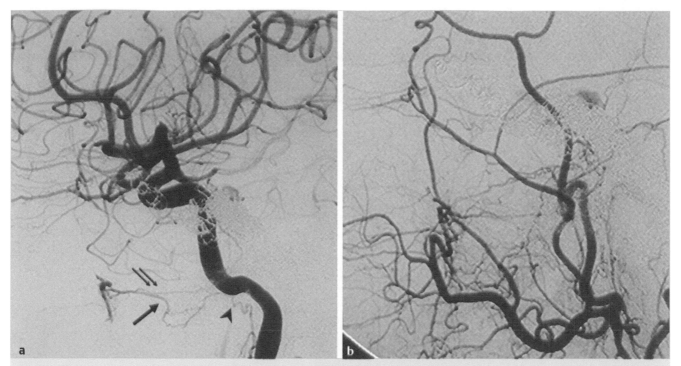

**Fig. 26.6** Right ICA (a) and right ECA (b) angiograms in lateral view posttransvenous coiling of a cavernous DAVF demonstrate the anastomosis between the vidian artery (*thin double arrows*) from the distal IMA to the vidian branch of the mandibular artery. The vidian artery has a characteristic horizontal course on the lateral view that differentiates it from the more inferior course of the pterygovaginal artery (*arrow*), which also anastomoses with a branch of the mandibular artery, and the pharyngeal artery (*arrowhead*) around the eustachian tube.

The MMA and accessory meningeal artery provide major anastomotic routes through the ILT to the cavernous ICA. The MMA gives off cavernous branches after exiting the foramen spinosum to join with the superior or tentorial branch of the ILT. The orbital branches of the MMA also anastomose with the anteromedial branch of the ILT within the superior orbital fissure. The petrosquamous or posterior branch of the MMA connects with the marginal artery of the tentorium, which can arise from the ILT, the ophthalmic artery, or the meningohypophyseal trunk of the ICA. The superior division of the accessory meningeal artery enters the cavernous sinus through the foramen ovale to join the posteromedial branch of the ILT and also supplies cranial nerve V3.

The distal IMA anastomoses with the ICA through several routes. The first is the artery of the foramen rotundum, which, as implied by its name, runs through the foramen rotundum and is best seen in the lateral view, where it can be identified by its corkscrew appearance, connecting with the anterolateral branch of the ILT (▶ Fig. 26.3) or, in rare cases, with the lateral clival artery (▶ Fig. 26.4). The vidian artery has a distinctly horizontal course, which can be easily identified on the lateral view from the distal IMA through the vidian canal to the foramen lacerum, where it anastomoses with the corresponding vidian branch of the mandibular artery of the petrous ICA. The pterygovaginal artery, which often originates adjacent to the vidian artery, has a more inferior course through the pterygovaginal canal along the roof of the nasopharynx, ending at the anastomotic circle around the eustachian tube.

## 26.3 Clinical Impact

The intracranial–extracranial anastomoses have an important role when embolizing in the region of the skull base. Particles and liquid embolic materials are the two most commonly used embolization materials in the external carotid artery (ECA) system. Although the penetration capacity of particles is dependent on the size, liquid embolic materials can open and enter small anastomotic channels that are not visualized on the initial angiograms and, therefore, should be used with increased caution. In general, nonvisualized anastomotic arteries range from 50 to 80 µm; therefore, particles that are larger than 150 µm will not penetrate these anastomoses and will avoid potential embolic complications. The visualization of an anastomotic channel is not a contraindication for embolization of the particular artery. There are several techniques that can be used to prevent embolic material from entering the collaterals, including simple proximal mechanical blockage of the collateral branch with large particles or coils before the embolization, or flow-reversal methods using a proximal balloon occlusion in the target ECA vessel, which leads to flow redirection from the ICA to the ECA territory. If the anastomoses serve as major collaterals to the ICA, embolization or injury to the ECA branches should be avoided.

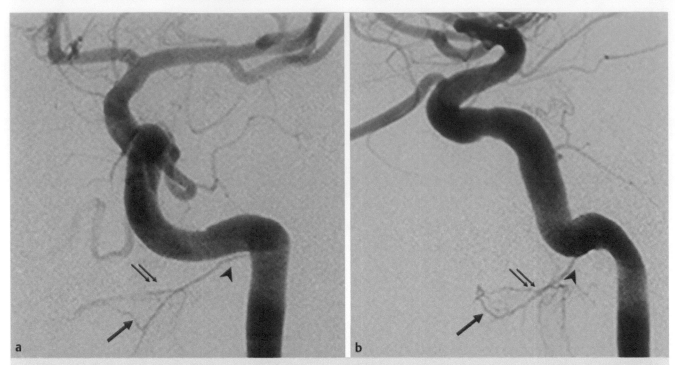

**Fig. 26.7** Left ICA angiograms in anteroposterior (a) and lateral (b) views demonstrate the anastomosis between the mandibular branch of the ICA (*arrowhead*) and the pterygovaginal artery (*arrow*), which anastomoses with a mandibular artery (*thin double arrows*) of the pharyngeal artery around the eustachian tube.

## Pearls and Pitfalls

- When performing embolization in the external carotid artery, in general, particles larger than 150 μm can be considered safe in the distribution of nonvisualized anastomotic channels.
- If the anastomoses are serving as intracranial collaterals, embolization or injury to the ECA branches should be avoided.

## 26.4 Additional Information and Cases

See ▶ Fig. 26.5, ▶ Fig. 26.6, and ▶ Fig. 26.7.

# Further Reading

[1] Geibprasert S, Pongpech S, Armstrong D, Krings T. Dangerous extracranial-intracranial anastomoses and supply to the cranial nerves: vessels the neurointerventionalist needs to know. AJNR Am J Neuroradiol 2009; 30: 1459–1468

[2] Lasjaunias P, Berenstein A, ter Brugge KG. Surgical neuroangiography. Vol. 1. 2nd ed. Berlin: Springer; 2006

[3] Lasjaunias P, Moret J, Mink J. The anatomy of the inferolateral trunk (ILT) of the internal carotid artery. Neuroradiology 1977; 13: 215–220

[4] Tubbs RS, Hansasuta A, Loukas M et al. Branches of the petrous and cavernous segments of the internal carotid artery. Clin Anat 2007; 20: 596–601

[5] Willems PW, Farb RI, Agid R. Endovascular treatment of epistaxis. AJNR Am J Neuroradiol 2009; 30: 1637–1645

# 27 The "Dangerous" Anastomoses III: Upper Cervical Anastomoses

## 27.1 Case Description

### 27.1.1 Clinical Presentation

A 65-year-old woman with a past history of coronary and peripheral vascular arterial disease, hypertension, and type 2 diabetes presented with dizziness and one episode of blackout. Vertebro-basilar insufficiency was suspected.

### 27.1.2 Radiographic Studies

See ▶ Fig. 27.1.

### 27.1.3 Diagnosis

Right ECA occlusion with retrograde reconstitution of the ECA through the upper cervical anastomoses from the VA.

## 27.2 Embryology and Anatomy

The ascending pharyngeal artery (APhA) corresponds to the remnant of the embryonic hypoglossal artery (HA). The HA originates from the third aortic arch and contributes to the development of the most proximal aspect of the cervical ICA. It is one of the embryonic carotid–vertebrobasilar anastomoses, originating from the proximal cervical ICA, slightly distal to the carotid bulb, and enters the posterior cranial fossa via the hypoglossal canal. The relationship between the third aortic arch and the HA can result in various anastomoses between their adult homologs, the ICA, and the APhA, with the most extreme of the spectrum being the persistent HA. See also Case 4.

In the adult, the APhA forms part of the pharyngo-occpital system, a vascular network in the suboccipital region through which the cervical vertebral and carotid arteries are connected by four routes: the occipital, ascending pharyngeal, vertebropharyngeal (C3), and C4-collateral routes.

The APhA originates most commonly from the posterior wall of the proximal ECA and anastomoses with the VA, typically at two levels. The more proximal one occurs laterally between the musculospinal branch of the APhA and the C3 radicular anastomotic branch of the VA. The distal one is the prevertebral branch via the odontoid arch, which usually arises from the HA and follows the same path as the persistent HA, serving as one of the collateral routes in cases of proximal ECA or VA occlusion, as seen in the index case.

The occipital artery is a remnant of the embryologic type 1 and type 2 proatlantal arteries, which correspond to the C1 and C2 segmental arteries, respectively. In an adult, the occipital artery still retains its connection from the ECA to the VA through the posterior anastomotic radicular routes via the musculocuta-

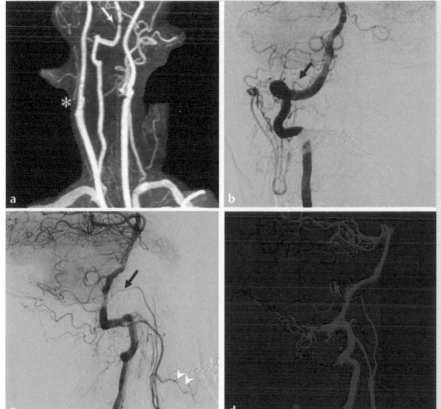

**Fig. 27.1** MRA of the neck (a) shows a high-grade stenosis of the proximal intracranial right VA or V4 segment (*white arrow*). Incidentally, there is a right ECA occlusion (*asterisk*). Right VA angiogram in anteroposterior (AP) (b) and lateral (c) views and a three-dimensional reconstruction image (d) show contrast filling of both the occipital artery and the APhA through an anastomosis via the artery of the hypoglossal canal (*arrows*) and musculocutaneous branches from the C1 segment. There is retrograde flow down to the origin of the ECA and opacification of the facial artery (*arrowheads*).

neous branches, which arise from the horizontal portion of the occipital artery at the C1 and C2 levels. These anastomotic channels are rather large and can be seen during selective injections of the occipital artery. They serve as the major collaterals from the VA in case of common carotid artery or ECA ligation or occlusion. The stylomastoid artery, originating either from the occipital or posterior auricular arteries, supplies the meninges of the posterior fossa and anastomoses with other meningeal

arteries, including the posterior meningeal artery from the distal cervical, i.e. suboccipital VA. For further information regarding the meningeal supply refer to Case 31.

The ascending and deep cervical arteries anastomose with the VA at the C2 to C4 levels. Both arise from the subclavian artery: the ascending cervical artery from the thyrocervical trunk and the deep cervical artery from the costocervical trunk. These arteries typically enlarge and serve as major collaterals in case of proximal VA occlusion.

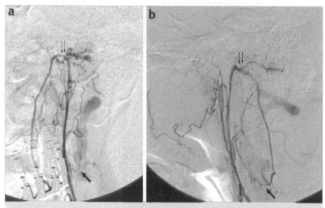

**Fig. 27.2** Left APhA angiograms in AP (a) and lateral (b) views demonstrate anastomoses of the musculospinal branch at the C3 level (*arrows*), with the VA with additional contributions from the odontoid arch (*thin double arrows*).

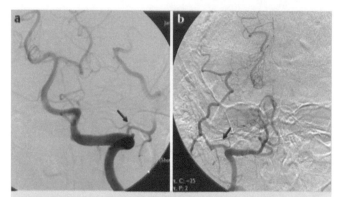

**Fig. 27.3** Left (a) and right (b) VA angiograms in AP view demonstrate C1 collaterals to the occipital arteries bilaterally (*arrows*).

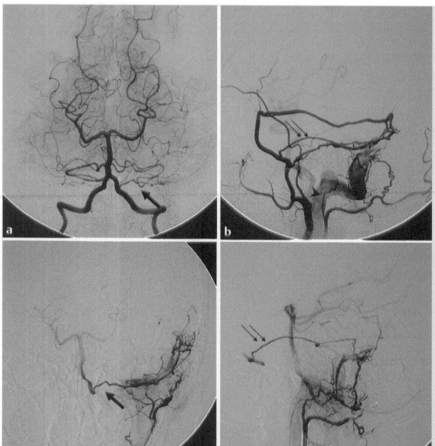

**Fig. 27.4** Left VA angiogram in AP view (a), left ECA angiogram in lateral view (b), and left occipital artery angiograms in AP (c) and lateral (d) views postembolization of a left transverse-sigmoid sinus dural arteriovenous fistula demonstrate the transmeningeal anastomoses to a posterior meningeal branch of the VA (*arrows*) and through the facial arcade to the petrous branch of the middle meningeal artery (*thin double arrows*) from the stylomastoid branches of the occipital artery (*arrowhead*).

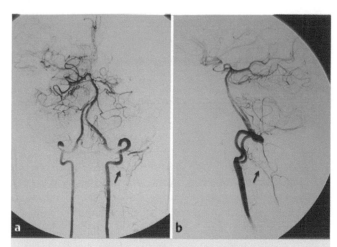

**Fig. 27.5** Left VA angiograms in AP (a) and lateral (b) views demonstrate the anastomoses between the VA and deep cervical artery at the C2 level (*arrows*).

## 27.3 Clinical Impact

The APhA has multiple anastomoses with the intracranial circulation, via internal carotid and vertebral arteries, as discussed in Case 30. The main complications, if the anastomoses are not promptly recognized, are seen in embolization procedures with small particles or liquid embolic materials. In the specific case of the VA/APhA anastomosis via the hypoglossal canal artery, an external artery particle injection may result in embolic strokes in the posterior circulation. The use of liquid embolic material could result in occlusion of the vasa nervorum of the hypoglossal nerve, supplied by the artery of the hypoglossal canal, with subsequent 12th cranial nerve palsy. As the anastomosis is located proximal to the origin of the anterior spinal artery, a potential risk of anterior spinal artery ischemia exists.

The occipital and cervical arteries also have several anastomoses with the vertebral arteries. Caution must be used when embolizing within these territories with small particles and liquid embolic materials to avoid posterior fossa infarctions. Occasionally, the anterior spinal artery may arise from the ascending and deep cervical arteries.

## 27.4 Additional Information and Cases

See ▶ Fig. 27.2, ▶ Fig. 27.3, ▶ Fig. 27.4, and ▶ Fig. 27.5.

## Further Reading

[1] Cavalcanti DD, Reis CV, Hanel R et al. The ascending pharyngeal artery and its relevance for neurosurgical and endovascular procedures. Neurosurgery 2009; 65 Suppl: 114–120, discussion 120

[2] Geibprasert S, Pongpech S, Armstrong D, Krings T. Dangerous extracranial-intracranial anastomoses and supply to the cranial nerves: vessels the neurointerventionalist needs to know. AJNR Am J Neuroradiol 2009; 30: 1459–1468

[3] Hacein-Bey L, Daniels DL, Ulmer JL et al. The ascending pharyngeal artery: branches, anastomoses, and clinical significance. AJNR Am J Neuroradiol 2002; 23: 1246–1256

[4] Houseman ND, Taylor GI, Pan WR. The angiosomes of the head and neck: anatomic study and clinical applications. Plast Reconstr Surg 2000; 105: 2287–2313

[5] Lasjaunias P, Berenstein A, ter Brugge KG. Surgical Neuroangiography. Vol. 1. 2nd ed. Berlin: Springer; 2006

[6] Lasjaunias P, Théron J, Moret J. The occipital artery. Anatomy—normal arteriographic aspects—embryological significance. Neuroradiology 1978; 15: 31–37

[7] Strub WM, Leach JL, Tomsick TA. Left vertebral artery origin from the thyrocervical trunk: a unique vascular variant. AJNR Am J Neuroradiol 2006; 27: 1155–1156

# 28 The Cranial Nerve Supply

## 28.1 Case Description

### 28.1.1 Clinical Presentation

An 82-year-old, right-handed woman presented with a several-month history of falls and gait ataxia, worse on the left side, which prompted further imaging.

### 28.1.2 Radiologic Studies

See ▶ Fig. 28.1, ▶ Fig. 28.2.

### 28.1.3 Diagnosis

Dural arteriovenous fistula (dAVF) of the petrous ridge with cortical venous reflux. The dAVF is fed by the middle meningeal artery (MMA), including its petrosal branch and the stylo-mastoid branch of the posterior auricular artery (i.e., the facial arcade).

## 28.2 Anatomy

Under normal conditions, the caliber of the arteries that supply the cranial nerves (the vasa nervorum) is between 100 and 300 µm, and they are, therefore, in most instances only visible on conventional angiography during superselective injections. Nevertheless, knowledge of their origin, their anastomoses, and their potential variations is paramount for safe embolization of a variety of skull base lesions, including dAVF and hypervascularized tumors.

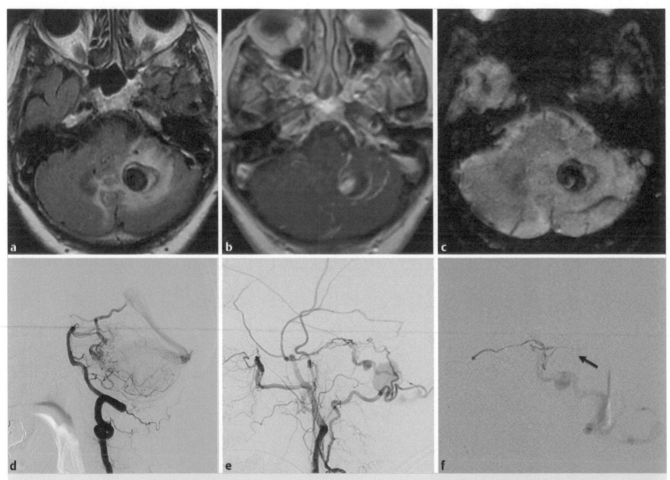

**Fig. 28.1** MRI axial fluid-attenuated inversion recovery (a), T1 contrast-enhanced (b), and susceptibility (c) weighted images demonstrate a vascular pouch in the left inferior cerebellum with significant perifocal edema, as well as abnormal sulcal vessels. Left vertebral artery angiogram in lateral view (d) reveals a cerebellar arteriovenous malformation, the imaging characteristics of which cannot explain the visualized pouch on MR. Subsequent injection into the left ECA (e) demonstrates a dural arteriovenous fistula along the petrous ridge, with arterial filling via the meningohypophyseal trunk and the facial arcade and multiple venous pouches and venous stenoses. After embolization of the distal MMA with glue deposition into the venous segment, minimal residual flow was visualized via the petrosal branch of the MMA (injection in f). From this vessel, transient opacification of a normal distal branch was seen that connected to the stylomastoid branch of the posterior auricular artery (*arrow*). As glue had been deposited in the foot of the vein, we only ligated the petrosal branch of the MMA with concentrated glue to ensure that the supply to the facial nerve was not compromised and the flow to the fistula was further reduced, which was supposed to facilitate further thrombosis. Case continued in ▶ Fig. 28.2.

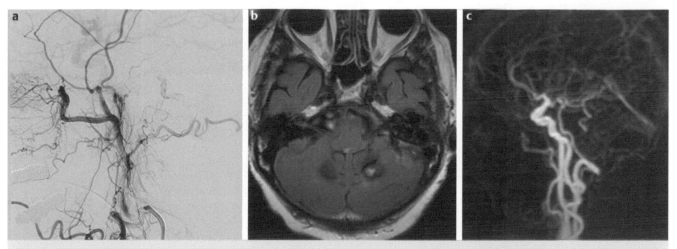

**Fig. 28.2** Immediate control angiogram (a) demonstrated residual very slow filling of the shunt via the stylomastoid branch of the posterior auricular artery. Upon follow-up MR 2 weeks later (b), the patient had thrombosed her venous pouch, the edema was no longer visualized, and only the arteriovenous shunting related to the cerebellar arteriovenous malformation was noted on the dynamic contrast-enhanced magnetic resonance angiography, with no further shunting visualized from the dural branches. (c) Clinically, she did very well, with no new neurological deficits and reversal of her presenting symptoms.

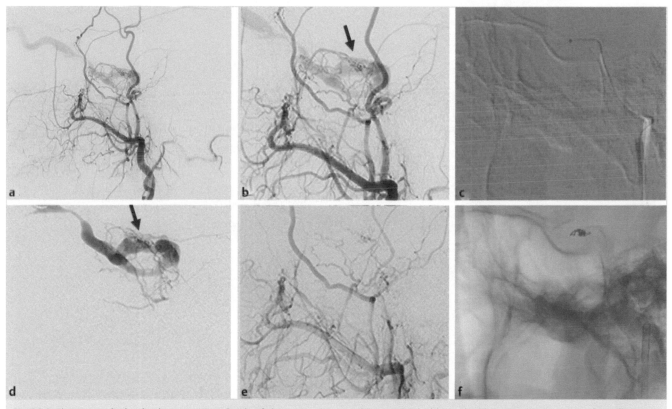

**Fig. 28.3** This patient had a dural arteriovenous fistula of the cavernous sinus that was supplied by multiple interconnecting internal maxillary branches that all converged into a single artery (*arrows*) at the superior roof of the cavernous sinus, as seen on the left ECA angiogram in lateral view (a,b). We opted for a transvenous approach through the inferior petrosal sinus (c), and the microcatheter could be placed via the cavernous sinus retrogradely into the feeding artery. Contrast injection (d) to verify the position shows both the cavernous sinus with its outflow and, retrogradely, the arterial network converging into the single fistulous zone. The fistula could be treated by a few coils that were deposited transvenously into the arterial common trunk, followed by retrograde coiling into the superior portion of the cavernous sinus (e,f). This case indicates the rich anastomotic network of dural branches that supply the cranial nerves of the cavernous sinus arising from the ECA and anastomosing with the ICA. Treating these fistulas either transarterially or transvenously with a liquid embolic agent that penetrates deep into this anastomotic network puts the patient at risk for ophthalmoplegia or embolic events in the ICA territory.

## 28.2.1 Cranial Nerves I and II

Being outpouchings of the brain, rather than true cranial nerves, the olfactory and optic nerves are not considered peripheral nerves and will be described only briefly: the olfactory nerve is supplied by the olfactory artery and ethmoidal branches of the ophthalmic artery, and the optic nerve is supplied by the proximal ophthalmic artery.

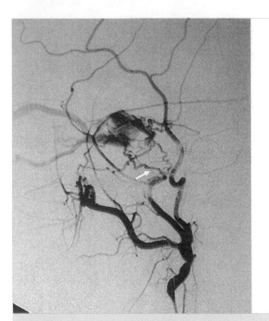

**Fig. 28.4** The branches of the trigeminal nerve are supplied as they course through the foramina of the skull base by the artery of the foramen ovale (mandibular branch; *white arrow*) from the MMA or accessory meningeal artery, whereas the maxillary nerve is supplied by the artery of the foramen rotundum (*black arrow*), a branch of the distal internal maxillary artery. Both branches anastomose with the ILT.

## 28.2.2 Cranial Nerves III, IV, and VI

In its cisternal segment, the oculomotor nerve receives arterial supply in the vicinity of the posterior perforating substance from the basilar or the posterior cerebral artery.

Once it extends forward from the brainstem, the trochlear nerve is supplied by the superior cerebellar artery and additional circumferential arteries of the P1 segment of the posterior cerebral artery, with which it courses through the ambient cistern.

The abducens nerve is supplied by the clival dural network along its course anterior to the pons, including the medial and lateral clival arteries from the hypoglossal and jugular branch of the neuromeningeal trunk of the ascending pharyngeal artery and, more cranially, the medial and lateral clival arteries from the meningohypophyseal trunk.

These dural arteries also contribute to the supply of cranial nerves III, IV, and V in their dural and transosseous course. The

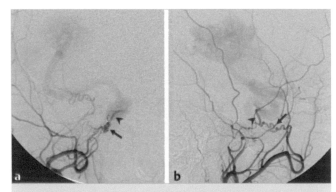

**Fig. 28.5** ECA injection, anteroposterior (a) and lateral (b) views, in a patient with a pial brain arteriovenous malformation of the fistulous type with significantly increased flow through the ICA. The ECA, with its artery of the foramen rotundum (*arrow*) that connects to the ILT (*arrowhead*) of the ICA, is "sumped" into the ICA.

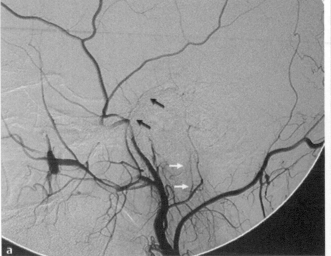
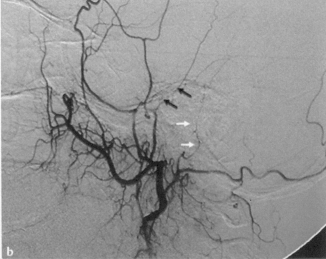

**Fig. 28.6** The "facial arcade" supplying the facial nerve is demonstrated in two patients. Left ECA angiograms (a,b) in lateral view demonstrate the facial arcade supply through the petrous branch of the MMA (*black arrows*) and the stylomastoid branch (*white arrows*), which arose from the posterior auricular artery in one patient (a) and from the occipital artery in the other patient (b).

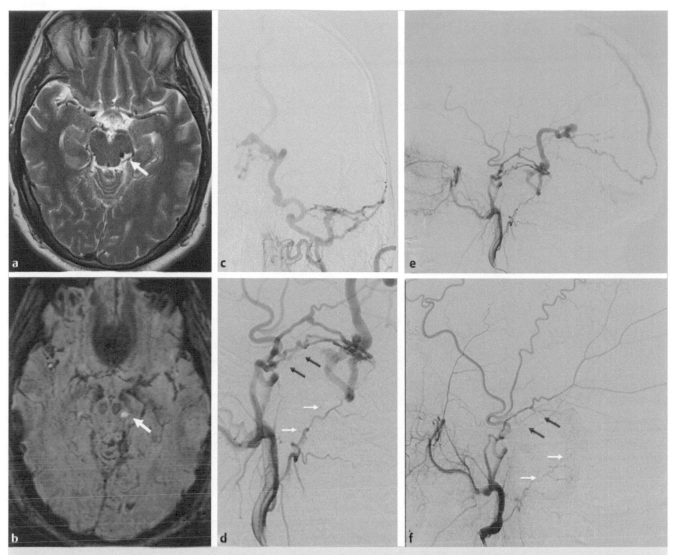

**Fig. 28.7** MRI with T2-weighted (a) and susceptibility-weighted (b) images demonstrates a dilated and arterialized lateral mesencephalic vein (bright signal on susceptibility-weighted imaging), indicating an arteriovenous shunt (*arrows*). Left ECA angiograms in anteroposterior (c) and lateral (d,e) views verify the shunt that is supplied by the facial arcade through the petrous branch of the MMA (*thin black arrows*) and the stylomastoid branch of the posterior auricular artery (*thin white arrows*). After complete obliteration of the fistula, the follow-up digital subtraction angiography (f) demonstrates persistent filling of the facial arcade, which is now of normal size.

third and fourth cranial nerves are supplied by the artery of the free margin of the tentorium on the roof of the cavernous sinus. This artery may arise from the meningohypophyseal trunk, directly off the internal carotid artery (ICA), but also from the MMA, the ophthalmic or lacrimal artery, or the inferolateral trunk (ILT). Further distally (i.e., in the cavernous sinus and the superior orbital fissure), the anteromedial branch of the ILT supplies nerves III, IV, and VI (▶ Fig. 28.3).

## 28.2.3 Cranial Nerve V

After the trigeminal nerve exits from the pons, it is supplied by the vestigial artery of the trigeminal artery that arises from the basilar artery. After the trigeminal nerve enters Meckel's cave, the Gasserian ganglion is supplied by the posteromedial and posterolateral branches of the ILT and may receive additional

supply from cavernous branches from the MMA. V2 is supplied by the artery of the foramen rotundum, which, in turn, is fed by the anterolateral branch of the ILT that arises from the cavernous horizontal segment of the ICA and by the artery of the foramen rotundum of the distal maxillary artery. V3 and the motor root of the trigeminal nerve have a common course through the foramen ovale and are supplied by the accessory meningeal artery, which anastomoses with the posteromedial branch of the ILT and the cavernous branches from the MMA (▶ Fig. 28.4; ▶ Fig. 28.5).

## 28.2.4 Cranial Nerves VII and VIII

In their cisternal course from the brainstem to the medial part of the internal acoustic meatus, the facial and vestibulocochlear nerves are supplied by the internal auditory artery of the cere-

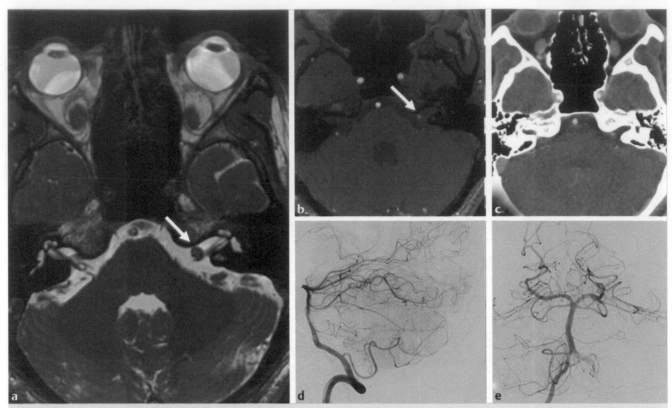

**Fig. 28.8** The labyrinthine artery that supplies the vestibulocochlear nerve arises from the distal anterior inferior cerebellar artery. This patient had an acute onset of headache followed by unilateral hearing loss and ataxia. On exam, he presented with a nonfunctioning vestibulocochlear nerve on the left. MRI, including heavily weighted T2 (a), and contrast-enhanced T1 with fat suppression (b) and axial CTA (c) revealed what was believed to be a dissecting (i.e., fusiform) aneurysm from the left anterior inferior cerebellar artery that, as it had not to hemorrhage, was followed conservatively and regressed over the course of the next 2 months (d,e). The eighth cranial nerve, however, did not regain its function.

bellolabyrinthine branch arising from the anterior inferior cerebellar artery. The internal auditory artery is also supplying the first labyrinthine segment of the facial nerve, proximal to the geniculate ganglion.

The second (tympanic) and third (mastoid) segments of the facial nerve are supplied by the "facial arcade" (i.e., an anastomotic circle that derives its supply anteriorly from the petrosal branch of the MMA and posteriorly from the stylomastoid branch of the posterior auricular artery). The stylomastoid branch can also arise from a common trunk of the posterior auricular artery and occipital artery, a variation seen in 50% of patients. The petrosal branch originates from the MMA distal to the foramen spinosum and courses posteriorly along with the superficial petrosal nerve to join the geniculate ganglion. The arcade toward the stylomastoid artery follows the intrapetrous facial nerve in the facial canal, horizontally at the tympanic portion, and then vertically at the mastoid portion.

The petrous branch of the MMA represents the dominant supply in the vast majority of cases; however, in some cases of dAVF in this region, both arteries are able to supply the facial nerve (refer also to Case 5's ▸ Fig. 5.4 for an example). Other arterial supply to the tympanic cavity may anastomose with the facial arcade and may be involved in dural arteriovenous shunts along the petrous ridge, including the infratympanic artery (branch of the ascending pharyngeal artery), the anterior tympanic artery (branch of the maxillary artery), and the caroticotympanic artery (branch of the ICA). Classically, there is no anastomosis between the internal auditory artery and the petrous branch of the MMA (▸ Fig. 28.6; ▸ Fig. 28.7; ▸ Fig. 28.8).

## 28.2.5 Cranial Nerves IX, X, XI, and XII

In their intraforaminal course, the nerves coursing through the pars nervosa of the jugular foramen (IX and X) are supplied by the jugular branch of the neuromeningeal trunk of the ascending pharyngeal artery, which anastomoses with the lateral clival artery of the meningohypophyseal trunk. The accessory spinal nerve is supplied from the musculospinal branch from the neuromeningeal trunk that originates before entering the foramen magnum, and proximal to the odontoid arch. At the level of the hypoglossal canal, the twelfth cranial nerve is supplied by the hypoglossal branch of the neuromeningeal trunk of the ascending pharyngeal artery. This artery anastomoses with the arcade of the dens that derives its supply from the C3 portion of the vertebral artery (▸ Fig. 28.9).

## 28.3 Clinical Impact

Particles and liquid embolic materials are the two most commonly used embolization materials employed in the external carotid artery (ECA) system. While the penetration capacity of particles (the most commonly used are Gelfoam, Gelfoam

often larger than the potential anastomoses and range from 100 to 300 µm, and may therefore be seen on superselective injections.

Few pathologies may lead to specific involvement of the vascularization of the cranial nerves. Diabetes or viral infections may be responsible for vasculitis of these small vessels and subsequent nerve ischemia and deficit. This is described, for example, in Bell palsy, where the viral involvement is responsible for a breakdown of the hematonervous barrier, resulting in gadolinium enhancement on MRI.

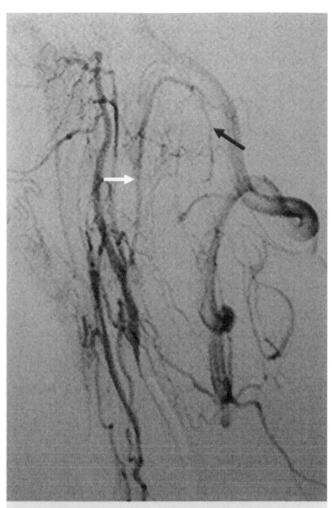

**Fig. 28.9** The lower cranial nerves are supplied by the ascending pharyngeal artery though its posteriorly directed neuromeningeal trunk (*white arrow*) that anastomoses with the arcade of the dens (*black arrow*) at the level of the hypoglossal canal.

---

### Pearls and Pitfalls

- Vasa nervorum are larger than most of the "dangerous" extracranial–intracranial anastomoses and may be visualized on superselective arterial injections. The major risk is that most of the cranial nerves are supplied by networks of vessels that are in hemodynamic equilibrium, the best example of which is the facial arcade. Embolization of one of the supplying vessels may still result in sufficient blood flow to the cranial nerve via the other channel, unless an embolic agent is used that polymerizes slowly, and therefore penetrates deeply into the entire network of vessels, potentially supplying a cranial nerve.
- Transarterial embolization of lesions in the cavernous sinus region requires exquisite knowledge of the arterial supply to cranial nerves III, IV, V, and VI to avoid cranial nerve palsies after liquid embolic embolization in this region.

## Further Reading

[1] Blunt MJ. The blood supply of the facial nerve. J Anat 1954; 88: 520–526
[2] El-Khouly H, Fernandez-Miranda J, Rhoton AL, Jr. Blood supply of the facial nerve in the middle fossa: the petrosal artery. Neurosurgery 2008; 62 Suppl 2: ONS297–ONS303, discussion ONS303–ONS304
[3] Geibprasert S, Pongpech S, Armstrong D, Krings T. Dangerous extracranial-intracranial anastomoses and supply to the cranial nerves: vessels the neurointerventionalist needs to know. AJNR Am J Neuroradiol 2009; 30: 1459–1468
[4] Krisht A, Barnett DW, Barrow DL, Bonner G. The blood supply of the intracavernous cranial nerves: an anatomic study. Neurosurgery 1994; 34: 275–279, discussion 279
[5] Ozanne A, Pereira V, Krings T, Toulgoat F, Lasjaunias P. Arterial vascularization of the cranial nerves. Neuroimaging Clin N Am 2008; 18: 431–439xii.

powder, and polyvinyl alcohol particles) is dependent on their respective sizes, the liquid embolic materials can open and enter not only the small anastomotic channels that are not visualized on the initial angiograms but also the vasa nervorum that supply the cranial nerves, as outlined here. They are

# 29 The Vascular Anatomy of the Nose

## 29.1 Case Description

### 29.1.1 Clinical Presentation

A 23-year-old patient with a known family history of recurrent epistaxis presented to the otolaryngology department with recurrent epistaxis. Within the last 24 hours, his hemoglobin level had dropped from 14.6 to 8.5 g/dL despite posterior packing at an outside institution. Given the significant blood loss, an emergency angiography was performed with the intent to embolize.

### 29.1.2 Radiologic Studies

See ▶ Fig. 29.1.

### 29.1.3 Diagnosis

Nosebleeds resulting from multiple mucocutaneous telangiectasias of the distal sphenopalatine arteries, suggestive of hereditary hemorrhagic telangiectasia (HHT).

## 29.2 Anatomy

The vascular supply to the nasal fossa involves both external and internal carotid arterial contributions, with four major contributing vessels involved on each site.

First, the sphenopalatine artery is the major contributor for the posteromedial and posterolateral supply to the nasal fossa.

This vessel is the most important source of supply to the mucoperiosteum of the nose. It originates from the pterygopalatine segment of the maxillary artery. The sphenopalatine artery exits from the superomedial aspect of the pterygopalatine fossa via the sphenopalatine foramen and enters the nasal fossa behind and slightly above the middle concha. It has two major groups of branches: posterior lateral nasal and posterior medial (or septal) branches. The posterior lateral nasal arteries supply the conchae and can anastomose with the anterior and posterior ethmoidal arteries superiorly. After the posterior lateral nasal artery has branched off the sphenopalatine artery, its main trunk courses medially along the posterior roof of the nasal cavity. Once the vessel has reached the septum, it gives origin to the posterior medial (or septal) branches that run anteriorly along the midline. The inferior septal branch courses as the nasopalatine artery through the incisive canal to anastomose with the greater palatine artery. Superiorly, small branches run toward the cribriform plate and anastomose with nasal branches of the ethmoidal arteries (▶ Fig. 29.2).

Second, the anterior and posterior ethmoidal arteries supply the superior aspect of the nasal fossa. Both arteries arise from the ophthalmic artery and send numerous small branches through the cribriform plate that anastomose medially and laterally with nasal branches of the sphenopalatine artery and provide a potential collateral pathway between the internal and external carotid circulations, which may be a cause for failed control of epistaxis after external carotid artery (ECA) embolization.

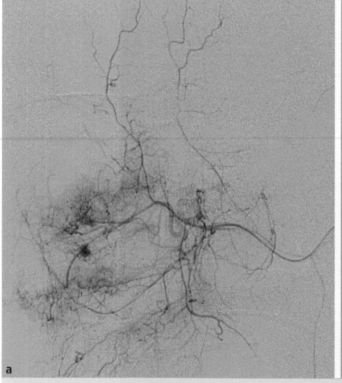
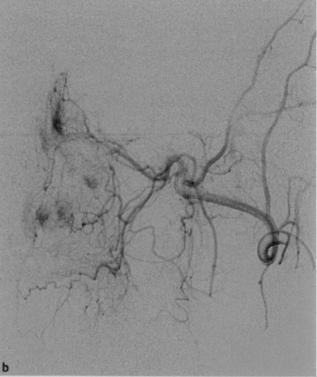

**Fig. 29.1** Selective sphenopalatine injection in lateral (a) and anteroposterior (AP) (b) views demonstrates multiple telangiectasias of the nasal mucosa, as classically seen in HHT. They are fed by the medial (septal) and lateral (conchal) arteries of the distal sphenopalatine artery.

Third, the terminal branch of the greater palatine artery supplies the inferior medial and lateral part of the nasal cavity. It enters the incisive foramen and anastomoses with the nasopalatine artery (i.e., the inferior septal branch of the sphenopalatine artery).

Finally, the septal branch of the superior labial artery that originates from the facial artery supplies the medial inferior wall of the nasal cavity. At the anteroinferior medial wall, the superior labial artery anastomoses with both the sphenopalatine artery (via the nasopalatine artery) and the distal greater palatine artery. This area is also known as locus Kiesselbachii and is the most common culprit region for anterior epistaxis.

## 29.3 Clinical Impact

### 29.3.1 Epistaxis

Given the anatomical considerations, the protocol used for embolization in patients with epistaxis depends mainly on the localization of the bleed. If no source of bleeding can be identified, our protocol consists of bilateral injections into the internal carotid artery (ICA) to determine whether normal supply to the eye is present, the contribution of the ethmoidal arteries (the larger the contribution, the lesser the likelihood that pure ECA injections will be successful to control the epistaxis), and whether ICA-related sources of epistaxis are present. This is followed by distal catheterization of the bilateral ECA branches that supply the nose and particle embolization to devascularize transiently the supply to the nasal mucosa: the sphenopalatine artery (medial and lateral branches), the greater palatine artery, and the distal facial artery (▶ Fig. 29.3).

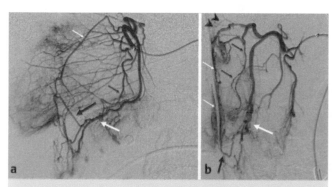

Fig. 29.2 Anatomy of the internal maxillary artery branches supplying the nose in lateral (a) and AP (b) views. The sphenopalatine artery has medial septal (*small white arrows*) and lateral conchal (*small black arrows*) branches. At the midline, the superior medial branches anastomose through the cribriform plate with the ethmoidal branches (*arrowheads*) of the ophthalmic artery. The inferior medial branch anastomoses with the greater palatine artery (*large white arrow*) as it courses as the nasopalatine artery (*large black arrow*) through the incisive canal.

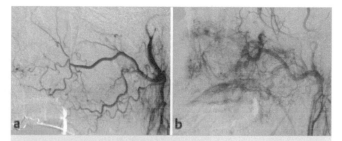

Fig. 29.3 In idiopathic epistaxis, there is often diffuse hyperemia within the nasal cavity, as seen on the ECA angiogram in arterial (a) and late capillary (b) phases.

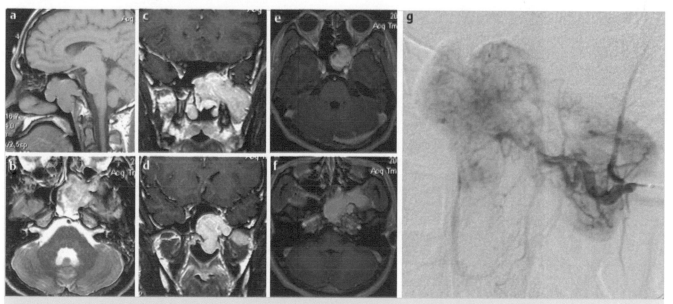

Fig. 29.4 MRI with sagittal T1 precontrast (a), axial T2 (b), and coronal (c,d) and axial (e,f) T1 postcontrast images in a 14-year-old boy who presented with recurrent epistaxis and a stuffy nose. The study demonstrated a densely enhancing mass in the nasal cavity suggestive of a juvenile angiofibroma. The sphenopalatine artery injection in the AP view (g) demonstrates multiple tumor vessels that mainly arise from the superior and medial septal branches, which will invariably anastomose with the ethmoidal arteries of the ophthalmic artery.

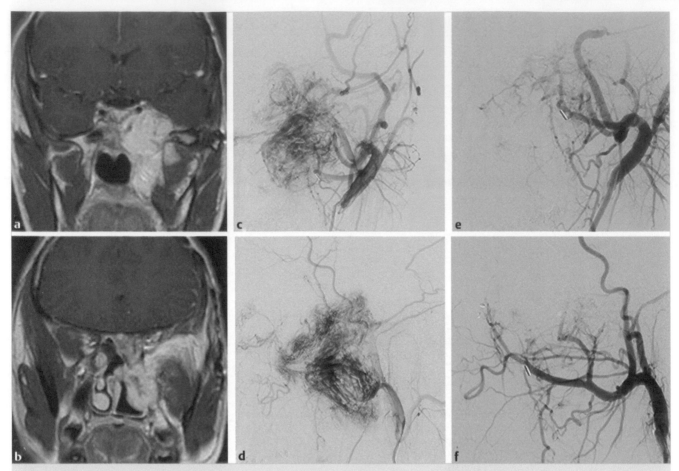

**Fig. 29.5** A companion case to the patient in ▶ Fig. 29.4 with a juvenile angiofibroma, seen on coronal T1 postcontrast MRI (a,b). Embolization before surgery was requested (c,d). After polyvinyl alcohol particle embolization, significant devascularization is seen (e,f).

## 29.3.2 HHT

HHT was first recognized in the 19th century as a familial disorder causing recurrent nosebleeds. The present diagnostic criteria require three of the following four clinical symptoms to be present in an individual to make the diagnosis of "definite" HHT: spontaneous recurrent nosebleeds; mucocutaneous telangiectasia at characteristic sites (lips, oral cavity, fingers, or the nose); visceral involvement, such as pulmonary, hepatic, or central nervous system arteriovenous malformations; and an affected first-degree relative, according to these criteria. Spontaneous recurrent nosebleeds from telangiectasia of the nasal mucosa are the most common clinical manifestation of HHT and can occur occasionally or on a daily basis. On selective angiographies, characteristic telangiectasias in the nose are seen and can be targeted by embolization. Choice of particles in these patients has to be larger, as within the telangiectasias, shunts are present that can lead to embolization of pulmonary vessels or, if additional shunts are present in the lungs, even to paradoxical brain embolism.

## 29.3.3 Tumors

As certain tumors of the nasal fossa are hypervascularized, preoperative embolization may be required, or they may present with nosebleeds as their first manifesting symptom. The typical

example is the juvenile nasopharyngeal angiofibroma that derives its blood supply from all potential sources (including the embryonic intersegmental arteries of the ICA), hypertrophied branches of the sphenopalatine artery, and the ethmoidal branches of the ophthalmic artery and the accessory middle meningeal and the ascending pharyngeal artery (▶ Fig. 29.4, ▶ Fig. 29.5), depending on the tumor extension through the skull base. In these tumors, multiple anastomoses between the ICA and the ECA are present, which is why we do not recommend direct puncture and liquid embolic embolization in most cases. Other vascular tumors involving the nasal fossa are hemangiopericytomas, hemangioendotheliomas, cavernous hemangiomas of the cavernous sinus, esthesioneuroblastoma, or neuroepitheliomas.

## 29.3.4 Collaterals

The anterior and posterior ethmoidal arteries of the ophthalmic artery penetrate the cribriform plate to anastomose with nasal branches of the sphenopalatine artery. Particles smaller than 80 μm may pass through these collaterals and lead to inadvertent embolization of the ophthalmic artery territory. In addition to these nasal branches, the distal internal maxillary artery can anastomose with the ophthalmic artery via the anterior deep temporal artery, which may connect to the inferior branch of the lacrimal artery of the ophthalmic artery (see Case 25's ▶ Fig. 25.1).

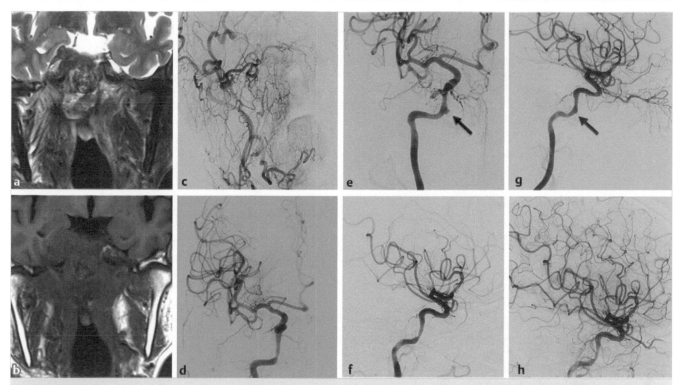

**Fig. 29.6** This 63-year-old man with a known nasopharyngeal cancer with skull base involvement seen on coronal T1- and T2-weighted (a,b) MRI, presented acutely with arterial bleeding from nose and mouth. Right ECA angiogram in AP view (c) demonstrates the tumor-supplying vessels, but no source of hemorrhage can be identified. It was only after injection into the ICA (d,e) that the source of hemorrhage was found: a pseudoaneurysm of the ICA (*arrow*) caused by tumor destruction of the bone and vessel wall invasion of the ICA, which was successfully treated with a covered stent graft (f,g,h).

## Pearls and Pitfalls

- In patients with posterior epistaxis and prominent ethmoidal branches, embolization may fail to control the bleeding, as the ethmoidal branches may reconstitute the supply to the nasal mucosa and, therefore, lead to continued epistaxis. Surgical ligation is the treatment method of choice in these cases.
- Because the diameter of the anastomoses between the ethmoidal arteries and the septal arteries is less than 80 μm, embolization of these branches with particles greater than this size is considered to be safe.
- With nasal packing in place, the majority of patients will show normal angiographic anatomy and no extravasation.
- The use of larger particles in HHT is recommended, as the shunts within the mucosa may be larger, and therefore, smaller particles may penetrate into the venous pulmonary bed. As patients with HHT are also prone to have arteriovenous fistulas in the lungs, this could theoretically lead to inadvertent paradoxical brain emboli.
- One must always inject the ICAs in patients with epistaxis to rule out a potential source of the bleeding from the ICA (▶ Fig. 29.6).
- In juvenile angiofibromas, all potential dangerous anastomotic pathways with the ICA will be open and have to be taken into consideration when embolizing the ECA branches.

## 29.4 Additional Information and Cases

See ▶ Fig. 29.6.

## Further Reading

[1] Koh E, Frazzini VI, Kagetsu NJ. Epistaxis: vascular anatomy, origins, and endovascular treatment. AJR Am J Roentgenol 2000; 174: 845–851

[2] Lasjaunias P, Marsot-Dupuch K, Doyon D. The radio-anatomical basis of arterial embolisation for epistaxis. J Neuroradiol 1979; 6: 45–53

[3] Osborn AG. The nasal arteries. AJR Am J Roentgenol 1978; 130: 89–97

[4] Willems PW, Farb RI, Agid R. Endovascular treatment of epistaxis. AJNR Am J Neuroradiol 2009; 30: 1637–1645

# 30 The Ascending Pharyngeal Artery

## 30.1 Case Description

### 30.1.1 Clinical Presentation

A 68-year-old woman presented with a painless cervical mass lesion.

### 30.1.2 Radiologic Studies

See ▶ Fig. 30.1.

### 30.1.3 Diagnosis

Carotid body paraganglioma.

## 30.2 Anatomy

The ascending pharyngeal artery (APhA) typically arises from the medial posterior wall of the proximal external carotid artery (ECA; ~80% of the cases). In the other 20% of cases, the origin may be from the occipital artery (as a branch or as a common trunk), from a common trunk with the lingual and facial arteries, from the carotid bifurcation, and even from the proximal cervical internal carotid artery (ICA), distal to the carotid bulb. In addition, the pharyngeal trunk and the neuromeningeal trunk may have separate origins. These variable patterns can be explained by the fact that the APhA has a separate origin from the ECA in the embryo, as part of the pharyngo-occipital system, rather than the ventral pharyngeal artery (ECA precursor). After its origin, the APhA courses superiorly, following the posterolateral wall of the pharynx, ventral to the ICA and dorsal to the ECA.

The APhA has two main branches, the pharyngeal trunk and the neuromeningeal trunk, and also gives rise to a third smaller but functionally important branch, the inferior tympanic artery.

The pharyngeal trunk supplies the mucosa of the posterior and lateral walls of the pharynx. It has three main branches: the superior, middle, and inferior pharyngeal arteries. There is a rich network of anastomotic vessels with the contralateral APhA and the distal branches of the internal maxillary artery. From an endovascular perspective, it plays a significant role in the treatment of posttonsillectomy hemorrhage (inferior pharyngeal artery) and in refractory epistaxis (middle pharyngeal artery). From the three pharyngeal arteries, the superior pharyngeal artery is the most important source of potentially dangerous anastomoses, as discussed later.

The neuromeningeal trunk has two main branches: the jugular and the hypoglossal branches. The jugular branch enters the skull base through the jugular foramen and runs posterolaterally. It supplies the vasa nervorum of the IX, X, and XI cranial nerves, as well as the posterior fossa dura mater and the walls of the sigmoid and petrosal sinus. The jugular branch plays a significant role in the supply of dural arteriovenous fistulas and is a reason why injections showing the APhA are mandatory in the diagnostic workup of this disease. The hypoglossal branch enters through the hypoglossal canal and supplies the XII cranial nerve and the meninges of the posterior cranial fossa. It also contributes to the odontoid arch through a descending branch. Both branches are involved in the supply of dural-based tumors such as meningiomas, and may be a target for superselective preoperative embolization. See also Cases 28 and 31.

The inferior tympanic artery commonly arises from the proximal neuromeningeal trunk but can arise from the pharyngeal trunk or as a separate branch between both main trunks. It enters the skull through the inferior tympanic canaliculus, together with the tympanic branch of cranial nerve IX (Jacobsen nerve), and gives supply to the vasa vasorum of the ICA. It may also contribute to the supply of cranial nerve VII through connections with the facial arcade. The main importance of the inferior tympanic artery is that it serves as a collateral route to reconstitute the petrous ICA in cases of segmental agenesis of the cervical ICA, better known as the "aberrant ICA" (see Case 3). It plays a significant role in the blood supply to glomus tympanicum and jugulotympanicum tumors.

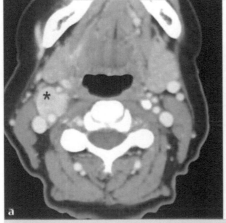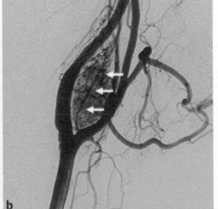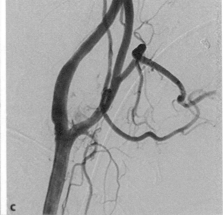

**Fig. 30.1** Axial contrast-enhanced CT (a) shows a right hypervascular cervical mass splaying the carotid bifurcation. A preembolization common carotid artery angiogram (b) shows a hypervascular tumor between the ECA and ICA. The main supply is derived from the APhA (*arrows*), which in this case was the first ECA branch, as well as the occipital artery. A postprocedure angiogram (c) shows complete devascularization of the lesion.

**Table 30.1** List of Potential Anastomoses of the APhA and Their Anastomotic Branches.

| APhA Branch | Anastomotic Branch | Connecting Artery | Parent Vessel |
|---|---|---|---|
| **Pharyngeal Trunk** | | | |
| Superior Pharyngeal Artery | Eustachian Branch | Pterygovaginal Artery | Petrous Internal Carotid Artery |
| | Recurrent Foramen Lacerum Branch | Foramen Lacerum Branch (Infero-lateral Trunk) | Petrous Internal Carotid Artery |
| Musculospinal Branch | | C3 Radicular Branch | Vertebral Artery |
| **Inferior Tympanic Artery** | | | |
| Inferior Tympanic Artery | Anterior Branch | Caroticotympanic Branch | Petrous Internal Carotid Artery |
| | Posterior Branch | Stylomastoid Artery | Facial Arcade |
| | Ascending Branch | Petrosal Artery (MMA) | Facial Arcade |
| **Neuromeningeal Trunk** | | | |
| Hypoglossal Branch | Medial Clival Branch | Medial Clival Artery (MHT) | Cavernous Internal Carotid Artery |
| | Pre-Vertebral Branch | Odontoid Arcade (C1-C2) | Vertebral Artery |
| | Descending Branch | Odontoid Arcade (C3) | Vertebral Artery |
| Jugular Branch | Lateral Clival Branch | Lateral Clival Branch (MHT) | Cavernous Internal Carotid Artery |

MMA = middle meningeal artery; MHT = meningohypophyseal trunk

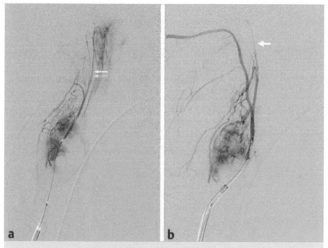

**Fig. 30.2** Superselective microcatheter injections of the APhA (a) and the occipital artery (b) in a patient with a glomus tumor show a separate origin of the pharyngeal trunk (*thin double arrows*) and neuromeningeal (*arrow*) trunk. The neuromeningeal trunk arises from the occipital artery.

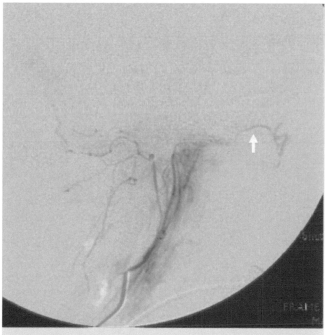

**Fig. 30.3** Right APhA angiogram reveals anastomosis of the superior pharyngeal artery with the distal internal maxillary artery through the pterygovaginal artery (*arrow*) around the eustachian tube.

## 30.3 Clinical Impact

The APhA is a route for multiple anastomoses with the ICA, branches of the ECA, and the vertebral arteries. ▶ Table 30.1 lists the "dangerous anastomoses" that may lead to focal neurological deficits and/or cranial nerve palsies during endovascular procedures in its territory.

The middle pharyngeal artery gives branches that connect to the ascending palatine and greater palatine arteries, branches of the facial artery, and the sphenopalatine arteries, which can be involved in posttonsillectomy hemorrhages. In addition, connections exist between the APhA and the occipital artery, ascending

cervical artery, and deep cervical artery, which may serve as indirect routes for anastomoses with the vertebral artery.

Before considering selective embolization of the APhA, the anatomy and potential anastomoses should be well known and properly imaged. The use of small particles (< 150 μm) should be avoided, as they have a higher risk of going through small anastomotic channels causing subsequent brain emboli. They also carry a higher risk of damaging the vasa nervorum, with

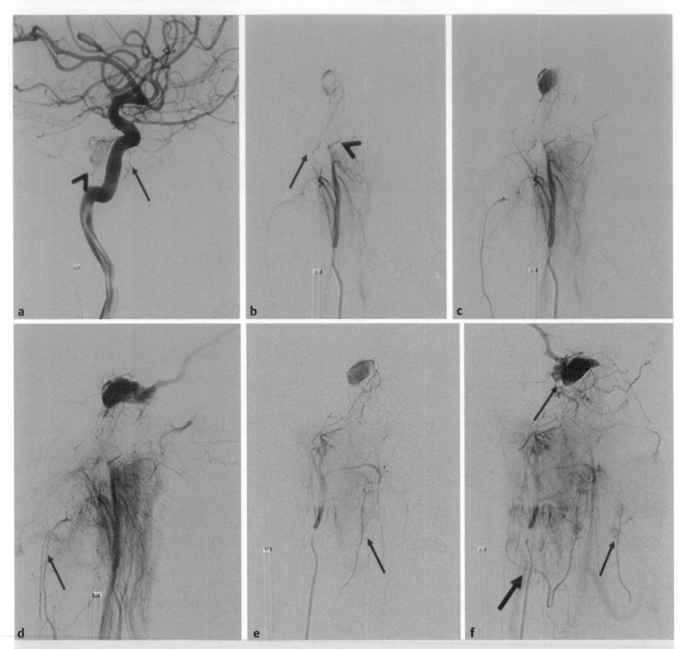

**Fig. 30.4** A 53-year-old man presented with a right proptosis and chemosis, and with increased intraocular pressures. Noninvasive angiographic imaging suggested a right cavernous DAVF. Right internal carotid artery injection in the lateral view (a) demonstrates filling of the fistula via the meningohypophyseal trunk (*arrow* in a) and the inferolateral trunk (*arrowhead* in a). Right APhA injections in lateral views (early, intermediate, and late phase: b,c,d) and anteroposterior views (in early and late phases: e,f) demonstrate the DAVF fed by the artery of the foramen lacerum (*arrowhead* in b), which anastomoses with the inferolateral trunk. There is also supply from the hypoglossal branch of the neuromeningeal trunk via the medial clival arteries (*arrow* in b) that anastomoses with the meningohypophyseal trunk. In addition, there is filling of the dens arcade (*arrows* in d,e,f) via the hypoglossal branch, which anastomoses with the vertebral artery (*thick black arrow*).

resultant cranial nerve palsies. Liquid embolic materials in the APhA should be avoided unless there is a distal safe position and sufficient safety margin. Reflux should be avoided. Endovascular occlusion of small APhA branches during a transarterial approach to treat a dural arteriovenous fistula (DAVF) can cause paralysis of cranial nerves IX, X, XI, and XII and even a facial nerve palsy.

Overlooking the APhA involvement in dural-based skull tumors, epistaxis, and posttonsillectomy hemorrhage can result in failure of the preoperative or therapeutic embolization. In addition, during the workup of DAVFs, failure to demonstrate or adequately opacify the APhA can result in a false-negative angiogram.

The APhA is invariably involved in the supply to paragangliomas of the head and neck region. As these tumors may be multiple (in up to 10% of sporadic forms and up to 40% of familial paragangliomas), it is our policy to always inject the contralateral APhA to exclude further paragangliomas. The additional angiographic protocol in paragangliomas for dependent on the location and extent of the tumor.

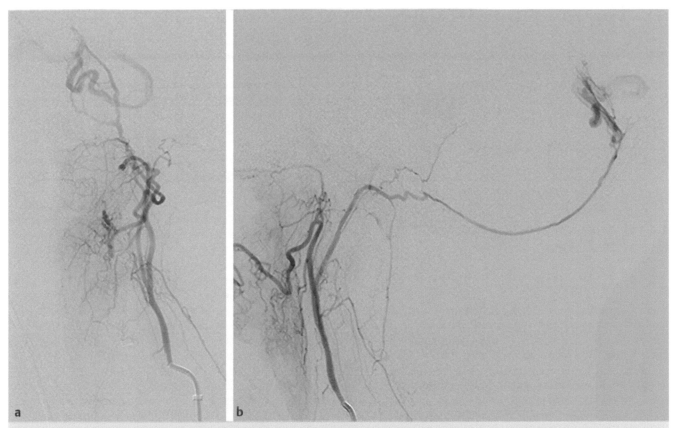

**Fig. 30.5** APhA injection in anteroposterior (a) and lateral views (b) in a 65-year-old patient with a DAVF of the posterior fossa. The DAVF was exclusively fed by a posterior meningeal branch that arose from the neuromeningeal trunk of the APhA indicating the potential role the APhA, can play in supplying the dura of the posterior fossa.

## Pearls and Pitfalls

- The APhA artery has a different embryologic origin than the ECA, which explains the variable origins this artery may show.
- The APhA is a source of multiple "dangerous" anastomoses with the ICA, VA, and facial arcade.
- The APhA provides direct supply to the lower cranial nerves (IX, X, XII, and XII). Damage to the vasa nervorum during embolization can result in cranial nerve palsies.
- In cases of posttonsillectomy hemorrhage, the APhA may be the only source of bleed. Failure to recognize it may result in an ineffective embolization procedure.
- During diagnostic angiograms, the APhA should be always demonstrated. Failure to do so may result in a false-negative exam, especially in DAVFs.

Of note is that the vasa vasorum of the carotid artery originate from the APhA.

## 30.4 Additional Information and Cases

See ▶ Fig. 30.2, ▶ Fig. 30.3, ▶ Fig. 30.4, and ▶ Fig. 30.5.

## Further Reading

[1] Cavalcanti DD, Reis CV, Hanel R et al. The ascending pharyngeal artery and its relevance for neurosurgical and endovascular procedures. Neurosurgery 2009; 65 Suppl: 114–120, discussion 120
[2] Geibprasert S, Pongpech S, Armstrong D, Krings T. Dangerous extracranial-intracranial anastomoses and supply to the cranial nerves: vessels the neurointerventionalist needs to know. AJNR Am J Neuroradiol 2009; 30: 1459–1468
[3] Hacein-Bey L, Daniels DL, Ulmer JL et al. The ascending pharyngeal artery: branches, anastomoses, and clinical significance. AJNR Am J Neuroradiol 2002; 23: 1246–1256
[4] Houseman ND, Taylor GI, Pan WR. The angiosomes of the head and neck: anatomic study and clinical applications. Plast Reconstr Surg 2000; 105: 2287–2313
[5] Lasjaunias P, Berenstein A, ter Brugge KG. Surgical Neuroangiography. Vol. 1. 2nd ed. Berlin: Springer; 2006
[6] Opatowsky MJ, Browne JD, McGuirt Jr WF, Jr, Morris PP. Endovascular treatment of hemorrhage after tonsillectomy in children. AJNR Am J Neuroradiol 2001; 22: 713–716
[7] Sato Y, Kashiwagi N, Nakanishi K, Yoshino K, Tomiyama N. Ascending pharyngeal-vertebral anastomosis demonstrated by computed tomography angiography of the ascending pharyngeal artery: a case report. Acta Radiol 2011; 52: 951–953

# 31 The Meningeal Supply

## 31.1 Case Description

### 31.1.1 Clinical Presentation

A 53-year-old woman presented with a history of seizures.

### 31.1.2 Radiologic Studies

See ▶ Fig. 31.1, ▶ Fig. 31.2.

### 31.1.3 Diagnosis

Meningioma fed by two separate branches of the middle meningeal artery (MMA).

## 31.2 Anatomy

There is considerable variation in the supply to the dura. We limit our description to the "classical" dural arterial anatomy and some of the more common arterial variations. There will be some overlap with other cases regarding the descriptive anatomy of the vessels supplying the dura; however, the major focus of this case is to describe the arteries that are involved in the supply of the dura mater and that, therefore, may play a role both in the embolization of dural arteriovenous fistulas (dAVF) and in the preoperative devascularization of cranial meningiomas. See also Cases 3, 5, 7, 25, 26, 27, 28, and 30.

The MMA arises from the internal maxillary artery and is the most important source of cranial dural supply. It enters the cranium via the foramen spinosum and makes a sharp turn as it enters the middle cranial fossa. It has frontal, temporal squamous, petrous, cavernous-ophthalmic, and parietal branches. Posterior branches course toward the sigmoid sinus and the transverse sinus and contribute medially to the supply of the tentorium. Cranially, the MMA anastomoses at the level of the superior sagittal sinus with the anterior falcine artery.

The accessory meningeal artery arises either from a common trunk with the MMA or distal to the MMA. It courses more medially and anteriorly compared with the MMA, toward the cavernous sinus region, where it anastomoses with the inferolateral trunk (ILT) at the level of the foramen ovale and (despite its name) supplies only a very small portion of the dura in this region.

The neuromeningeal trunk of the ascending pharyngeal artery supplies, via the hypoglossal and the jugular branches, the dura surrounding the respectively named foramina. At the level of the hypoglossal canal, the hypoglossal artery connects to the odontoid arcade, which interconnects to the C3 branches of the vertebral artery system, thus supplying the dura around the foramen magnum and dens. The hypoglossal artery may give rise to the artery of the falx cerebelli and the posterior meningeal artery (see Case 30's ▶ Fig. 30.5 for an example). Its clival branches supply the inferior clivus and anastomose with the internal carotid artery (ICA). The jugular branch supplies the dura of the jugular foramen and the lateral clivus and may extend cranially toward Dorello's canal (abducens nerve) and, further laterally, toward the sigmoid sinus, where it can anastomose with the MMA and the transosseous dural branches of the occipital artery.

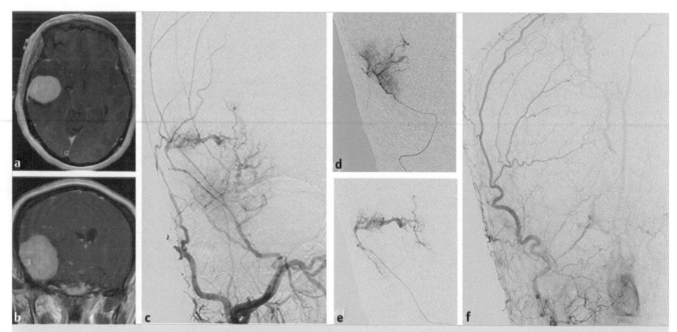

**Fig. 31.1** Axial (a) and coronal (b) contrast-enhanced T1-weighted MRIs demonstrate a right frontotemporal densely and homogeneously enhancing convexity meningioma with perifocal edema and midline shift. Neurosurgery requested a preoperative angiography to determine its vascularity with potential embolization if the tumor was deemed hypervascular. Right external carotid artery (ECA) angiogram in anteroposterior view (c) reveals two MMA branches with sunburst-type supply to the tumor. Both branches were subsequently injected (d,e). After polyvinyl alcohol particle embolization, complete devascularization of the tumor can be seen on the control angiogram (f).

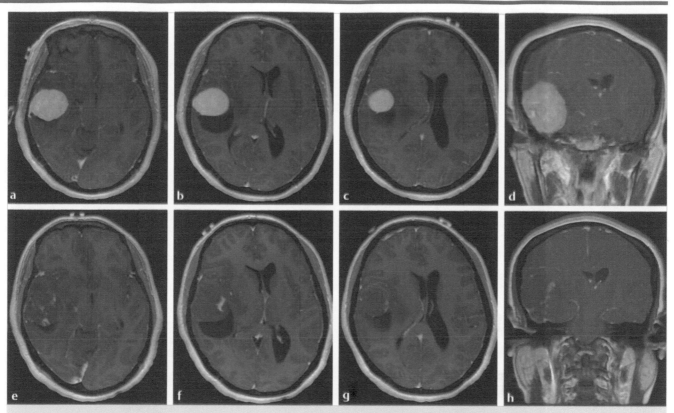

**Fig. 31.2** Preoperative (a–d) versus postoperative (e–h) contrast-enhanced T1-weighted MRIs demonstrate the effect of PVA embolization with intratumoral necrosis and significant decrease in contrast material uptake.

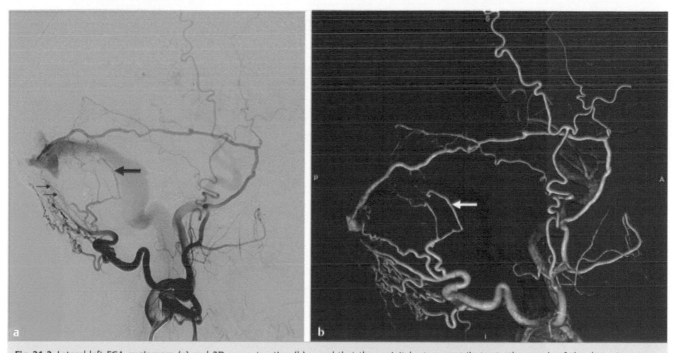

**Fig. 31.3** Lateral left ECA angiogram (a) and 3D reconstruction (b) reveal that the occipital artery contributes to the supply of the dura via transmastoidal (the stylomastoid branch, *arrow*) and transosseous (*small arrows*) branches that, in this case of a dural shunt, demonstrate anastomoses with the MMA.

The occipital artery usually supplies the dura of the posterior fossa via a transmastoid branch that runs through the bone into the lateral posterior fossa. Although this transmastoid artery may also arise from the ascending pharyngeal artery and the posterior auricular artery, it is most commonly seen to arise from the distal occipital artery (▶ Fig. 31.3). In rare cases, the occipital artery can give rise to the posterior meningeal artery or the artery of the falx cerebelli. In shunt-

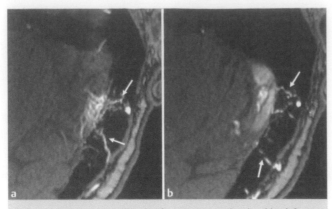

**Fig. 31.4** In a patient with a dural arteriovenous fistula of his left transverse sinus, time-of-flight MRA at 3 T (axial source data, a,b) demonstrates the osteodural contribution (*arrows*) from the occipital artery piercing the bone to contribute to the supply to the fistula. Given the fine network of these osteodural arteries in the supply of dural-based lesions, deep penetration of liquid embolic material is more difficult to achieve through these vessels then through the more direct feeder arising from the meningeal vessels. This is of particular importance when using embolic material that polymerizes quickly, such as glue.

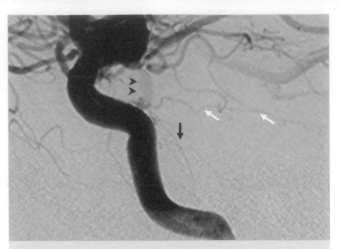

**Fig. 31.5** This ICA injection demonstrates the posteriorly directed artery of the free margin of the tentorium (*white arrows*) and the dorsal meningeal artery (*black arrow*) that courses downward to anastomose with the ascending pharyngeal artery along the clivus. Both arteries may arise from a common meningohypophyseal trunk that also leads to supply of the posterior pituitary (the *black arrowheads* point to the posterior pituitary blush).

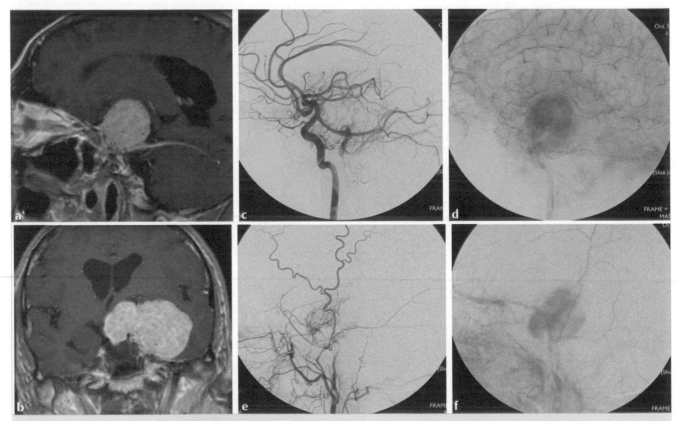

**Fig. 31.6** Tumors of the cavernous sinus region will have extensive supply from the ICA (via ILT and the meningohypophyseal trunk), the internal maxillary artery (via the MMA, accessory meningeal artery, and artery of the foramen rotundum and ovale), and the ascending pharyngeal artery via clival branches, as seen in this large clival meningioma on MRI (a,b), ICA (c,d), and ECA (e,f) angiograms. When embolizing these tumors, caution must be taken to respect the extracranial–intracranial anastomoses and the arterial cranial nerve supply.

ing dural lesions, small osteodural branches will be recruited that traverse through the bone. As they are typically—even in the presence of a shunt—very small and tortuous, it is unlikely that liquid embolic material with a short polymeriza-tion time will reach the shunt through these vessels (▶ Fig. 31.4).

Dural supply from the ICA is via the ILT, the meningohypo-physeal trunk, and the ophthalmic artery, as described in Cases

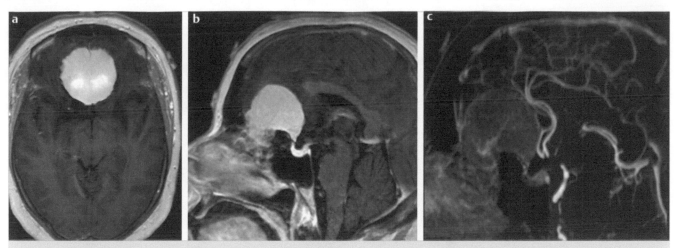

**Fig. 31.7** Olfactory groove meningioma: axial (a) and sagittal (b) contrast-enhanced T1 W MR sequences, and sagittal contrast-enhanced MRV source images (c). Tumors of the olfactory groove will be supplied by direct branches of the ophthalmic artery (i.e., the anterior and posterior ethmoidal arteries). Additional supply in this region can be derived from the recurrent meningeal branch of the ophthalmic artery and the MMA.

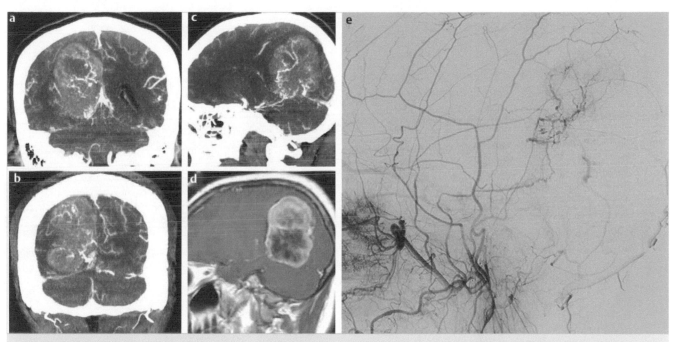

**Fig. 31.8** The MMA supplies the majority of the dura, including the posterior falx and the superior tentorium cerebelli, as in this case of a hypervascularized meningioma that presented with intratumoral hemorrhage, seen on the contrast-enhanced CT (a,b,c) and MRI T1-weighted image (d) related to the significant hypervascularization (e).

5 and 7. In brief, the meningohypophyseal trunk gives rise to the artery of the free margin of the tentorium that runs posterosuperiorly; the dorsal meningeal artery that courses inferiorly to Dorello's canal, where it anastomoses with clival branches of the ascending pharyngeal artery; and the basal tentorial artery, which runs posterolaterally along the superior aspect of the petrous bone (▶ Fig. 31.5).

The ILT will supply the cavernous sinus and the middle cranial fossa, including the dura surrounding the foramen ovale and rotundum. It is connected to the ophthalmic artery via its recurrent branch. The arterial system of this region can be regarded as a para-cavernous network that connects the MMA system with the accessory meningeal artery, the ICA, the ophthalmic artery, the marginal tentorial artery, and the ascending pharyngeal artery. Hypervascularized tumors in this region will therefore derive their supply from all of these potential sources, whereas arteriovenous shunting lesions will enlarge these pre-existing channels to contribute to the shunt (▶ Fig. 31.6).

The ophthalmic artery has two major subdivisions: the medial and the lateral groups (see Case 8). The lateral group can supply the dura via the recurrent meningeal artery, which anastomoses with the MMA. The medial group has a more significant dural supply: Via perforating branches through the cribriform plate, the anterior and posterior ethmoidal arteries supply the

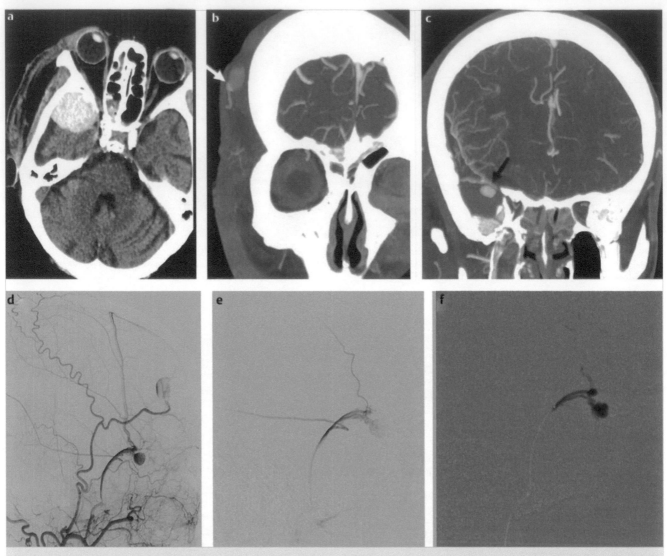

**Fig. 31.9** CT (a) and CTA (b,c) after trauma demonstrate an acute middle cranial fossa epidural hematoma and a subgaleal hematoma. The CTA shows traumatic pseudoaneurysms of the MMA (*arrow* in c) and the superficial temporal artery (*arrow* in b) that are confirmed during ECA angiography (d). A microcatheter was advanced to the distal MMA (e) (i.e., past the skull base entry through the foramen spinosum), and the vessel was sacrificed (glue cast in f). Vessel sacrifice of the MMA distal to the foramen spinosum can be safely performed, as the anastomoses and the cranial nerve supply occur in close relation to the skull base.

anterior cranial fossa. In addition, the distal anterior ethmoidal artery gives rise to the artery of the falx cerebri (anterior falcine artery) through the foramen cecum. This artery supplies the falx and anastomoses distally and cranially with the MMA (▶ Fig. 31.7).

The following intradural arteries can participate in the supply to the dura: Both the intradural vertebral artery (more commonly, however, from its extradural compartment) and the intradural posterior ICA can give rise to the artery of the falx cerebelli and the posterior meningeal artery to supply the dura of the posterior fossa. The superior cerebellar artery can give rise to a tentorial branch. This so-called medial dural tentorial artery is classically only visible in dural tentorial arteriovenous fistulas and will arise from the rostral trunk of the superior cerebellar artery in its lateral pontomesencephalic segment in the ambient cistern directly under the free margin of the tentorium. The posterior cerebral artery can give rise to small dural branches from both its distal cortical and its choroidal vessels. These have been coined the arteries of Davidoff and Schechter and are classically only seen in the setting of tumors or vascular malformations, as they are too small to be visualized on routine angiographies.

## 31.3 Clinical Impact

Endovascular presurgical treatments aim to decrease vascularity (less blood loss), induce necrosis (as a softer tumor will enable easier cleavage), and enable complete removal of certain deep-seated skull base tumors. Depending on the goal, different embolization materials/techniques and different times between embolization and surgery can be chosen. To lessen blood loss, one has to aim for deep feeders, and a ligation-type embolization may be sufficient if surgery is performed within the first 48 hours; however, if time between embolization and surgery is

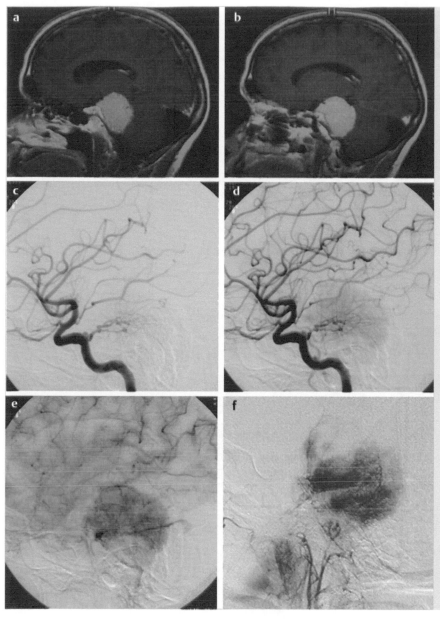

**Fig. 31.10** A 52-year-old woman presented with progressive facial hypesthesias, ataxia, and headaches. MRI with sagittal contrast-enhanced T1-weighted images (a,b) revealed a meningioma of the clivus. Tumors of the clivus will be supplied both from the neuromeningeal trunk of the ascending pharyngeal artery via the clival branches (f) and from the dorsal meningeal artery of the meningohypophyseal trunk of the ICA (c,d,e). This anastomosis has to be kept in mind when embolizing tumors in this region.

longer, dural anastomoses will reconstitute the ligated vessels. If one aims to induce tumoral necrosis, very small particles have to be used (45–150 μm). As necrotic tumors tend to expand slightly within the first day after embolization, one should wait for at least 72 hours and up to 1 week to have the best intraoperative results and to capitalize on the soft necrotic tumor. This technique is not indicated if one works close to "dangerous vessels," as the particles may penetrate through the anastomoses or occlude the vasa nervorum. In these cases, larger particles (300–500 μm) are safer, but revascularization will appear faster.

## 31.4 Additional Information and Cases

See ▶ Fig. 31.8, ▶ Fig. 31.9, ▶ Fig. 31.10, ▶ Fig. 31.11, and ▶ Fig. 31.12.

### Pearls and Pitfalls

- Intraventricular meningiomas are supplied by the choroidal arteries; therefore, distal catheterization and embolization are mandatory to avoid inadvertent embolization toward healthy territories.
- One must differentiate true dural supply arising from pial arteries (i.e., the medial dural tentorial artery of the superior cerebellar artery and the artery of Davidoff and Schechter of the posterior cerebral artery) from induced distal pial supply to dural arteriovenous fistulas: although the latter can lead to catastrophic hemorrhage if the dural arteriovenous fistula is occluded, the former will not.

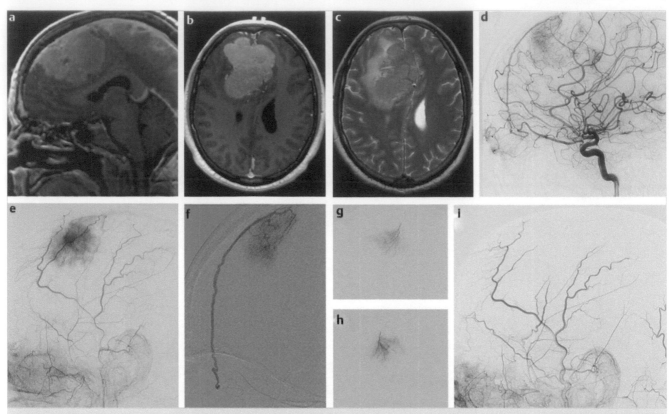

**Fig. 31.11** The anterior falx is supplied by the falcine artery, which arises from the anterior ethmoidal artery and from the MMAs. Sagittal (a) and axial (b) contrast-enhanced T1-weighted, and axial T2-weighted (c) MRIs demonstrate a large anterior falcine meningioma. Left ICA (d) and left ECA (e) angiograms in lateral view reveal supply from the falcine artery and branches of the MMAs with an intense tumoral blush. Compartmentalization of the tumor can be seen on the superselective injections of the feeding arteries (f,g,h), which were subsequently embolized with significant devascularization of the tumor on control angiogram (i).

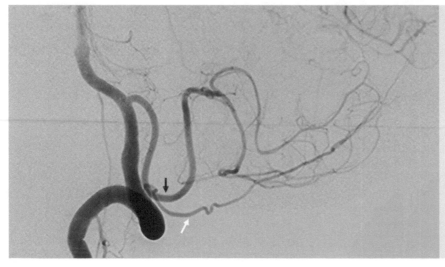

**Fig. 31.12** Considerable variations exist regarding the origin of the arteries supplying the meninges of the posterior fossa. They may arise from the vertebral artery, the occipital artery, the ascending pharyngeal or the posterior auricular artery, or, as seen in this figure, from a pial vessel (i.e., the posterior ICA; *black arrow*). The *white arrow* points to the posterior meningeal artery.

# Further Reading

[1] Banerjee AD, Ezer H, Nanda A. The artery of Bernasconi and Cassinari: a morphometric study for superselective catheterization. AJNR Am J Neuroradiol 2011; 32: 1751–1755

[2] Cavalcanti DD, Reis CV, Hanel R et al. The ascending pharyngeal artery and its relevance for neurosurgical and endovascular procedures. Neurosurgery 2009; 65 Suppl: 114–120, discussion 120

[3] Martins C, Yasuda A, Campero A, Ulm AJ, Tanriover N, Rhoton A, Jr. Microsurgical anatomy of the dural arteries. Neurosurgery 2005; 56 Suppl: 211–251

[4] Merland JJ, Bories J, Djindjian R. The blood supply of the falx cerebri, the falx cerebelli and the tentorium cerebelli. J Neuroradiol 1977; 4: 175–202

[5] Merland JJ, Théron J, Lasjaunias P, Moret J. Meningeal blood supply of the convexity. J Neuroradiol 1977; 4: 129–174

[6] Morris P. Practical Neuroangiography. Philadelphia: Wolters Kluwer Health; 2007

[7] Shukla V, Hayman LA, Ly C, Fuller G, Taber KH. Adult cranial dura I: intrinsic vessels. J Comput Assist Tomogr 2002; 26: 1069–1074

[8] Théron J, Lasjaunias P, Moret J, Merland JJ. Vascularization of the posterior fossa dura mater. J Neuroradiol 1977; 4: 203–224

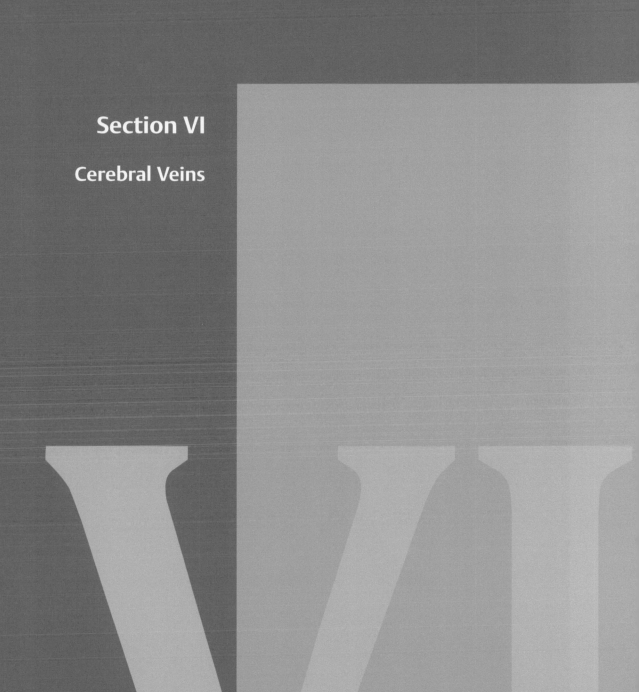

# Section VI

## Cerebral Veins

# 32 The Superior Sagittal and Transverse Sinuses

## 32.1 Case Description

### 32.1.1 Clinical Presentation

A 76-year-old man presented with progressive dementia for 1 year and recent new onset of seizures.

### 32.1.2 Radiologic Studies

See ► Fig. 32.1, ► Fig. 32.2, and ► Fig. 32.3.

### 32.1.3 Diagnosis

Malignant-type superior sagittal sinus (SSS) dural arteriovenous fistula (dAVF) with occlusion of the posterior SSS and rerouting of the shunt into transmedullary veins.

## 32.2 Embryology and Anatomy

In a 4-week embryo (4 mm), three meningeal venous plexuses (anterior, middle, and posterior) can be identified draining into the primitive head vein. By the 14-mm embryo stage, the primordium of the SSS, the sagittal plexus can be appreciated, formed from the midline coalescence of the anterior and middle venous plexuses. The numerous epidural plexuses, by

confluence of their lumen, will evolve to become what is in adult life seen as the SSS. The development of the brain and skull base leads to the adult configuration of the SSS by the 50-mm stage (9-week fetus), in which the SSS joins with the straight sinus to drain into the torcular herophili. During this development, asymmetrical growth of the SSS predisposes it to drain freely into one side more than another, usually to the right transverse sinus; the straight sinus typically prefers the left transverse sinus.

Several variations of the SSS may be encountered. The most extreme form includes absence of the posterior SSS and drainage of the anterior portion of the brain through an anterior-dominant sinus pericranii via a midline vein at the forehead. If no posterior outlet for the SSS exists, occlusion of this vein must be avoided to prevent cerebral venous infarctions. Posteriorly, there may be a high division of the SSS, with two separate channels going to each transverse sinus.

This so-called duplication of the SSS is likely related to incomplete midline fusion of the plexuses that form the SSS. In its incomplete form, if the dural sinuses retain some of their embryologic plexiform pattern, septations within the SSS may be seen (more frequently in the posterior aspect; ► Fig. 32.4).

Cavernous spaces located within the walls of the dural sinuses, including the SSS, have been reported. On occasion, these spaces may also bulge into the lumen of the dural sinus. Small

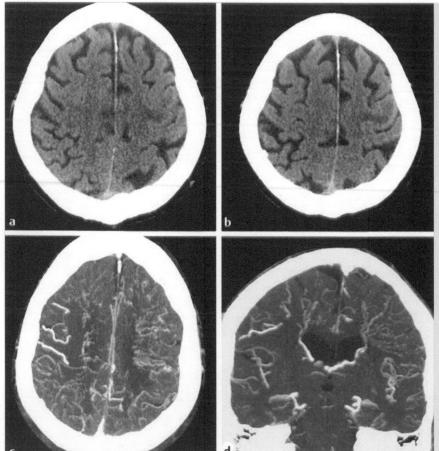

**Fig. 32.1** Unenhanced axial CT (a,b) demonstrates an area of white matter hypodensity at the high left frontoparietal region. Contrast-enhanced axial (c) and coronal CT (d) reveal abnormal vessels along the cortical sulci and periventricular white matter in bilateral cerebral hemispheres. These findings are suggestive of venous hypertension with venous infarction, likely related to an underlying dAVF and/or venous thrombosis.

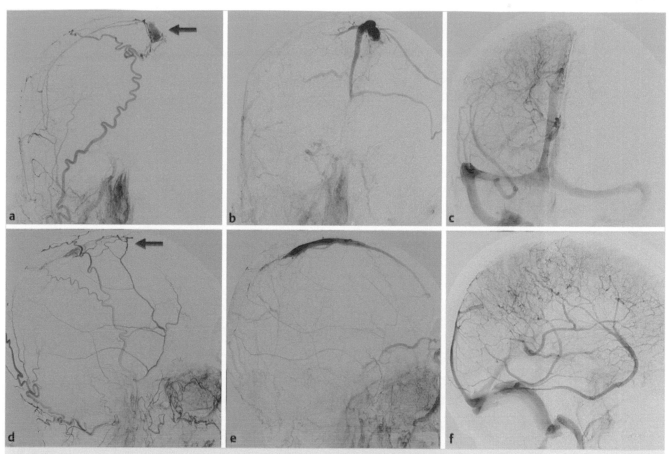

**Fig. 32.2** Right external carotid artery (ECA) angiogram in arterial (a,b) and venous (c,d) phases reveals a dAVF at an isolated SSS (arrows), with thrombosis of the posterior aspect. The shunt is mainly supplied by branches of the middle meningeal artery with reflux into the cortical veins. Right internal carotid artery (ICA) angiogram in late venous phase (e,f) shows no filling of the SSS, with rerouting of the drainage through the transmedullary veins into the deep venous system and vein of Labbé to the transverse sinus.

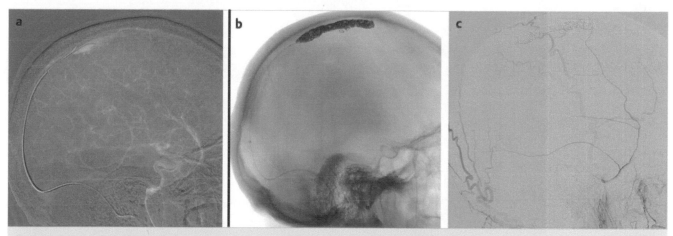

**Fig. 32.3** Subtraction roadmap image in lateral view (a) shows the position of the guidewire through the thrombosed segment of the SSS. Skull radiography in lateral view (b) reveals the coil meshwork, and right ECA angiogram in lateral view postembolization (c) demonstrates complete obliteration of the dAVF. The patient experienced significant improvement of his neurological symptoms.

arteries from the middle meningeal branches are also observed to terminate within these cavernous spaces; these may play a role in the formation of dAVFs and are presumably also related to the dural sinus malformations seen in childhood.

The SSS serves as a major drainage route for the superior convexity veins and the vein of Trolard. Most of the cortical veins draining into the SSS are usually 1 mm or less in size. In the anterior frontal region, they enter the SSS perpendicularly, but the angle becomes progressively more acute posteriorly. In the occipital region, they may even curve anteriorly before draining into the SSS and may sometimes be confused with developmental venous anomalies. In some cases, the SSS may be absent in the

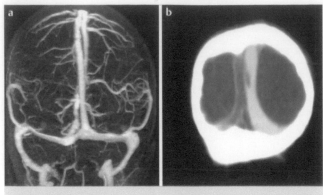

**Fig. 32.4** Venous 3D phase contrast MRA (a) and contrast-enhanced CT venography (b) in the same patient demonstrate thrombus within the right channel of the SSS close to the torcular. It is best seen on CT and is not as well appreciated on magnetic resonance because of the compartmentalization of the sinuses.

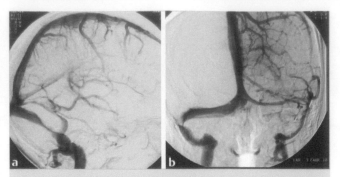

**Fig. 32.5** Left ICA injection in AP and lateral view in the venous phase demonstrates hypoplasia of the left transverse sinus with distal reconstruction of the sigmoid sinus, mainly via the vein of Labbé. The right transverse sinus demonstrates significant narrowing in its distal third. Although hypoplasia of one of the transverse sinuses is relatively common, the additional finding of stenosis of the contralateral site is typical for idiopathic intracranial hypertension or pseudotumor cerebri.

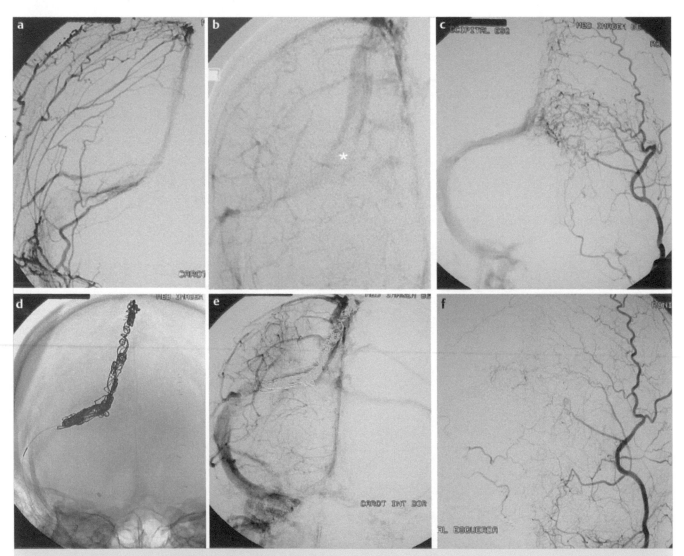

**Fig. 32.6** Right ECA (a) and left ECA (c) angiograms in AP view in arterial (a,c) phase and right ICA angiogram in AP view in venous (b) phase reveal a dAVF at the SSS and right transverse sinus. Note the filling defect within the SSS in the venous phase of the right ICA injection (*asterisk*), corresponding with the location of shunt drainage, suggesting compartmentalization. Skull radiography in AP view (d) shows location of the coils within the isolated compartment. Right ICA angiogram in venous phase (e) and left ECA angiogram (f) in arterial phase in AP views postembolization demonstrate complete obliteration of the dAVF with preservation of the SSS and right transverse sinus. (Used with permission from Piske RL, Campos CM, Chaves JB, et al. Dural sinus compartment in dural arteriovenous shunts: a new angioarchitectural feature allowing superselective transvenous dural sinus occlusion treatment. AJNR Am J Neuroradiol. 2005;26(7):1715–1722. © American Society of Neuroradiology.)

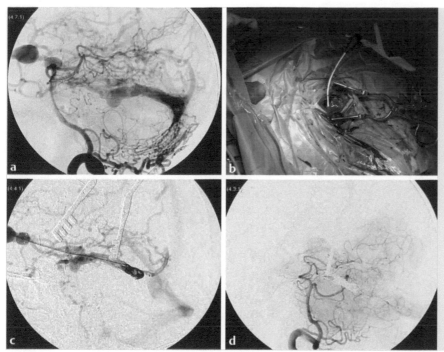

Fig. 32.7 Left VA angiogram in lateral view (a) demonstrates a dAVF at an isolated transverse sinus with significant cortical venous reflux. A catheter was placed into the diseased transverse sinus surgically (b). Contrast injection through the microcatheter (c) confirms the correct location. Postcoiling left VA angiogram in oblique view (d) reveals complete obliteration of the dAVF.

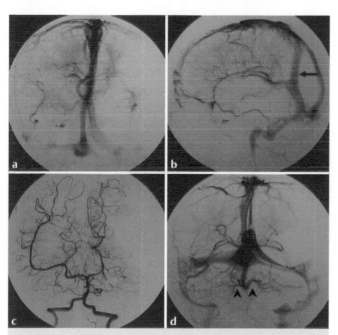

Fig. 32.8 Right ICA angiogram in AP (a) and lateral (b) views in the late venous phase demonstrate the presence of bilateral deep developmental venous anomalies and a falcine sinus (arrow) in a patient with a dAVF of a persistent petrosquamosal sinus. Variation of the right posterior cerebral artery territory (thin double arrows) and developmental venous anomalies within the posterior fossa (arrowheads) are also noted on the left VA angiogram in AP view in the arterial (c) and late venous (d) phases.

frontal region, anterior to the coronal suture. When this happens, the superior frontal veins typically take over the territory and converge more posteriorly to form the SSS.

The transverse-sigmoid sinus starts to appear by the 18-mm embryo stage as an anastomosing channel between the middle

and posterior venous plexuses, passing dorsal to the otic capsule and just lateral to the endolymphatic sac. The anterior and middle venous plexuses later merge to become only the anterior dural plexus, and its drainage route forms the transverse sinus. By the 50-mm stage, the distal end, from the entry point of the superior petrosal sinus down to the jugular fossa or the sigmoid portion of the sinus, consists of a large channel and is already similar to that in the adult, whereas the proximal portion or the transverse sinus is less well defined, with a large capillary network composed of several smaller channels. As the blood flow from the SSS and straight sinus become more established, the smaller venous plexuses coalesce, leaving only a larger channel. After the 50-mm stage, the transverse-sigmoid sinus gradually bends backward until it becomes perpendicular to the internal jugular vein in the adult.

In an adult, the transverse sinus receives blood from the inferior cerebellar hemispheric veins and veins from the inferior and lateral surfaces of the temporal and occipital lobes, including the vein of Labbé. As mentioned previously, the superior petrosal vein also enters the transverse sinus at its terminal end. On occasion, the transverse sinus may connect with nuchal and scalp veins via the mastoid emissary vein. The sigmoid sinus starts where the transverse sinus leaves the tentorial margin and drains into the jugular bulb inferiorly. It receives blood from the pons and medulla and may connect with the vertebral plexuses and suboccipital muscular and scalp veins via the mastoid and anterior and posterior condyloid emissary veins. Hypoplasia or aplasia of the transverse sinuses may be encountered in up to 20% of the population, with the left more commonly affected than the right side. The size of the jugular foramen usually correlates with the size of the transverse sinus and may be helpful in differentiating aplasia from thrombosis (▶ Fig. 32.5).

## 32.3 Clinical Impact

In the case of dAVFs with isolated pouches, either at the SSS or transverse sinus, the involved segment is no longer used for venous drainage of the brain and therefore can be sacrificed with-

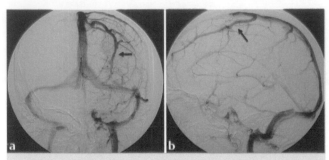

**Fig. 32.9** Left ICA angiogram in AP (a) and lateral (b) views in venous phase demonstrating the absence of the anterior aspect of the SSS, taken over by a large left frontal vein (*arrows*), entering the SSS posterior to the coronal suture, which is a normal variation and should not be mistaken for thrombosis.

out any complications. There are several approaches to reach the isolated segment. The reopening technique has been reported as a safe and effective method to gain access to isolated venous pouches and the cavernous sinus. The major alternatives to this approach are a transarterial approach or open surgery with direct puncture of the involved sinus.

In cases in which the dural sinus is still patent, sacrificing the involved segment may not be possible because of drainage of the superior convexity cortical veins and vein of Trolard into the SSS and vein of Labbé and inferior cerebellar hemispheric veins into the transverse sinus. Accidental occlusion of these veins may lead to venous infarction and hemorrhage, and therefore, transvenous embolization may be contraindicated. A venous approach may still be possible if there is compartmentalization of the sinus, with the fistula being present only in one distinct venous channel of the dural sinus. In the SSS, an oblique antero-posterior (AP) view on conventional angiogram, together with subtraction of the shunt feeder and internal carotid artery injections, is the best way to identify the presence of this compartment. The normal and abnormal/involved compartments will be opacified separately during selective injections into the internal and external carotid angiograms (▶ Fig. 32.6).

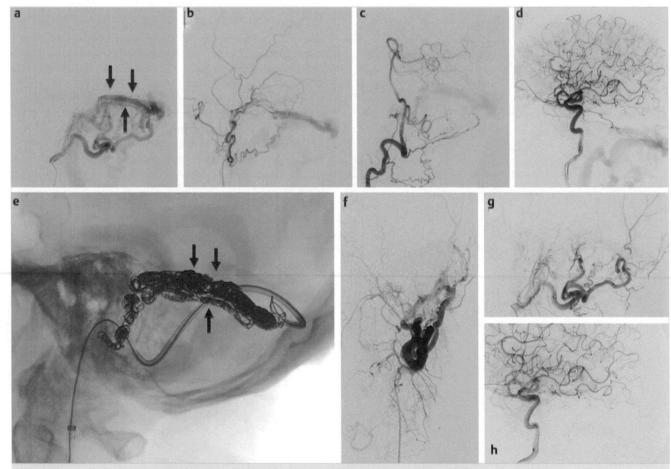

**Fig. 32.10** This patient with a widespread dAVF of the transverse sinus (filling from the occipital artery [a], the internal maxillary artery [b], the dural branches of the vertebral artery [c], and the artery of the free margin of the tentorium from the ICA [d]) demonstrated shunting into two separate channels, as best seen on the occipital artery injection (*arrows* in a). In these cases, both channels have to be occluded (see coil package in e); otherwise, the fistula will persist. This case highlights the fact that the sinuses are not simple pipes but are composed of multiple parallel channels. Dural fistulas can occur in any or multiple of these channels. Complete occlusion of the fistula after transvenous occlusion, as indicated by injections into the occipital artery (AP [f] and lateral [g]) and the ICA (h).

## Pearls and Pitfalls

- The dural sinuses are variable in size and configuration; their variation must be differentiated from sinus thrombosis.
- Major tributaries of the SSS include the superior convexity cortical veins and vein of Trolard; for the transverse sinus, they are the vein of Labbé and inferior cerebellar hemispheric veins.
- If a dAVF with an isolated pouch is encountered, it can be safely assumed that the isolated pouch can be sacrificed during treatment without risk of venous infarction.
- Compartmentalization of a dAVF should be looked for in case of a dAVF in a patent sinus. The normal and abnormal compartments will opacify separately on the external and internal carotid injections.

# 32.4 Additional Information and Cases

See ▶ Fig. 32.7, ▶ Fig. 32.8, ▶ Fig. 32.9, and ▶ Fig. 32.10.

# Further Reading

[1] Curé JK, Van Tassel P, Smith MT. Normal and variant anatomy of the dural venous sinuses. Semin Ultrasound CT MR 1994; 15: 499–519

[2] Lasjaunias P, Berenstein A, ter Brugge KG. Surgical Neuroangiography. Vol. 1. 2nd ed. Berlin: Springer; 2006

[3] Lekkhong E, Pongpech S, Ter Brugge K et al. Transvenous embolization of intracranial dural arteriovenous shunts through occluded venous segments: experience in 51 patients. AJNR Am J Neuroradiol 2011; 32: 1738–1744

[4] Piske RL, Campos CM, Chaves JB et al. Dural sinus compartment in dural arteriovenous shunts: a new angioarchitectural feature allowing superselective transvenous dural sinus occlusion treatment. AJNR Am J Neuroradiol 2005; 26: 1715–1722

[5] Streeter GL. The development of the venous sinuses of the dura mater in the human embryo. Am J Anat 1915; 18: 145–178

# 33 The Cavernous Sinus

## 33.1 Case Description

### 33.1.1 Clinical Presentation

An 81-year-old woman presented with history of left eye chemosis and proptosis. She also had increased ocular pressure on physical examination. There was no audible bruit.

### 33.1.2 Radiologic Studies

See ▶ Fig. 33.1, ▶ Fig. 33.2.

### 33.1.3 Diagnosis

Left cavernous dural arteriovenous fistula (dAVF).

## 33.2 Embryology and Anatomy

The cavernous sinus can be defined at around the 18-mm stage, arising from the anterior or trigeminal portion of the primitive head vein. At the 20-mm stage, it receives tributaries from the ophthalmic veins and a large cerebral vein draining the lateral wall of the diencephalon, as well as smaller tributaries from the network in the region of the semilunar ganglion. At this point, no tributaries are detected from the cerebral hemisphere, as the blood now flows in the opposite direction, toward the developing transverse sinus. The interruption between the cavernous sinus and the internal jugular vein (the trunk of the primitive head vein) is also complete, and the blood from the cavernous sinus flows upward through the petrosquamous

sinus (remnant of the trunk of the middle dural plexus that will usually regress or may persist as a connection between the cavernous sinus and the middle meningeal vein) into the transverse sinus.

The superior petrosal sinus initially forms as a tributary of the petrosquamous sinus and only later connects the cavernous sinus with the transverse sinus. A small plexiform inferior petrosal sinus can be seen at around the 14-mm stage, surrounding cranial nerves IX and X and becoming an apparent drainage pathway connecting the cavernous sinus to the internal jugular vein at around the 50-mm stage.

In the fetus, at around the 70–128-mm stages (13–18 weeks' gestation), the cavernous sinus is a complex network consisting of many fine tubular venous spaces (also known as the venous canals of Krivosic), which develop in the complex immature lateral sella mesenchyme. These spaces are formed only by an endothelial layer, with no smooth muscles, unlike the common venous walls. As the development progresses to around the 180-mm stage (23 weeks' gestation), these venous channels expand with progressive thinning of the immature mesenchyme, which is taken over by the development of the dura and collagen after the stage of 230 mm (28 weeks' gestation). Depending on the variations in further development, the cavernous sinus in an adult may therefore be a large sinusoidal venous space containing trabeculations or a venous plexus consisting of multiple venous channels.

Inferior draining pathways from the cavernous sinus connecting to the pterygoid plexus have been observed from the 70-mm stage (13 weeks' gestation). The number of these venous pathways abruptly increases after the 230-mm stage (28

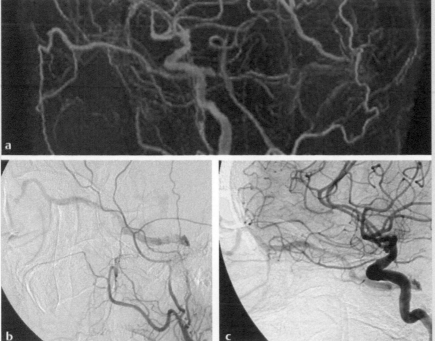

**Fig. 33.1** MRA (a) reveals a left cavernous dAVF, draining into the superior ophthalmic vein, further draining into the angular vein and common facial vein, respectively. No cortical venous reflux is identified. Left external carotid artery (ECA) (b) and left ICA (c) angiograms in lateral view show supply to the dAVF from the artery of the foramen rotundum, petrous branches of the middle meningeal artery, and the meningohypophyseal trunk of the ICA. Treatment was deemed necessary in this case, despite the benign type, because of the increased ocular pressure.

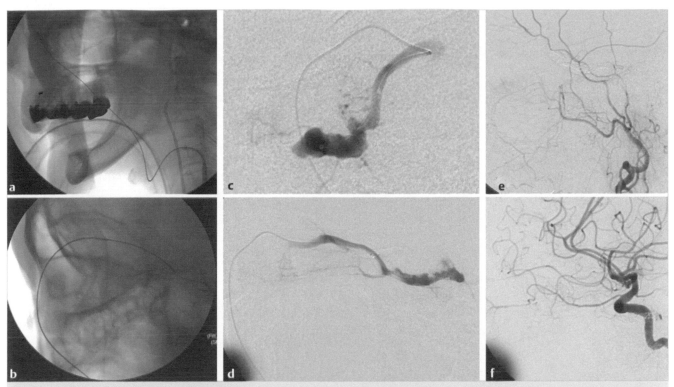

Fig. 33.2 Skull radiography in lateral views (a,b) demonstrates the approach from the internal jugular vein through the common facial vein into the superior ophthalmic vein to reach the cavernous sinus. Microcatheter injections in anteroposterior (AP) (c) and lateral (d) views confirm the location of the microcatheter within the cavernous sinus. Left ECA (e) and left ICA (f) angiograms in lateral view after coil embolization demonstrate complete obliteration of the cavernous dAVF.

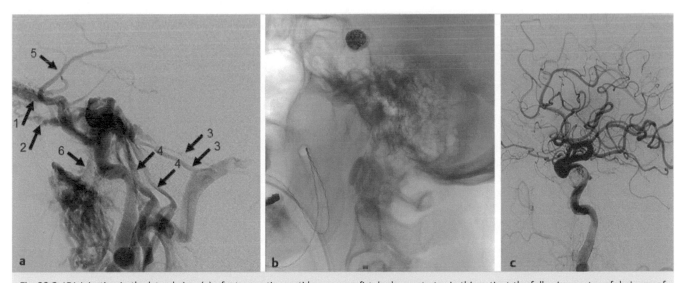

Fig. 33.3 ICA injection in the lateral view (a) of a traumatic carotid-cavernous fistula demonstrates in this patient the following routes of drainage of the cavernous sinus: anteriorly, there is drainage through the superior and inferior ophthalmic veins (1,2), and posteriorly and inferiorly, there is drainage to the bilateral superior (3) and inferior (4) petrous sinuses to the sigmoid sinus and jugular vein. Laterally and superiorly, there is drainage toward the superficial middle cerebral vein (5) to the cortical veins, and anteroinferiorly, there is drainage via the vein of the foramen ovale (6) to the pterygoid plexus. After a combination of coil and balloons (b), the fistula could be occluded (c).

weeks' gestation), likely related to the rapidly developing skull base and its neural foramina.

Two secondary intradural anastomoses involving the cavernous sinus usually occur postnatal or in the late fetal phase. The first one is between the embryonic tentorial sinus (draining the middle cerebral veins) and the anterior end of the cavernous sinus, near its junction with the common ophthalmic vein. This anastomosis will eventually link the superficial and deep

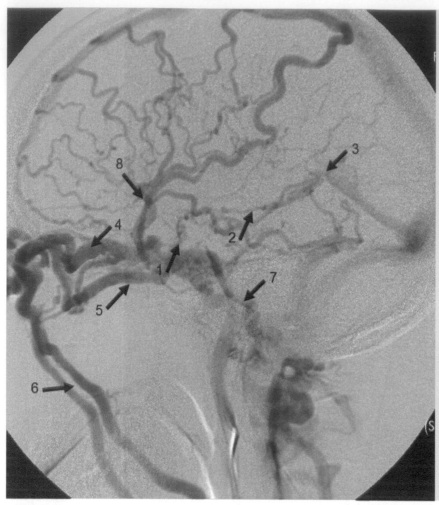

**Fig. 33.4** The ICA injection in the lateral view of this patient with a traumatic carotid-cavernous fistula demonstrates a superoposteriorly directed reflux into the deep middle cerebral vein/uncal vein (1) to the basal vein of Rosenthal (2), the vein of Galen, and the straight sinus (3). In addition, most of the routes identified in the previous patient are again identified: anteriorly, there is drainage through the superior (4) and inferior (5) ophthalmic veins into the angular and bilateral facial veins (6), and posteriorly and inferiorly, there is drainage to the superior and inferior petrous sinus (7) to the sigmoid sinus and jugular vein. Laterally and superiorly, there is drainage toward the superficial middle cerebral vein (8) toward the cortical veins and the superior sagittal sinus.

middle cerebral veins (i.e., the cerebral hemispheric drainage) with the cavernous sinus and, therefore, with the basal vein, respectively. This is also known as the "cavernous capture," which typically occurs during the first year of life. The second anastomosis, commonly dorsal to the fifth nerve root, is between the cavernous sinus and the superior petrosal sinus at the entrance of the great anterior cerebellar vein (or metencephalic vein).

In an adult, the cavernous sinus typically has the following connections (▶ Fig. 33.3; ▶ Fig. 33.4): First, superoanterior with the ophthalmic veins, middle cerebral vein, or superficial Sylvian vein, and from the same superior region but directed posteriorly, via the deep middle cerebral vein/uncal vein to the basal vein of Rosenthal; second, inferiorly with the pterygoid plexus through various neural foramina at the skull base, the most prominent of which being the vein of the foramen ovale; and third, posteriorly with the superior petrosal vein, which may connect with the petrosal vein of the posterior fossa; the inferior petrosal vein, which connects with the internal jugular vein; and the basilar plexus, which connects with the vertebral venous plexus. Finally, it connects medially with the contralateral cavernous sinus through at least two intercavernous anastomotic channels.

## 33.3 Clinical Impact

Because of its many drainage pathways and anastomoses, the cavernous sinus may play a major role in various diseases and situations.

A transvenous approach is, in our practice, the treatment of choice for most dAVFs of the cavernous sinus region because of the often small size of the feeding arteries and their potential dangerous anastomoses and cranial nerve supplies (see Case 28's ▶ Fig. 28.3).

There are many routes to reach the cavernous sinus in case of transvenous cavernous blood sampling or transvenous treatment of a dAVF. The major route most commonly used is through the inferior petrosal sinus, accessible through the jugular bulb. This route may still be used even though the inferior petrosal sinus (IPS) is not visualized on the angiogram. The so-called blind catheterization technique consists of using a larger guidewire, typically the 0.038- or 0.035-inch Glidewire (Terumo, Somerset, NJ), to predilate or create a tract with gentle rotation. When the cavernous sinus is reached, a blank roadmap is performed and the initial guidewire is retracted. This is then rapidly followed by insertion of a microcatheter into the newly reopened tract.

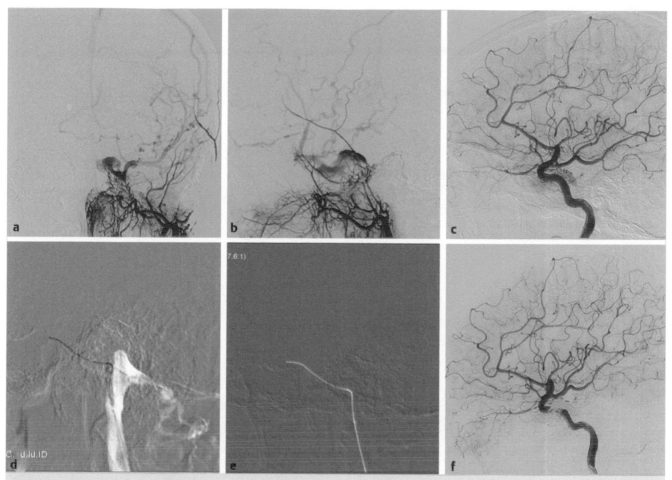

**Fig. 33.5** A 79-year-old woman presented with left eye chemosis and proptosis for 3 months before admission. Left ECA angiogram in AP (a) and lateral (b) views and left ICA in lateral view (c) demonstrate a left cavernous dAVF supplied by branches of the middle meningeal artery, accessory meningeal artery, artery of the foramen rotundum, meningohypophyseal trunk, and inferolateral trunk, draining into the sphenoparietal sinus to the middle cerebral vein with cortical venous reflux. Subtraction roadmap images (d,e) in lateral view show location of the guidewire through the thrombosed IPV from the jugular bulb. This is used to create a channel for the microcatheter. Left ICA angiogram in lateral view (f) posttransvenous coil embolization reveals complete closure of the dAVF.

Another important route is through the ophthalmic and angular veins. This can be achieved through two pathways. The first is through the common facial vein, which typically connects with the internal jugular vein. The second, which is slightly more tortuous, is through the anterior branch of the superficial temporal vein, which connects with the external jugular vein.

Other, smaller routes have also been described, including access through the pterygoid plexus, superior petrosal vein, superficial Sylvian vein, and basilar plexus. Apart from this, the cavernous sinus may also be accessed through direct puncture or through surgical exploration of the ophthalmic vein.

Because of its anatomical relationship with the cranial nerves in the lateral sella compartment, overextension of the cavernous sinus using various embolic material has been reported to cause cranial nerve palsy. In most instances, this is usually temporary and may be resolved with a short course of steroid treatment.

It should be noted that in cases of pediatric vein of Galen malformations and dural arteriovenous shunts that compromise the normal venous outflow of the brain, the cavernous sinus may play an important role as an alternative drainage route. Therefore, the presence of a bulging cavernous sinus with an intracranial shunt does not necessarily always point to a cavernous carotid fistula.

## 33.4 Additional Information and Cases

The most important differential diagnosis of a cavernous dAVF is a direct carotid-cavernous fistula (type A according to Barrow's classification), which is a direct shunt between the internal carotid artery and the cavernous sinus. These shunts are typically traumatic in origin, although some may occur spontaneously in patients with underlying vascular wall disease, such as Marfan syndrome, or with rupture of a preexisting cavernous internal carotid artery (ICA) aneurysm. Physical examination in these cases will usually reveal a carotid bruit overlying the orbit and/or temporal region, and dynamic imaging will show

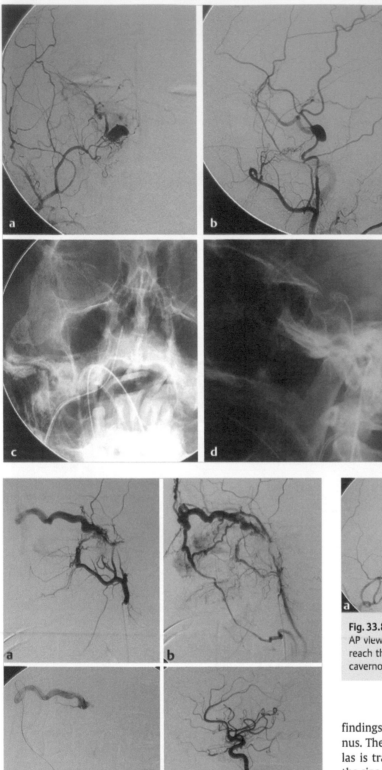

Fig. 33.6 Right ECA angiogram in AP (a) and lateral (b) views show a cavernous dAVF, draining only through the middle cerebral vein with cortical and deep venous reflux. Skull radiograph in AP (c) and lateral (d) views demonstrate the location of a guidewire through the thrombosed IPV, creating a channel for the microcatheter to reach the cavernous sinus that enabled complete obliteration.

Fig. 33.7 Left ECA angiograms (a,b) in lateral view in arterial and venous phases reveal a left cavernous dAVF, draining into the left superior ophthalmic vein, which further drains into the common facial and superficial temporal veins. A common facial vein approach is used to reach the cavernous sinus (c), and the dAVF is embolized using fibered coils. Left common carotid artery angiogram postcoiling in lateral view (d) shows complete obliteration of the dAVF.

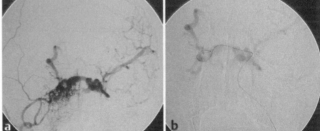

Fig. 33.8 Right ECA angiogram (a) and microcatheter injection (b) in AP view demonstrate the use of the intercavernous connection to reach the right cavernous sinus for transvenous coil embolization of a cavernous sinus dAVF with cortical venous reflux.

findings of a high-flow shunt from the ICA to the cavernous sinus. The treatment of choice for direct carotid-cavernous fistulas is transarterial balloon or coil embolization, depending on the size of the fistula.

Other differential diagnoses of an enlarged cavernous sinus on imaging include vascular causes (e.g., giant partially thrombosed aneurysm, cavernous sinus thrombosis), tumors (meningioma, pituitary adenoma, cavernous hemangiomas), and infections (fungal, meningitis). These can easily be excluded on CTA or MRA (▶ Fig. 33.5; ▶ Fig. 33.6; ▶ Fig. 33.7; ▶ Fig. 33.8; ▶ Fig. 33.9; ▶ Fig. 33.10; ▶ Fig. 33.11; ▶ Fig. 33.12).

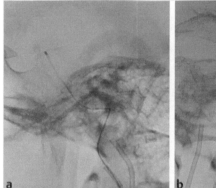
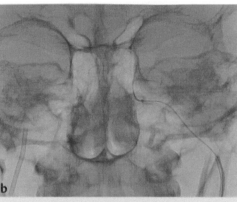
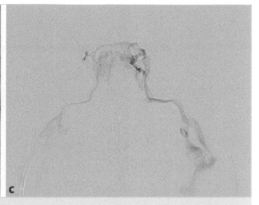

**Fig. 33.9** Normal cavernous sinus anatomy in a patient for whom bilateral cavernous sinus venous sampling was requested for suspected pituitary microadenoma. The plain radiographs (lateral and AP views: a,b) demonstrate the course of the microcatheter through the inferior petrosal sinus along the clivus into the cavernous sinus. The microcatheter injection (c) demonstrates the cavernous sinus anatomy, including the intercavernous sinus. To access the cavernous sinus, the easiest route is via the IPS, which can be accessed via the jugular vein with the guiding catheter pointing medially and posteriorly.

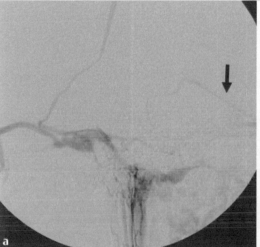
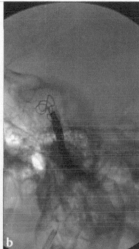
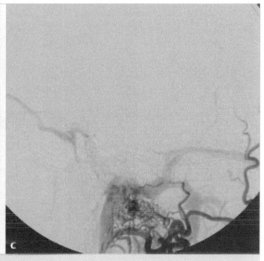

**Fig. 33.10** A 44-year-old man with a bruit related to an angiographically proven benign dural fistula located along the distal aspect of the transverse sinus on the left side presented with new symptoms of chemosis. Repeat angiography of the left ascending pharyngeal (lateral view, a) and occipital arteries revealed interval transformation of the benign dural shunt into a malignant one, with newly developed reflux through the inferior petrosal sinus into the cavernous sinus, and from there into the superficial middle cerebral vein and the deep venous system (*arrow* in a pointing to the straight sinus as an indicator for posterior deep drainage). As a transarterial treatment was deemed too dangerous for the lower cranial nerves, transvenous disconnection of the malignant reflux was performed with coils in the inferior petrosal sinus (b) and the cavernous sinus at its outflow routes to the deep veins and the superficial middle cerebral vein, leading to obliteration of the malignant reflux on postembolization angiography (c).

## Pearls and Pitfalls

- The cavernous sinus usually does not have any significant role in the venous drainage of the brain in an adult and may be sacrificed during an endovascular procedure.
- Several routes may be used to approach the cavernous sinus; however, a visualized route should be chosen first.
- The inferior petrosal sinus is the most direct route to the cavernous sinus and may be used even though it is not visualized or occluded. CT in the bone window may help to identify whether it is occluded or anatomically not present.

# Further Reading

[1] Harris FS, Rhoton AL. Anatomy of the cavernous sinus. A microsurgical study. J Neurosurg 1976; 45: 169–180

[2] Hashimoto M, Yokota A, Yamada H, Okudera T. Development of the cavernous sinus in the fetal period: a morphological study. Neurol Med Chir (Tokyo) 2000; 40: 140–150

[3] Lasjaunias P, Berenstein A, ter Brugge KG. Surgical Neuroangiography. Vol. 1. 2nd ed. Berlin: Springer; 2006

[4] Lekkhong E, Pongpech S, Ter Brugge K et al. Transvenous embolization of intracranial dural arteriovenous shunts through occluded venous segments: experience in 51 patients. AJNR Am J Neuroradiol 2011; 32: 1738–1744

[5] Padget DH. The cranial venous system in man in reference to development, adult configuration, and relation to the arteries. Am J Anat 1956; 98: 307–355

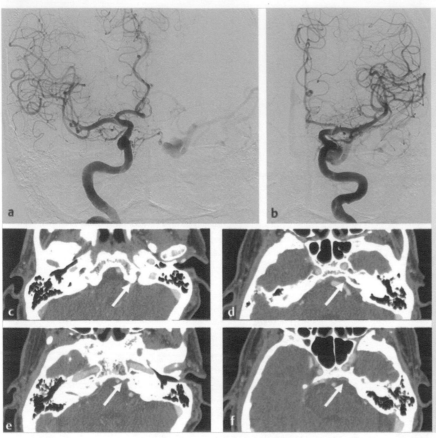

Fig. 33.11 This 59-year-old male patient harbored a dAVF of the cavernous sinus with cortical venous reflux via the sphenoparietal sinus seen on the right (a) and left (b) ICA angiograms in AP view. No venous outlet through the inferior petrosal sinus was seen. Before treatment, a contrast-enhanced axial computed tomography scan (c–f) was performed that demonstrated that the inferior petrosal sinus was anatomically present (*arrows*) but did not opacify (note the contrast-filled right IPS). Case is continued in ▶ Fig. 33.12.

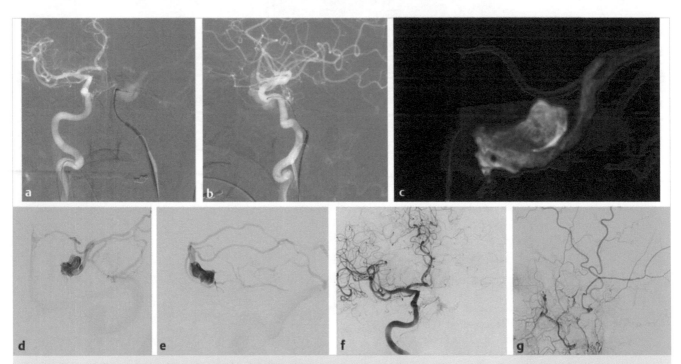

Fig. 33.12 Knowledge of the presence of a sizeable IPS allowed for safe reopening of the IPS with a 0.035-inch guidewire with which access to the cavernous sinus was gained (a,b). Once inside the sinus, contrast injection through the microcatheter (d,e) with three-dimensional rotational reconstruction (c) revealed the exact origin of the sphenoparietal sinus that was subsequently catheterized and occluded to avoid cortical venous reflux (f,g). On follow-up, the fistula was completely occluded.

# 34 The Superficial Cortical Veins

## 34.1 Case Description

### 34.1.1 Clinical Presentation

A 62-year-old woman with a known arteriovenous malformation (AVM) in the right frontoparietal lobe presented for embolization.

### 34.1.2 Radiographic Studies

See ▶ Fig. 34.1.

### 34.1.3 Diagnosis

Right frontal AVM with codominant vein of Trolard and superficial middle cerebral vein (SMV).

## 34.2 Embryology and Anatomy

The superficial venous draining system is composed of a network of subpial veins, which run underneath the arterial network, opening into larger subarachnoid venous collectors (typically called cortical draining veins) and finally drain into the dural venous sinuses. These veins drain the brain cortex and superficial white matter, including the U-fibers.

Anatomic variations are the norm, rather than the exception, and cortical veins vary in size, number, route, and drainage pathway. Naming individual veins according to their topographic location is not practical and has led to many different names, for inconstant arrangements. From a practical approach, the superficial venous system can be subdivided into three functional groups that are in hemodynamic equilibrium with each other and that may be interconnected. Each of these groups has its own major venous collector, which can provide an alternative anastomotic pathway to the other groups.

First is the mediodorsal group: It collects the high-convexity and midline cortical veins, opening preferentially into the superior sagittal sinus. The major venous collector for this group is the vein of Trolard.

Second is the posteroinferior group, which collects the parietotemporal region and opens preferentially into the transverse sinus. The venous collector for this group is the vein of Labbé.

Third is the anterior group. It collects the veins along the sylvian fissure and opercular region. The venous collector for this group is the SMV.

The vein of Trolard, also called the superior anastomotic vein, is by definition the largest anastomotic venous channel connecting the SMV with the superior sagittal sinus. It usually lies over the precentral, central, or postcentral sulcus but may be as far anterior as the anterior frontal veins or as far posterior as the anterior parietal veins. A "duplicated" vein of Trolard may be present, in which case two equal-sized anastomotic veins connect the SMV territory with the superior sagittal sinus.

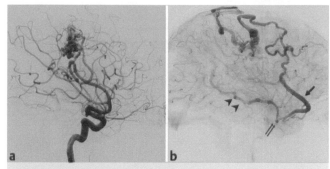

**Fig. 34.1** Right internal carotid artery (ICA) angiogram in lateral view in arterial (a) and late capillary (b) phases show a frontal AVM nidus with drains cranially to the superior sagittal sinus via the cranial segment of the vein of Trolard. Because of cranial venous outflow obstruction, the AVM also drains through the caudal segment of the vein of Trolard that connects to the superficial middle cerebral vein (*arrow*). This anastomosis allows the nidus to drain finally to the vein of Rosenthal (*arrowheads*) via the deep middle cerebral vein (*thin double arrows*).

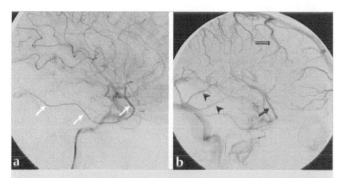

**Fig. 34.2** Balanced cortical venous system. Right ICA angiogram in lateral view in late arterial (a) and venous (b) phases demonstrates early filling of the inferior temporal vein, which drains into the superior petrosal sinus (*white arrows*). The venous phase (b) shows a balanced cortical venous system with an equal-sized vein of Trolard (*thin double arrows*), the SMV (*arrow*), and a duplicated vein of Labbé (*arrowheads*).

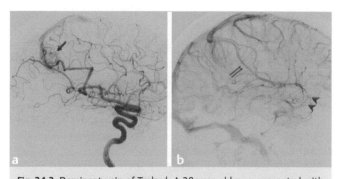

**Fig. 34.3** Dominant vein of Trolard. A 38-year-old man presented with a ruptured right superior parietal AVM. Right ICA angiogram in lateral view in arterial (a) and venous (b) phases shows an ill-defined nidus (*arrow*) with early filling of a superior parietal cortical draining vein. The venous phase shows a dominant vein of Trolard (*thin double arrows*), no vein of Labbé, and a SMV with preferential cranial drainage to the vein of Trolard (*arrowheads*).

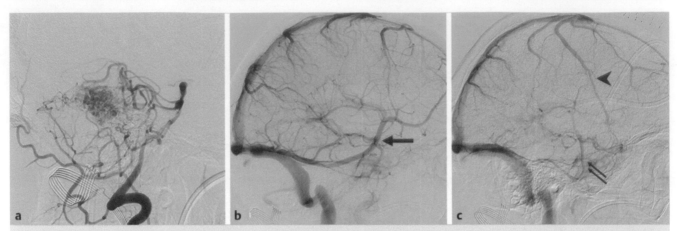

**Fig. 34.4** Dominant right vein of Labbé and left vein of Trolard. A 49-year-old woman presented with a ruptured posterior fossa AVM. Left vertebral artery angiogram in lateral view (a) reveals the right cerebellar AVM with multiple feeders from the ipsilateral anterior-inferior and postero-inferior cerebellar arteries. The ICA angiograms were performed to look for multiplicity. Right (b) and left (c) ICA angiograms in lateral views in venous phase show a right dominant vein of Labbé (*arrow*) and a left dominant vein of Trolard (*arrowhead*). Also note the presence of a small left SMV (*thin double arrows*), which drains into the pterygoid plexus and a small left vein of Labbé.

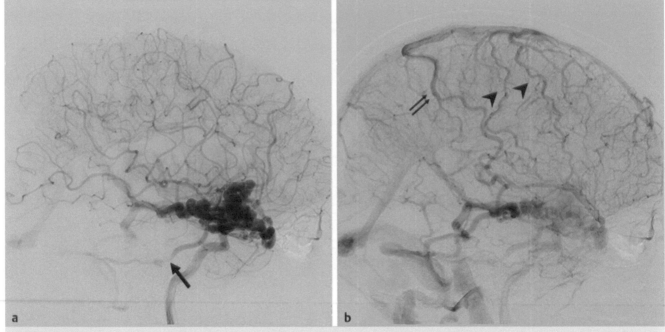

**Fig. 34.5** Dominant SMV with pseudophlebitic pattern. A 47-year-old man presented with a long-standing history of headaches and an unruptured right temporal AVM. Right ICA angiogram in lateral view in early capillary (a) and venous (b) phases demonstrates a large, diffuse AVM nidus that drains to the SMV and vein of Rosenthal. In this case, the SMV drains to the superior petrosal sinus via the inferior temporal vein, which has a focal stenosis as it enters the sinus (*arrow*). The venous phase shows a dominant SMV with absent vein of Labbé and a small vein of Trolard (*thin double arrows*). There is venous congestion with tortuous cortical draining veins giving a pseudophlebitic pattern (*arrowheads*).

The vein of Labbé, also known as inferior anastomotic vein, is by definition the largest venous channel connecting the SMV with the transverse sinus. Classically, it will course over the occipitotemporal sulcus, along the path of the middle temporal vein. Less frequently, it will course along the path of the anterior or posterior temporal veins. A "duplicated" vein of Labbé may be present, but the posterior vein will typically be larger.

The SMV, also called the superficial sylvian vein, overlies the sylvian fissure and drains the region of the operculum. Most frequently, it drains anteriorly through the venous sinuses of the sphenoid ridge into the cavernous sinus or the pterygoid venous plexus. It also may drain directly into the cavernous sinus or course around the temporal pole to drain into the superior petrosal sinus, through the inferior temporal vein. Superiorly, it may anastomose with the vein of Trolard, and posteroinferiorly, with the vein of Labbé. Two separate trunks of the SMV may be seen, but these will classically converge into a single channel more anteriorly. The central segment of the SMV may be absent. In this case, the anterior component will drain toward the sphenoid ridge sinuses and the posterior segment to the vein of Trolard, the vein of Labbé, or both.

The classic notion that the SMV drains into the so-called sphenoparietal sinus has recently been challenged. The sphenoparietal sinus actually corresponds to a combination of two separate venous structures: the parietal portion of the anterior branch of the middle meningeal veins and a dural channel located under the lesser sphenoid wing, called the sinus of the lesser sphenoid wing or sphenobasilar sinus wing. It was shown that the SMV never connected to the anterior branch of the middle meningeal veins or the sinus of the lesser sphenoid wing, although it might drain into the cavernous, paracavernous, and/or laterocavernous sinuses. This so-called cavernous capture of the SMV is not seen in the embryo or during early infancy and occurs during the first 6 to 12 months of age.

The three aforementioned venous groups with their respective anastomotic collector veins exist in a hemodynamic balance in a reciprocal relationship. The anatomic configuration of these veins can range from a balanced network of three separate or interconnected anastomotic draining veins to a dominant anastomotic vein, with the two others being hypoplastic. The vein of Trolard or Labbé may be completely absent, but the SMV, at least in part, will almost invariably be present.

## 34.3 Clinical Impact

The main complication of not recognizing a single dominant system is a venous infarct after surgery or endovascular procedures if the drainage route is inadvertently compromised. For example, in pterional craniotomies for clipping of middle cerebral artery aneurysms, patients with a dominant SMV are at a higher risk of venous infarct if the vein is occluded during surgery. In patients with a transvenous approach for dural arteriovenous fistulas of the transverse sinus, the opening of a dominant vein of Labbé should be preserved while occluding the sinus. If a transarterial approach is used, the operator should be careful to avoid "overshooting" the fistula (i.e., pushing too much liquid embolic material too deep into a dominant Trolard or Labbé vein).

## 34.4 Additional Information and Cases

When a cortical vein does not fill in the venous phase of a cerebral angiogram, the question is whether that vein is congenitally absent or is present, but filled with thrombus. Clinical presentation and ancillary findings in the noninvasive imaging studies are crucial to answering this question properly. From an angiographic point of view, it helps to assess the individual venous anatomy characteristics. If there is a clearly dominant single collector or two large collectors that are patent, the absent vein is probably hypoplastic or absent. If, in contrast, other patent venous collectors are small, the absent vein is more likely to be thrombosed. The exception would be the SMV, which, at least in part, is almost always present, so complete absence of the SMV in the venous phase is likely to be a venous thrombosis/occlusion (▶ Fig. 34.2; ▶ Fig. 34.3; ▶ Fig. 34.4; ▶ Fig. 34.5; ▶ Fig. 34.6).

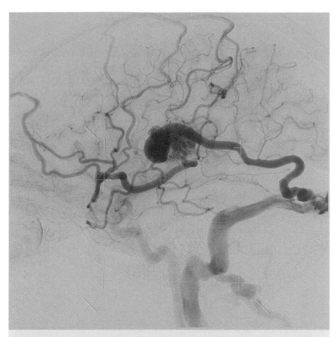

**Fig. 34.6** ICA injection lateral view in a patient with a brain AVM. The AVM is located in the tributary territory to both the Labbé vein and the middle superficial cerebral vein, and there is subsequent drainage into both. Because of venous obstruction involving the outlets of both major drainage routes, there is secondary rerouting into cranially directed veins, leading to widespread interference with normal venous drainage. This type of pattern has been associated to presentation with seizures resulting from venous congestion.

### Pearls and Pitfalls

- There are three main venous collectors for the cortical draining veins: the vein of Trolard, the vein of Labbé, and the SMV. These three collectors exist in a hemodynamic balance.

- If there is one single or two dominant collectors, the third one may be absent, with an exception made for the superficial middle cerebral vein (SMV), of which at least part will almost invariably be present.

- Nonvisualization of the vein of Labbé or Trolard during the venous phase may be normal, but if the SMV is not demonstrated, venous thrombosis or occlusion is likely.

- The occlusion of a dominant collector will almost invariably result in a venous infarct because of venous congestion, as there is no good collateral venous drainage. As such, occluding a large collector during surgery or endovascular procedures has to be avoided.

- The individual variability between size, configuration, and location of these collectors explains the high variability in the patterns of venous ischemia.

- Widespread venous congestion or a long pial course of the cortical draining vein has been implicated in clinical presentation with seizures in patients with brain AVMs.

# Further Reading

[1] Lasjaunias P, Berenstein A, ter Brugge KG. Surgical Neuroangiography. Vol. 1. 2nd ed. Berlin: Springer; 2006

[2] Rhoton AL, Jr. The cerebral veins. Neurosurgery 2002; 51 Suppl: S159–S205

[3] San Millán Ruíz D, Fasel JH, Rüfenacht DA, Gailloud P. The sphenoparietal sinus of Breschet: does it exist? An anatomic study. AJNR Am J Neuroradiol 2004; 25: 112–120

[4] Scott JN, Farb RI. Imaging and anatomy of the normal intracranial venous system. Neuroimaging Clin N Am 2003; 13: 1–12

[5] Shankar JJ, Menezes RJ, Pohlmann-Eden B, Wallace C, ter Brugge K, Krings T. Angioarchitecture of brain AVM determines the presentation with seizures: proposed scoring system. AJNR Am J Neuroradiol 2013; 34: 1028–1034

# 35 The Transmedullary Veins

## 35.1 Case Description

### 35.1.1 Clinical Presentation

A 61-year-old previously healthy man came to medical attention because of mild cognitive deficits and slight subjective gait instability.

### 35.1.2 Radiological Studies

See ▶ Fig. 35.1, ▶ Fig. 35.2, and ▶ Fig. 35.3.

### 35.1.3 Diagnosis

Choroidal arteriovenous malformation (AVM) with reflux into transmedullary veins leading to hydrocephalus.

## 35.2 Embryology and Anatomy

The transcerebral veins are also called medullary or anastomotic veins, as they interconnect the superficial with the deep venous systems. Embryologically, these veins become apparent in the 40-mm embryo as a plexus of fine, straight veins that pass from the ependymal layer to the surface of the cortex, where they drain into pial collectors. There are two transcerebral venous systems present that may interconnect with each other via deep-seated venular anastomoses: the superficial and the deep medullary veins. While the former drain the white matter toward the surface from a depth of 1–2 cm, the latter drain the remainder of the white matter toward the ventricle centripetally into the subependymal veins of the lateral sinuses. Direct anastomotic veins between the superficial cortical and deep subependymal systems may be present.

The deep veins of the frontal and parietal lobes have a fan-shaped organization and converge at the superolateral angle of the lateral ventricle, with frontal veins joining the septal and anterior caudate veins and the parietal veins draining toward the thalamostriate veins. The occipital lobe veins join the lateral atrial veins, whereas the temporal lobe transmedullary veins take an ascending direction to join the inferior ventricular veins.

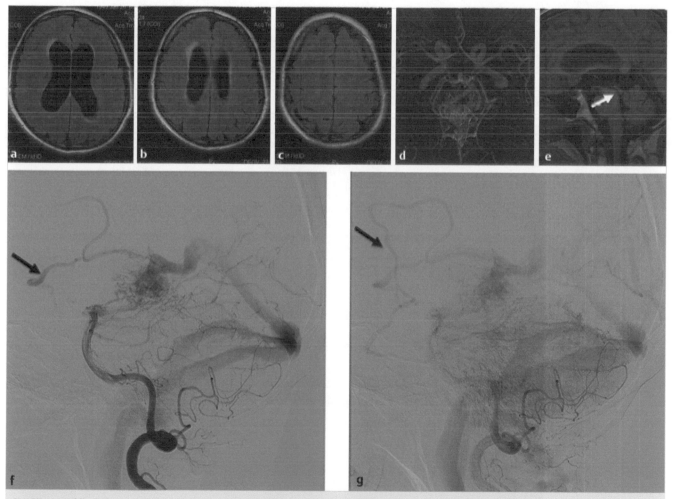

**Fig. 35.1** Axial fluid-attenuated inversion recovery (FLAIR) weighted scans in multiple cuts (a,b,c) demonstrate mild hydrocephalus with increased size of the ventricles, decreased width of the sulci, and periventricular FLAIR hypersignal as a sign for decreased transependymal CSF reabsorption. The time-of-flight MRA (d) shows a choroidal AVM, and the midsagittal T1-weighted scan (e) proves patency of the aqueduct (arrow). No other cause for the patient's hydrocephalus was identified. Conventional angiography (vertebral artery injection, lateral views on early and late phases f,g) revealed the AVM, which drained not only toward the straight sinus but also into the transmedullary veins (*arrows* in f,g). Case continued in ▶ Fig. 35.2.

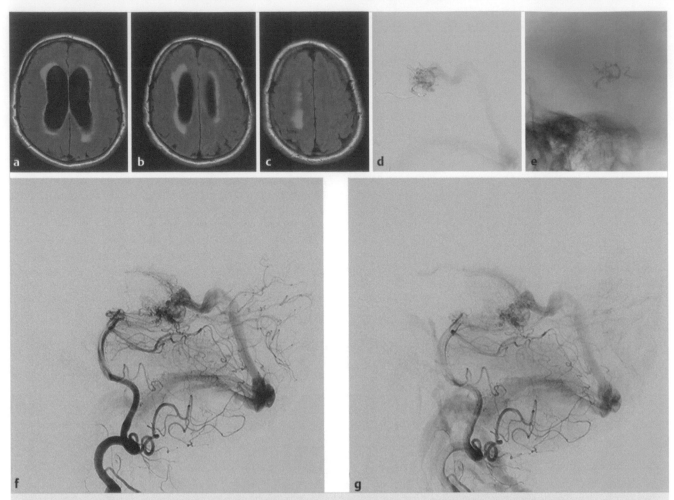

**Fig. 35.2** Within the next 5 months, the patient's symptoms became worse, with significant impairment of cognitive function and corresponding worsening of his hydrocephalus (axial FLAIR weighted scans, a,b,c), with ventricular widening and increased interstitial edema suggesting further decreased transependymal CSF reabsorption. There was no evidence for obstruction of the ventricular system, and it was proposed that the hyperpressure in his transependymal veins after arterialization was related to an impaired CSF reabsorption through the transmedullary veins. After partial embolization ([d] microcatheter position in the posterior lateral choroidal artery; [e] glue cast) that led to obliteration of the transmedullary drainage (conventional angiography postembolization, lateral view [f,g]), the symptoms reversed. Case is continued in ▶ Fig. 35.3.

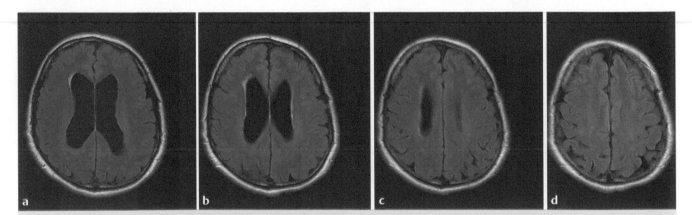

**Fig. 35.3** MR follow-up 3 weeks after the embolization demonstrated marked improvement of the transependymal CSF reabsorption on various axial FLAIR sections (a–d). The hydrocephalus had decreased, indicating it was indeed the arterialization of the transmedullary veins that could be held responsible for the decreased CSF reabsorption.

Angiographically, these vessels are typically not seen; however, they will be visualized in the setting of arterialization of the veins (because of an arteriovenous shunt), significant outflow restrictions, or in the presence of developmental venous anomalies (DVAs). It was Pierre Lasjaunias who pointed out that these DVAs are, in fact, extreme variations of the normal trans-

medullary veins that are necessary for the drainage of white and gray matter. They consist of converging dilated medullary veins that drain centripetally and radially into a transcerebral collector that opens into either the superficial subcortical or deep pial veins. They serve as normal drainage routes of the brain tissue, as the habitual venous drainage of their territory is absent. Their etiology and mechanism of development are unknown, but it is currently accepted that they act as a compensatory system of cerebral parenchymal venous drainage because of an early failure, abnormal development, or intrauterine occlusion of normal capillaries or small transcerebral veins.

## 35.3 Clinical Impact

The aforementioned considerations, as well as the described clinical case, indicate that transmedullary veins may play a role in two different types of clinical scenarios: disorders of reabsorption of cerebrospinal fluid (CSF) and in patients with DVAs. Concerning the former, CSF is absorbed not only via arachnoid granulations (pacchionian bodies), as in the widely accepted bulk flow theory, but also via physiological transependymal flow at the level of the brain capillaries. Increased venous pressures in the periventricular and transmedullary veins, as a consequence of arteriovenous shunting toward periventricular and transmedullary veins, as seen in the index patient, will therefore impede efficient CSF absorption by reducing the pressure gradient between the capillary bed and surrounding CSF spaces. Drainage into the transmedullary veins is, however, rare and is typically seen only if deep or superficial venous systems are overloaded (because of downstream narrowing or very high flow) or if normal drainage pathways are occluded or nonfunctional (e.g., in babies with vein of Galen AVMs). In these instances, the collateral transcerebral anastomotic outlets will have to be recruited. In patients with vein of Galen AVMs, the often-visualized hydrocephalus is therefore related to the same

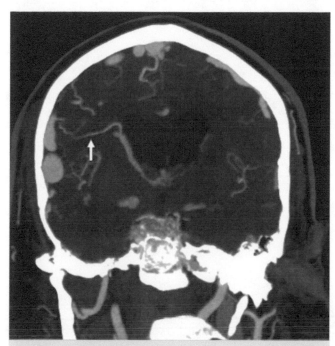

Fig. 35.4 In a patient with a high-flow pial arteriovenous fistula with multiple venous pouches, drainage is directed in part into the deep venous system (note the different caliber of the thalamostriate veins on both hemispheres) through a dilated transmedullary vein (*arrow*). If in these scenarios hydrocephalus is present, it is believed to be related to decreased CSF reabsorption via the transmedullary veins.

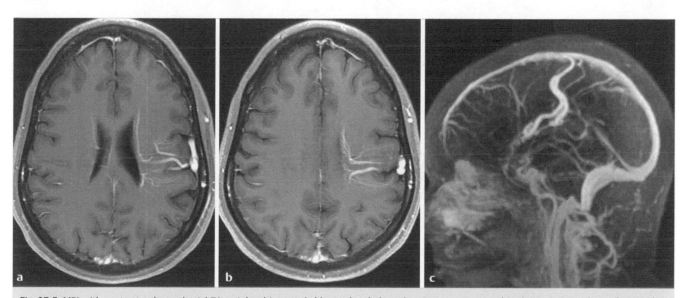

Fig. 35.5 MRI with contrast-enhanced axial T1-weighted images (a,b) reveals tubular enhancing structures within the periventricular and cortical regions of the left frontoparietal lobe with a caput medusae-like appearance. Contrast-enhanced MR venography (c) in sagittal view confirms the presence of a deep- to superficial-type DVA, draining into the superior sagittal sinus. Note the missing connection of the deep periventricular veins on the left to the ventricular atrial and thalamostriate veins, which are present on the unaffected right side.

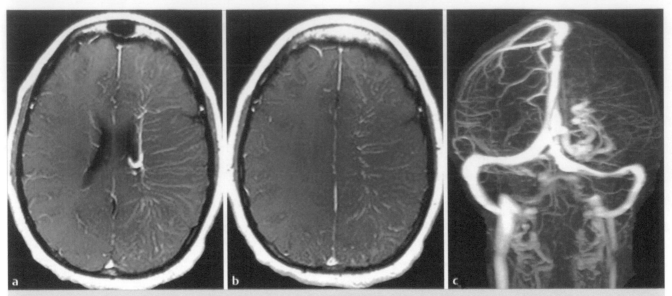

**Fig. 35.6** MRI with contrast-enhanced axial T1-weighted images (a,b) reveal tubular enhancing structures within the periventricular and cortical regions of the left cerebral hemisphere, with a collecting vein at the left lateral ventricle. MR venography (c) in coronal view confirms the presence of a superficial- to deep-type DVA, draining into the deep venous system. Note the paucity of the superficial cortical venous system on the left compared with on the right.

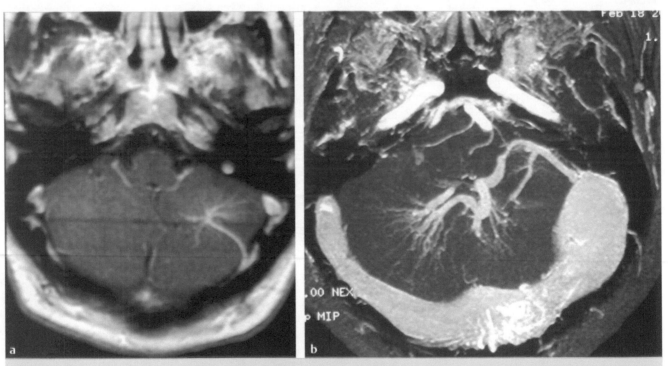

**Fig. 35.7** Contrast-enhanced axial T1-weighted images in two different patients (a,b) reveal posterior fossa DVAs. The larger lesion in the second patient (b) is also associated with a dural sinus malformation. The larger the lesion, and the bigger the territory affected by the misbalanced venous drainage, the higher the likelihood for these lesions to become symptomatic.

pathomechanical concept as in our index patient, which explains why extraventricular drainage will not ameliorate the hydrocephalus in these vascular shunts.

Concerning the clinical significance of transcerebral veins in DVAs, it has to be first pointed out that DVAs are benign anatomical variations and are, therefore, usually incidentally discovered. It is only rarely that they become symptomatic. As DVAs are extreme variations of normal venous drainage, a single collector drains an abnormally large parenchymal territory. This can lead to a more fragile venous outflow system, as the single venous collector can be overloaded, accounting for the dilated medullary veins. Therefore, AVMs employing a DVA as their venous outflow are more likely to rupture as compared to AVMS that can drain into both the deep and the superficial venous systems.

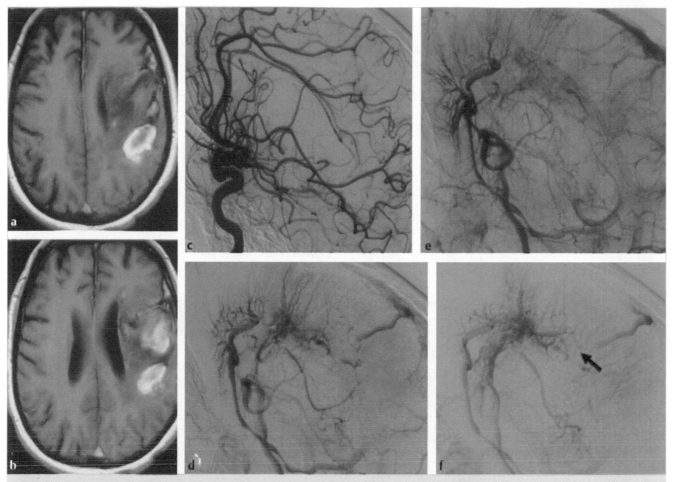

Fig. 35.8 T1-weighted scans (a,b) in this patient with acute onset of hemiparesis and headache demonstrate a left frontoparietal hemorrhage. On conventional angiography (c–f, lateral view of left internal carotid artery injection at arterial and capillary early and late venous phases), a complex DVA is seen in with acute thrombosis in a posteriorly located collecting vein (*arrow* in f).

## Pearls and Pitfalls

- Transmedullary veins connect the deep and superficial venous systems.
- They are usually "dormant" channels that may be recruited in postnatal life if an arteriovenous shunt has overloaded either the deep or the superficial system because of high flow or associated outflow obstructions.
- In patients with DVAs, these anastomoses are no longer present, as either the deep system drains superficially or vice versa. Patients with a DVA, therefore, have less compensatory capabilities of their venous system.

## Further Reading

[1] Ebinu JO, Matouk CC, Wallace MC, Terbrugge KG, Krings T. Hydrocephalus secondary to hydrodynamic disequilibrium in an adult patient with a choroidal-type arteriovenous malformation. Interv Neuroradiol 2011; 17: 212–216

[2] Geibprasert S, Pereira V, Krings T, Jiarakongmun P, Lasjaunias P, Pongpech S. Hydrocephalus in unruptured brain arteriovenous malformations: pathomechanical considerations, therapeutic implications, and clinical course. J Neurosurg 2009; 110: 500–507

[3] Jimenez JL, Lasjaunias P, Terbrugge K, Flodmark O, Rodesch G. The trans-cerebral veins: normal and non-pathologic angiographic aspects. Surg Radiol Anat 1989; 11: 63–72

[4] Lasjaunias P, Burrows P, Planet C. Developmental venous anomalies (DVA): the so-called venous angioma. Neurosurg Rev 1986; 9: 233–242

[5] Pereira VM, Geibprasert S, Krings T et al. Pathomechanisms of symptomatic developmental venous anomalies. Stroke 2008; 39: 3201–3215

# 35.4 Additional Information and Cases

See ▶ Fig. 35.4, ▶ Fig. 35.5, ▶ Fig. 35.6, ▶ Fig. 35.7, and ▶ Fig. 35.8.

# 36 The Deep Venous System I: Internal Cerebral Veins, Tributaries, and Drainage

## 36.1 Case Description

### 36.1.1 Clinical Presentation

A 64-year-old woman presented with seizures and progressive headaches. Outside computed tomography revealed a large mass centered at the tentorial incisura, and she presented to neurosurgery.

### 36.1.2 Radiologic Studies

See ▶ Fig. 36.1, ▶ Fig. 36.2, and ▶ Fig. 36.3.

### 36.1.3 Diagnosis

Tentorial incisura meningioma with occlusion of the straight sinus and rerouting of the deep venous drainage.

## 36.2 Embryology and Anatomy

The deep venous system consists of the internal cerebral veins (ICVs) and their tributaries and, morphologically speaking, the basal vein of Rosenthal system, which is discussed in Case 37. During embryogenesis, the first vein to drain the developing brain is the median prosencephalic vein (MPV; or vein of Markowski), a single, temporary midline vein that drains the

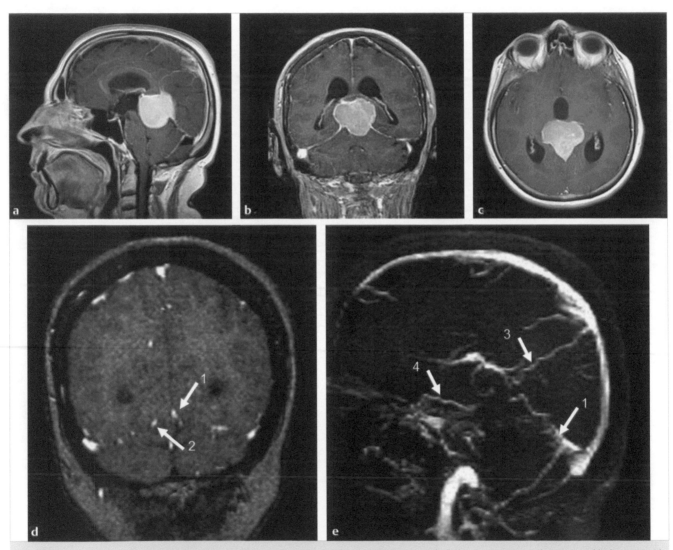

**Fig. 36.1** In this patient with a tentorial incisura meningioma (a–c; T1-weighted postcontrast MRI), the major question to be answered before surgical removal is whether the straight sinus is functional and, if not, how the deep brain drains, as this will determine which veins to spare during surgery and which approach to take. Coronal MR venography (d) with sagittal reconstructions (e) suggests occlusion of the vein of Galen with a straight sinus stump (1), persistence of a left-sided tentorial sinus (2), superior drainage into a medial parietal vein (3), and anterior drainage of the right basal vein of Rosenthal (4). Digital subtraction angiography was performed to further elucidate these findings. Case continued in ▶ Fig. 36.2.

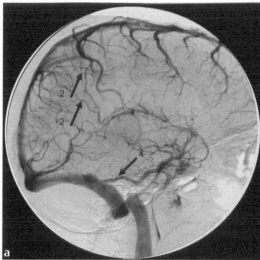

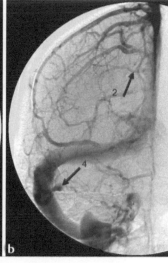

**Fig. 36.2** Right internal carotid artery injection lateral (a) and AP (b) in the venous phase demonstrates drainage of the ICVs, rather than in the vein of Galen, craniomedially into two medial parietal veins (2) toward the superior sagittal sinus. The basal vein of Rosenthal is seen to drain laterally via the inferior temporal vein (4) toward the transverse sinus. The small white arrows denote the collateral pathways. Case continued in ▶ Fig. 36.3.

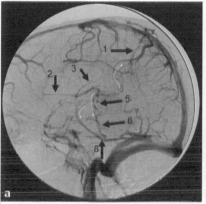

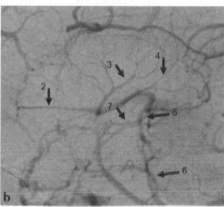

**Fig. 36.3** Left internal carotid artery injection in the venous phase in lateral view (a, enlarged view in b) demonstrates drainage to the medial parietal veins (1) toward the superior sagittal sinus, but also drainage from the septal veins (2), the thalamostriate veins (3), and the posterior atrial veins (4) into the ICVs, and from there, via an inferior thalamic vein (5) to the lateral mesencephalic vein (6), which opens to the superior petrosal vein. This "epsilon" shape of the venous drainage is typically seen in vein of Galen AVMs, where the deep venous system has not gained access to a normally developed straight sinus drainage. Additional drainage of the basal vein of Rosenthal (7) in the present case is through the inferior temporal vein (8). The small curved white arrows denote the collateral pathways.

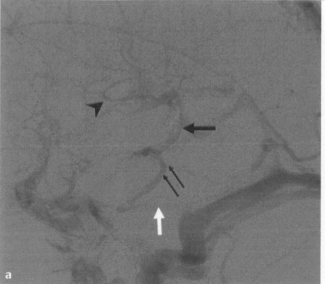

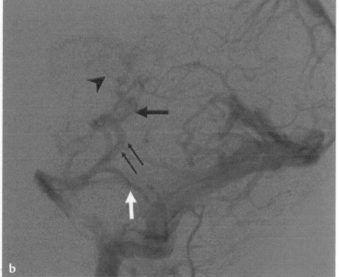

**Fig. 36.4** The epsilon-shaped drainage of the deep venous system in two different patients (a,b). The thalamostriate veins (*arrowhead*) drain via the inferior thalamic vein (*black arrow*) toward the lateral mesencephalic vein (*small black arrows*), which drains via the superior petrosal sinus (*white arrow*) into the sigmoid sinus. Note the absence of the straight sinus in (b).

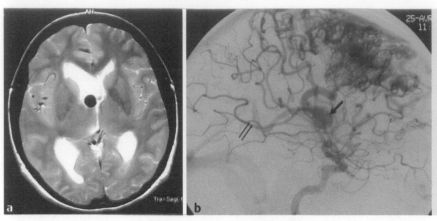

**Fig. 36.5** Axial T2-weighted MRI (a) and lateral view of a right internal carotid artery injection (b). Hydrocephalus in a patient with an unruptured AVM due to occlusion of the foramen of Monro by a venous pouch related to a focally dilated anterior thalamostriate vein that served as drainage route of a right frontal anterior cerebral artery–fed AVM. Note the deep venous drainage of this AVM, as indicated by early opacification of the vein of Galen (*double arrow*).

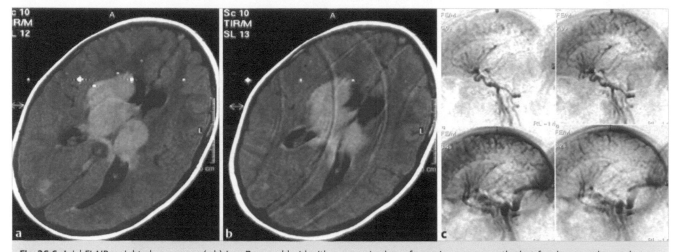

**Fig. 36.6** Axial FLAIR weighted sequences (a,b) in a 7-year-old girl with progressive loss of consciousness over the last few hours and a newly developed anisocoria demonstrates edematous changes bilaterally in the thalamus and in the right caudate. Contrast-enhanced, time-resolved MRA on sagittal cuts demonstrates the absence of the straight sinus, the ICVs, and the basal vein of Rosenthal, indicating extensive internal cerebral venous thrombosis with significant venous congestion. The patient had complained about headaches over the course of the last 4 days and was severely dehydrated because of repeated vomiting. The thalamus is drained by multiple routes: its anterior portion can join the thalamostriate vein, the superior thalamic vein enters the ICV directly, and the posterior and inferior thalamic veins enter into the basal vein of Rosenthal or the lateral mesencephalic vein. The significant venous congestion seen in this child indicates widespread deep venous system thrombosis.

choroid plexus and the surrounding neural parenchyma. Progression of arterial supply and growth of neural structures will lead to formation of the paired ICVs and subsequent regression of the median prosencephalic veins as the ICV annexes the drainage of the choroid plexus. The most caudal part of the MPV persists as the vein of Galen. If an arteriovenous shunt has formed, however, between the choroidal arteries and the MPV prior to this annexation, the arterialization of the MPV will prevent its regression, and the MPV will persist as the major drainage of the so-called vein of Galen arteriovenous malformation (AVM), which is in fact a choroidal AVM that is draining through the embryonic precursor of the vein of Galen (i.e., the MPV). In these cases, the ICV will not connect to the deep venous system (i.e., the vein of Galen) and will have to find alternate drainage pathways.

In normal development, the ICV will drain most of the deep subependymal and choroid venous system. The ICV is formed at the foramen of Monro by the confluence of the septal and thalamostriate veins (the venous angle) as the most consistent and largest tributaries of the ICV. The septal veins drain the deep structures of the frontal lobe, the septum and the fornix. The

medial surface of the caudate head is drained by the anterior caudate vein, which opens into the thalamostriate vein, which receives additional supply from the transmedullary veins of the posterior frontal and anterior parietal lobes and the internal capsule. Despite its name, it does not play a major role in drainage of the thalamus. Along its posterior course within the tela choroidea, close to the midline, the ICV will receive the choroidal veins and additional subependymal inflow from the atrial veins and the superior thalamic vein, the vein of the corpus callosum, and the habenular veins. Both ICVs merge to form the vein of Galen between the pineal gland and the inferior aspect of the splenium. The vein of Galen is subarachnoid in location and will receive multiple other sources of venous drainage, acting as a true collecting vein with multiple potential venous outlets. It will connect bilaterally to the basal vein of Rosenthal (opening an anteromedial drainage route to the cavernous sinus and an anterolateral route to the temporal cortex via the inferior temporal vein). Superiorly, the vein of Galen will connect with the splenial and occipital veins, as well as the inferior sagittal sinus. Its major drainage route is through the straight sinus.

## Pearls and Pitfalls

- The primary vein to drain the deep brain is the median vein of the prosencephalon, which is a transitory vein that regresses into the proximal portion of the vein of Galen after its territory is annexed by the ICVs. In cases of arteriovenous shunting, it will not regress but, rather, prohibits the normal outflow routes of the ICV to form (i.e., the vein of Galen). This condition will lead to the so-called vein of Galen AVMs.

- The adult vein of Galen is a collector at the crossroads of multiple drainage pathways, including the cerebellum and the basal ganglia. It can distribute its drainage anteriorly to the cavernous sinus via the basal vein of Rosenthal, laterally toward the inferior temporal vein, and posteriorly toward the straight sinus.

- Because of these anastomotic interconnections, only simultaneous obstruction of veins of Galen and basal veins will obstruct deep venous outflow. This can occur in the tentorial incisura from swelling or displacement of the midbrain because of brain edema or hematoma, or as a result of widespread thrombosis.

- The ICV is formed by two rather constant veins, the septal veins and the thalamostriate veins, at the level of the foramen of Monro in the venous angle, which serves as an important anatomic landmark. Its major additional tributaries are the choroidal and atrial veins.

## 36.3 Clinical Impact, Additional Information and Cases

See ▶ Fig. 36.4, ▶ Fig. 36.5, and ▶ Fig. 36.6.

## Further Reading

[1] Alvarez H, Garcia Monaco R, Rodesch G, Sachet M, Krings T, Lasjaunias P. Vein of Galen aneurysmal malformations. Neuroimaging Clin N Am 2007; 17: 189–206

[2] Andeweg J. Consequences of the anatomy of deep venous outflow from the brain. Neuroradiology 1999; 41: 233–241

[3] Ono M, Rhoton AL, Jr, Peace D, Rodriguez RJ. Microsurgical anatomy of the deep venous system of the brain. Neurosurgery 1984; 15: 621–657

[4] van den Bergh WM, van der Schaaf I, van Gijn J. The spectrum of presentations of venous infarction caused by deep cerebral vein thrombosis. Neurology 2005; 65: 192–196

[5] Youssef AS, Downes AE, Agazzi S, Van Loveren HR. Life without the vein of Galen: Clinical and radiographic sequelae. Clin Anat 2011; 24: 776–785

# 37 The Deep Venous System II: The Basal Vein of Rosenthal and the Venous Circle

## 37.1 Case Description

### 37.1.1 Clinical Presentation

A 53-year-old woman presented with history of long-standing headaches and, more recently, left pulsatile tinnitus.

### 37.1.2 Radiologic Studies

See ▶ Fig. 37.1.

### 37.1.3 Diagnosis

Right temporal arteriovenous malformation (AVM) draining through the venous circle of Trolard.

## 37.2 Anatomy

The basal vein of Rosenthal (BVR) originates at the junction between the anterior cerebral vein and the deep middle cerebral vein, just anterior to the midbrain near the anterior perforated substance. It courses superior and medial to the posterior cerebral artery around the midbrain, traversing the prepeduncular, ambient and quadrigeminal cisterns to finally open into the vein of Galen. In some cases, it may drain into the straight sinus or the internal cerebral veins. Alternatively, the BVR may be discontinuous, with the anterior part draining anteriorly to the cavernous sinus or posteriorly to the superior petrosal sinus via the lateral mesencephalic vein, and the posterior part to the vein of Galen. In addition, the BVR may keep its "embryonic" pattern and drain to a tentorial sinus, or even a temporal cortical vein.

The BVR is a venous efferent that forms late during embryogenesis and serves as a longitudinal anastomosis between telencephalic, diencephalic, and mesencephalic veins, serving as a connection between the deep middle cerebral vein and the vein of Galen. As the BVR is primarily not involved in the drainage of the subependymal venous network, embryologically speaking it cannot be regarded as part of the deep venous system, even though it is located in the depth of the brain. It anastomoses medially with its contralateral homolog through the venous circle (see following), and inferiorly with the petrosal vein via the lateral mesencephalic vein. Each of these channels constitutes an alternative outlet in case of venous obstruction or venous overflow (as seen in venous thrombosis or in regional AV shunts). The relatively late appearance of the BVR and the numerous tributaries account for the multiple variations encountered in the basal vein. The extent of the venous territories connecting to the BVR accounts for its unfavorable hemodynamic effects when it participates in the drainage of an AV shunt. Its

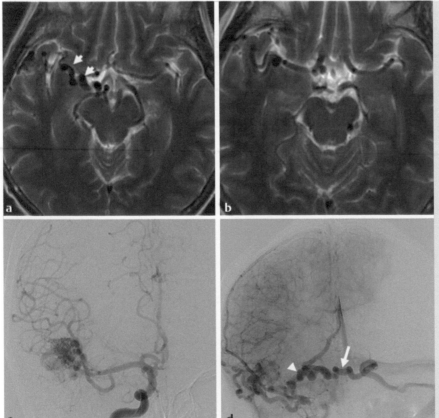

**Fig. 37.1** T2-weighted axial images of a brain MRI (a,b) and conventional angiography (right internal carotid artery injection; anteroposterior [AP] view, early and late phase [c,d]) show a right temporal AVM nidus draining mainly via the deep middle cerebral vein (*small arrows*) into the right basal vein of Rosenthal (BVR). The posterior communicating vein (*arrow* in d) and the contralateral BVR are also enlarged and open into the left superior petrosal sinus, via the left lateral mesencephalic vein. This drainage pattern explains the left pulsatile tinnitus, even though the AVM is located in the right hemisphere.

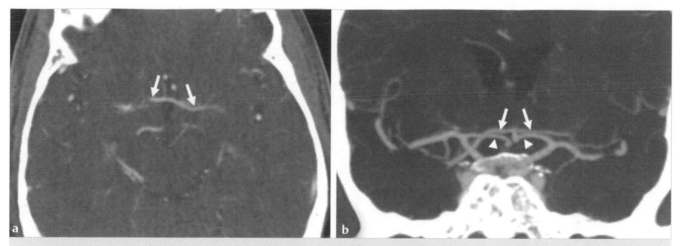

Fig. 37.2 The anterior communicating vein (*arrows*) in a patient being investigated for stroke with CTA (axial [a] and coronal [b] reformats) is seen to run in close spatial relation to the A1 segments (*arrowheads*) along the lamina terminalis and above the optic chiasm.

**Table 37.1** Tributaries of the basal vein of Rosenthal

| Telencephalic Group | Diencephalic Group | Bridging Tegmental Group | Tectal Group |
|---|---|---|---|
| Uncal vein | Peduncular vein | Lateral mesencephalic vein | Tectal vein |
| Inferior striate vein | Hypothalamic vein | Posterior mesencephalic vein (or accessory basal vein) | Tectogeniculate vein |
| Optic chiasm vein | Hippocampal vein | | Superior vermian vein |
| Anterior communicating vein | Inferior thalamic vein | | Precentral vein |
| Inferior frontal vein | Inferior ventricular vein | | |
| Olfactory vein | Anterior pontomesencephalic vein | | |
| | Posterior communicating vein | | |
| | Infratemporal vein | | |

Data from Lasjaunias P, Berenstein A, ter Brugge KG, Raybaud C. Intracranial venous system. In: Lasjaunias P, Berenstein A, ter Brugge KG. Surgical Neuroangiography: Vol. 1 Clinical Vascular Anatomy and Variations. 2nd ed. Berlin: Springer; 2001: 631–713.

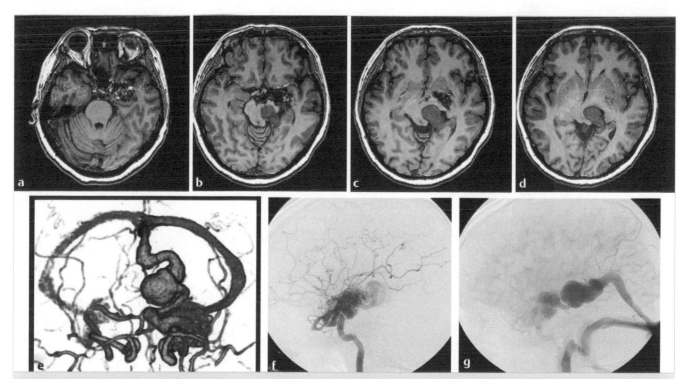

Fig. 37.3 Axial T1-weighted MRIs at various levels (a–d) in a patient with progressive hemiparesis demonstrates a left anterior mesial temporal lobe AVM with a giant outpouching in the ambient cistern, compressing the cerebral peduncle. CTA with 3D reconstruction (e) and left ICA injection in early arterial (f) and capillary phases (g) demonstrate an anterior temporal AVM draining into the basal vein of Rosenthal that harbors a large venous pouch in its ambient segment.

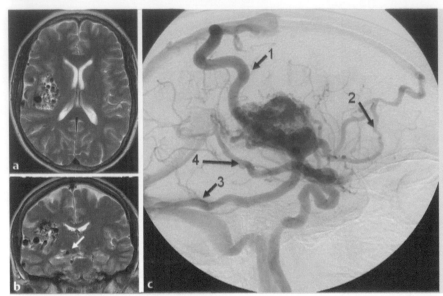

**Fig. 37.4** Right insular AVM in a patient presenting with seizures. Axial (a) and coronal (b) T2-weighted scans demonstrate an insular AVM. On magnetic resonance, a dilated BVR is seen (*arrow* in b). Lateral view of right ICA injection (c) demonstrates the AVM draining superficially toward the vein of Trolard (1), anteriorly towards the middle superficial cerebral vein (2), infero-laterally into the vein of Labbé (3), and antero-inferiorly via the inferior temporal vein into the BVR (4).

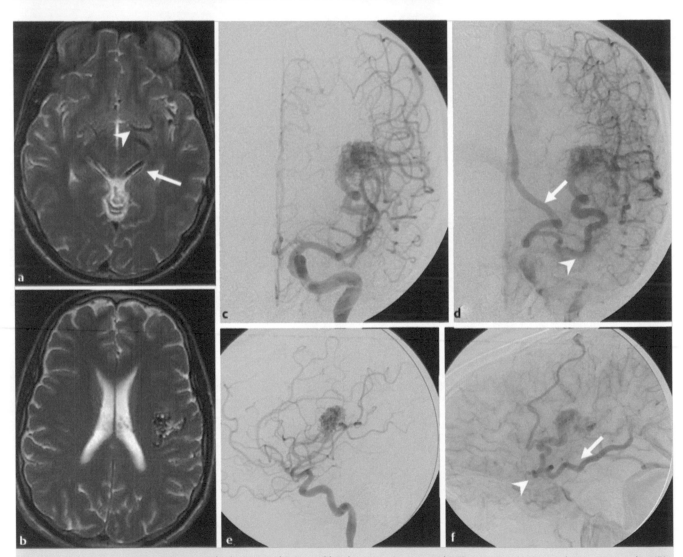

**Fig. 37.5** A 24-year-old patient came to medical attention because of head trauma. On an outside CT scan, prominent vessels were seen and a MRI was performed that demonstrates, on T2-weighted scans (a,b), a posterior insular AVM. Note the prominent left deep middle cerebral vein (*arrowhead*) and BVR (*arrow*). Angiography of the left ICA in AP (c,d) and lateral (e,f) views in early and later phases demonstrate the insular AVM that drains superficially into the vein of Trolard and inferior-anteriorly via the deep middle cerebral vein (*arrowheads* in d,f) and the uncal vein into the BVR (*arrows* in d,f).

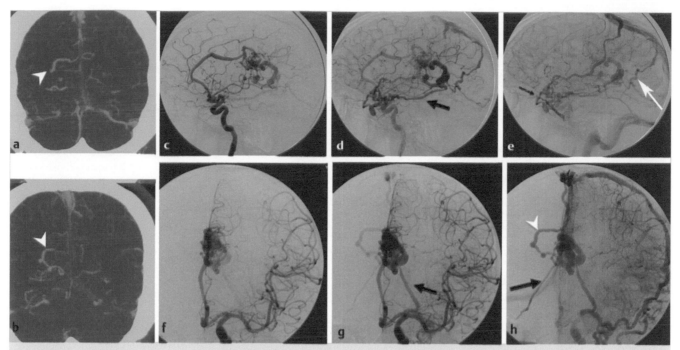

**Fig. 37.6** Distal pericallosal AVM in a patient with occlusion of the straight sinus (see coronal CTA on a,b). Conventional angiography of the left ICA in early arterial (c,f), early venous (d,g), and late venous (e,h) phases in lateral and AP views demonstrate the alternate drainage pathways via the bilateral BVR (*large arrows* in d,g,h) that drains via the deep middle cerebral vein (*small arrow* in e,h) to the superficial venous system and via a right occipital vein to a right median parietal vein (*arrowheads* in a,b,e,h).

drainage territory encompasses the orbital surface of the frontal lobe, the insula and mesial temporal lobe structures, the hypothalamus, parts of the striatum and thalamus, and the midbrain.

The venous circle, or circle of Trolard, connects the anterior afferents to the BVR in the chiasmatic region anteriorly and the ventral midbrain region posteriorly. Both anterior cerebral veins are connected medially by the anterior communicating vein, present in ~50% of the population (▶ Fig. 37.2). This vein parallels the anterior communicating artery as it courses along the lamina terminalis above the optic chiasm. It may have a plexiform configuration, with multiple small channels rather than a single vessel. The medial afferent branches that contribute to the anterior venous circle include the septal veins, callosal veins, anterior cerebral veins, chiasmatic veins, and olfactory veins near the midline. The lateral afferents include the inferior striate veins, insular veins, and uncal veins.

The posterior venous circle connects the BVRs via the peduncular veins, through the posterior communicating vein. This vein is located in the interpeduncular fossa, posterior to the basilar artery, and is a fairly constant vessel. It is generally larger than the anterior communicating vein. The afferents that contribute to the posterior venous circle include the hypothalamic veins medially and the ventral mesencephalic veins laterally. The venous circle outflow is via the deep sylvian veins into the cavernous sinus anteriorly and into the petrous vein and superior petrosal sinus posteriorly, via the lateral mesencephalic vein and the medial pontine vein (▶ Table 37.1).

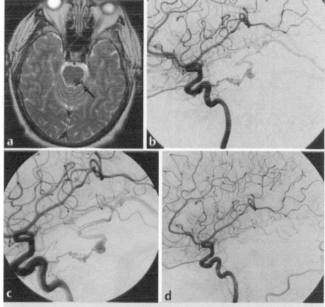

**Fig. 37.7** A 59-year-old man presented with a right posterior fossa hemorrhage. On T2-weighted MRI (a), a dilated lateral mesencephalic vein (*arrow*), as well as dilatation of the BVR, was seen. Angiography (left ICA, lateral view, b) demonstrates a dural AVF fed by the artery of the free margin of the tentorium that had a direct communication with the lateral mesencephalic vein that subsequently opens into the BVR. The patient was treated via a transvenous approach through the deep venous system (microcatheter in c), with subsequent complete occlusion of the fistula (d).

Pearls and Pitfalls

- Even though deeply located, the basal vein of Rosenthal (BVR) cannot be regarded as part of the deep venous system since it is not involved in the drainage of the subependymal venous network.
- The BVRs have a relatively large venous territory, which explains the adverse hemodynamic effects when involved in the drainage of AV shunts.
- The venous circle connects the BVRs anteriorly in the chiasmatic region and posteriorly in the interpeduncular fossa via the anterior and posterior communicating veins, respectively.
- The presence of the venous circle may explain symptoms remote and even contralateral from the location of the shunt.

# 37.3 Clinical Impact, Additional Information and Cases

See ▶ Fig. 37.3, ▶ Fig. 37.4, ▶ Fig. 37.5, ▶ Fig. 37.6, and ▶ Fig. 37.7.

# Further Reading

[1] Cullen S, Demengie F, Ozanne A et al. The anastomotic venous circle of the base of the brain. Interv Neuroradiol 2005; 11: 325–332
[2] Daenekindt T, Wilms G, Thijs V, Demaerel P, Van Calenbergh F. Variants of the basal vein of Rosenthal and perimesencephalic nonaneurysmal hemorrhage. Surg Neurol 2008; 69: 526–529, discussion 529
[3] Lasjaunias PL, Berenstein A, ter Brugge K, Raybaud CA. Intracranial venous system. In: Surgical Neuroangiography: 1 Clinical Vascular Anatomy and Variations. Berlin: Springer; 2001:631–713
[4] Tubbs RS, Loukas M, Louis RG, Jr et al. Surgical anatomy and landmarks for the basal vein of rosenthal. J Neurosurg 2007; 106: 900–902
[5] van der Schaaf IC, Velthuis BK, Gouw A, Rinkel GJE. Venous drainage in perimesencephalic hemorrhage. Stroke 2004; 35: 1614–1618

# 38 The Infratentorial Veins

## 38.1 Case Description

### 38.1.1 Clinical Presentation

A 39-year-old man presented with a long-standing history of headaches. CTA revealed a right cerebellar arteriovenous malformation (AVM) nidus. He was referred for elective angiogram.

### 38.1.2 Radiologic Studies

See ▶ Fig. 38.1.

### 38.1.3 Diagnosis

Cerebellar AVM with drainage toward the torcular and focal stenosis of one of the draining veins.

## 38.2 Anatomy

The infratentorial veins can be divided into four separate groups: the superficial, deep, brainstem, and bridging veins.

### 38.2.1 Superficial Veins

The superficial infratentorial veins drain the cortical surfaces of the cerebellum and are grouped according to the cerebellar surface they drain (tentorial, petrosal, or suboccipital) and whether they are involved in the venous drainage of the hemisphere or the vermis.

The tentorial surface drains via two main veins: the superior vermian and the superior hemispheric veins. The superior ver-

mian veins drain the superior vermis and medial aspect of the tentorial surface of the cerebellar hemispheres. They are subdivided in two groups: the anterior group, which will ultimately drain into the vein of Galen via the superior vermian vein proper and that courses through the quadrigeminal cistern, and the posterior group, which will ultimately drain into the torcular. The latter can drain into the torcular alone or after joining the inferior vermian vein. The superior hemispheric veins are further subdivided into an anterior and a posterior group and a much smaller lateral group. The anterior group will drain via the cerebellomesencephalic fissure vein or the superior vermian vein. The posterior group drains into the torcular, superior petrosal, transverse, or tentorial sinuses via bridging veins. They usually form a common trunk with the inferior hemispheric veins from the suboccipital surface before draining into the sinuses. The lateral group drains directly or indirectly into the superior petrosal sinus.

The suboccipital surface drains via three main veins: the inferior vermian, the inferior hemispheric, and the superficial tonsillar veins. The inferior vermian vein is usually a paired structure that runs along the cerebellovermian fissure and drains to the torcular or the transverse sinus directly or indirectly via a tentorial sinus. The inferior vermian veins drain the inferior vermis and medial aspect of the suboccipital surface of the cerebellar hemispheres. The inferior hemispheric veins can run longitudinally or transversely. Most of the longitudinal veins ascend to join the superior hemispheric veins and subsequently empty into a dural or tentorial sinus. The transverse veins are in relation to the cerebellar fissures, and most of them drain medially into the inferior vermian vein. The superficial tonsillar veins are subdivided into retrotonsillar, medial, and lateral groups. The

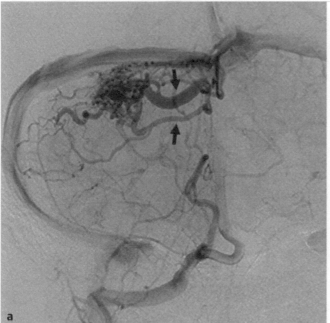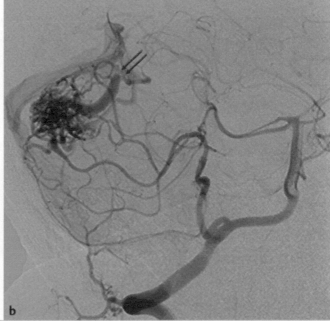

**Fig. 38.1** Right vertebral artery angiograms in anteroposterior (AP) (a) and oblique (b) views demonstrate a compact right cerebellar AVM nidus with supply from both the posterior inferior cerebellar artery and the superior cerebellar artery. There are two superior hemispheric veins draining toward the torcular (*arrows*). The more dilated draining vein shows a focal narrowing before entering the torcular (*thin double arrows*).

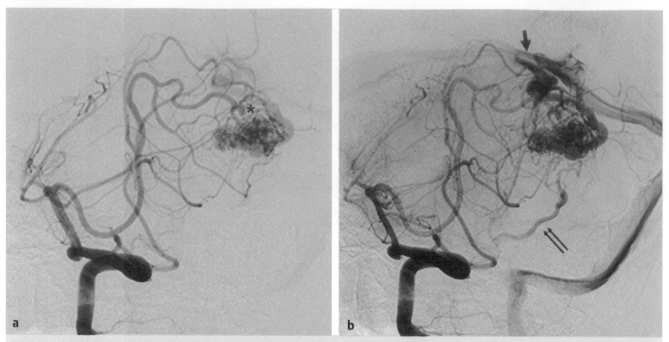

**Fig. 38.2** A 19-year-old woman presented with a left cerebellar hematoma secondary to a ruptured cerebellar AVM. Left vertebral angiograms in early (a) and late (b) arterial phases in oblique view show a compact AVM nidus with a small prenidal aneurysm (*asterisk* in a). The venous drainage is through superior hemispheric veins, one from the posterior group that drains into the straight sinus via a tentorial sinus (*arrow*) and one from the lateral group that drains into the superior petrosal sinus via the petrosal vein (*thin double arrows*).

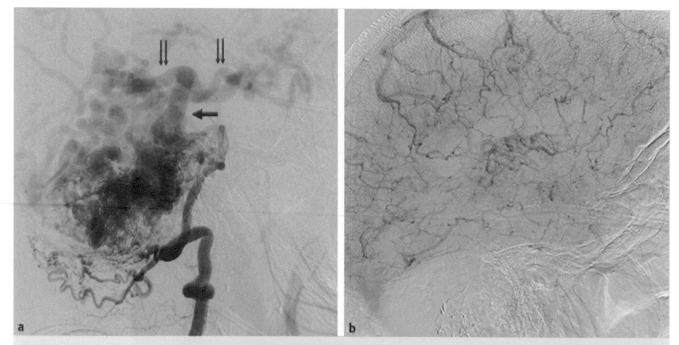

**Fig. 38.3** A 72-year-old man presented with a ruptured left cerebellar AVM. Left vertebral artery angiogram in lateral view (a) shows a diffuse nidus with marked dilatation of the lateral mesencephalic vein (*arrow*) with venous reflux to the basal vein of Rosenthal and, subsequently, to both deep and superficial supratentorial draining veins (*thin double arrows*). (b) Left internal carotid artery (ICA) angiogram in lateral view in venous phase (b) shows a "corkscrew" appearance of the cortical draining veins, with a pseudophlebitic pattern characteristic of chronic venous congestion.

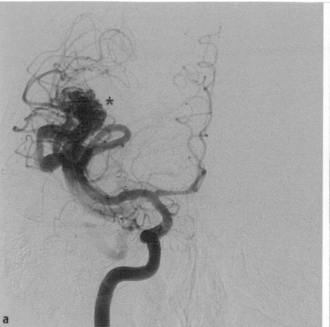
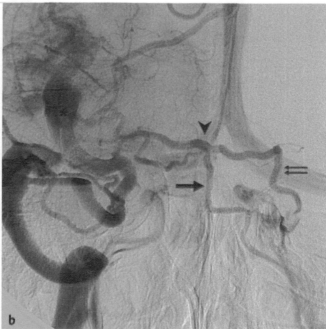

**Fig. 38.4** A 36-year-old man presented with an unruptured right frontal opercular AVM for gamma knife planning. Right ICA angiograms in arterial (a) and venous (b) phases in AP view demonstrate the right-sided AVM nidus (*asterisk*) with drainage to the basal vein of Rosenthal (via the uncal or deep middle cerebral vein). There is drainage toward the infratentorial veins via the pontomesencephalic and median anterior pontine vein (*arrow*) that connects with the posterior communicating vein (*arrowhead*). There is also drainage to the contralateral lateral mesencephalic vein (*thin double arrows*), which drains to the superior petrosal sinus via the petrosal vein.

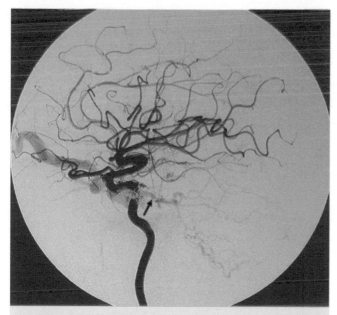

**Fig. 38.5** Left ICA angiogram in lateral view shows a partially treated malignant cavernous sinus dural arteriovenous fistula, with infratentorial cortical venous reflux through the superior petrosal sinus (*arrow*) via the petrosal vein to the anterior cerebellar veins.

medial and lateral veins drain into the retrotonsillar veins, which subsequently converge to form the inferior vermian veins.

The petrosal surface is drained mainly by anterior hemispheric veins. These are subdivided into superior, middle, and inferior groups, which converge in the region of the flocculus to form the vein of the cerebellopontine fissure. This vein will ultimately drain into the superior petrosal sinus.

## 38.2.2 Deep Veins

The main deep veins run longitudinally and are located within the three fissures in the cerebellum. They are divided into two groups: the veins of the fissures and the veins of the cerebellar peduncles.

The veins running along the fissures include the cerebellomesencephalic vein, cerebellopontine vein, and cerebellomedullary vein. They act mainly as collectors for the cerebellar hemispheric veins and the veins of the cerebellar peduncles.

The veins of the superior and inferior cerebellar peduncles run along the posterior surface of their respective peduncles, within the cerebellomesencephalic and cerebellomedullary fissures. The vein of the middle cerebellar peduncle runs on the lateral surface of the peduncle in the anterior part of the cerebellopontine fissure.

## 38.2.3 Veins of the Brainstem

For conceptual purposes, the veins of the brainstem can be divided according to the segment they drain and the direction in which they course.

The main transversely oriented veins are from cranial to caudal: the peduncular veins, which join in the midline to form the posterior communicating vein (see Case 37); the transverse pontine vein; the pontine-medullary sulcal vein; and the transverse medullary vein.

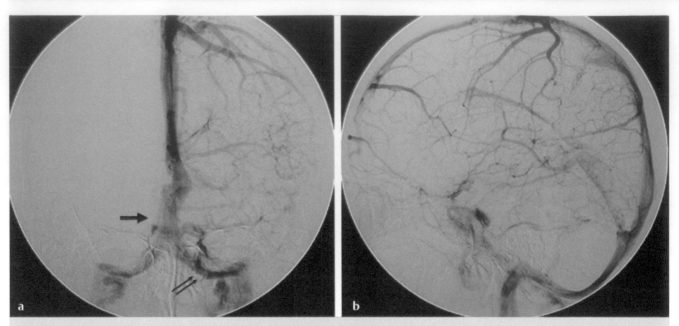

**Fig. 38.6** Left ICA angiogram in AP (a) and lateral (b) views in late venous phase for a patient sent for investigation of subarachnoid hemorrhage. Note the presence of a median occipital sinus (*arrow*), connecting with the marginal sinuses (*thin double arrows*) bilaterally. The transverse-sigmoid sinuses could not be identified in this injection and are likely to be severely hypoplastic or aplastic.

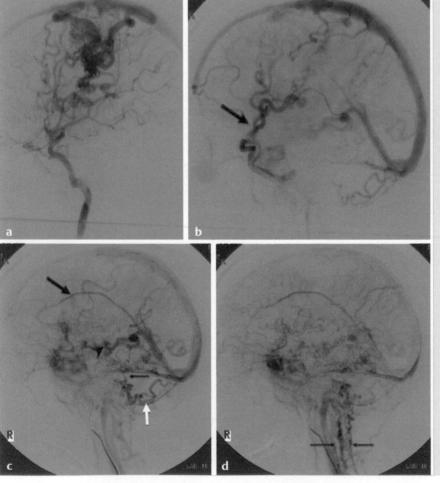

**Fig. 38.7** A 23-year-old woman presented with progressive ascending paraplegia and sluggish speech. Right ICA injection in lateral views at early arterial (a), capillary (b), and early (c) and late (d) venous phases demonstrates a prerolandic AVM that drains primarily toward the superior sagittal sinus (a). There is secondary rerouting via a rather small middle superficial cerebral vein (*arrow* in b) toward the cavernous sinus region with some outflow to the pterygoid fossa. Because of bilateral transverse sinus occlusion, however, the major drainage is directed retrograde into the straight sinus. Early venous phases demonstrate flow from the straight sinus to the inferior sagittal sinus (*arrow* in c) and into the deep venous system, including the basal vein of Rosenthal (*arrowhead* in c), the lateral mesencephalic vein (*thin arrow* in c), and the cerebellar veins (*white arrow* in c). As the only potential outflow route, blood is further redirected via the inferior fossa anastomotic venous network into the perimedullary veins (*thin arrows* in d), which are causing venous congestion of the cervical cord and therefore are responsible for the symptoms in this patient.

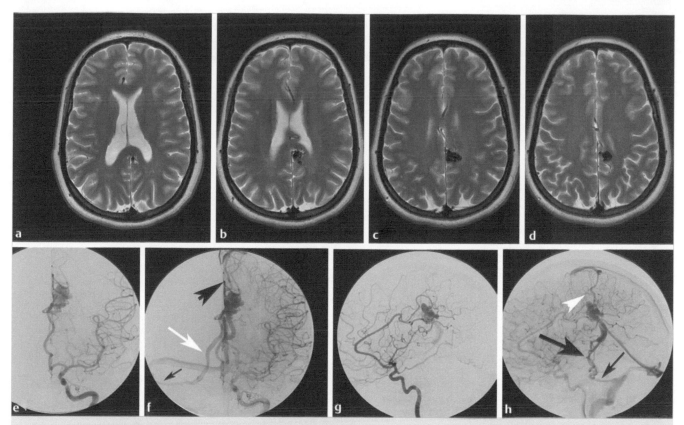

**Fig. 38.8** Axial T2-weighted scans (a–d) and left ICA injection in arterial and early venous phases AP and lateral (e–h) demonstrate a posterior cingulate AVM with an abnormal small straight sinus that leads to rerouting of venous drainage into the median parietal vein cranially toward the superior sagittal sinus (*arrowheads*) and inferiorly via the lateral mesencephalic vein (*arrow*) and the superior petrosal sinus (*small arrows*) to the transverse sinus.

The longitudinal veins are divided into a midline and a lateral group. The midline veins run as an anastomotic venous channel composed of the median anterior pontomesencephalic vein, the median anterior pontine vein, and the median anterior medullary vein, which is continuous with the anterior spinal vein. The venous blood flow can run cranially to the posterior communicating vein or the peduncular veins or caudally toward the spinal veins. The lateral veins are the lateral anterior pontomesencephalic, mesencephalic, and medullary veins, which anastomose with each other and the midline veins. A particularly important vein in this group is the lateral mesencephalic vein, which connects the basal vein of Rosenthal with the lateral brainstem veins and the vein of the medullary fissure. When the basal vein of Rosenthal is discontinuous, the anterior segment will drain posteriorly to the infratentorial veins via the lateral mesencephalic vein. In addition, in patients with a vein of Galen malformation, the lower part of the epsilon sign seen in lateral angiograms represents the lateral mesencephalic vein, which serves as a collateral venous drainage route between the deep venous system and the extracranial veins.

## 38.2.4 Bridging Veins

The bridging veins cross-connect the subarachnoid and subdural spaces to reach the dural venous sinuses. These bridging veins collect into the vein of Galen superiorly, to the torcular and tentorial sinuses posteriorly, and to the superior petrosal sinus via the petrosal vein laterally. Small bridging veins between the brainstem veins and the cavernous sinus can also be rarely seen in angiography.

## 38.2.5 The Persistent Occipital Sinus

Of the three embryologic meningeal venous plexuses, the posterior plexus undergoes the fewest changes, simply extending to become the occipital sinus by the 50-mm stage. It serves as a connection between the torcular and the marginal sinus (at the level of the foramen magnum) and is continuous with the dorsal internal vertebral venous plexus. The occipital sinus is often prominent in the newborn and slowly decreases in size as the jugular bulb maturation occurs during the first year of life.

The presence of an occipital sinus can explain the combination of a hypoplastic transverse sinus with a normal-sized or even large jugular bulb, as the occipital sinus will use the jugular bulb to drain.

## 38.3 Clinical Impact, Additional Information and Cases

See ▶ Fig. 38.2, ▶ Fig. 38.3, ▶ Fig. 38.4, ▶ Fig. 38.5, ▶ Fig. 38.6, ▶ Fig. 38.7, and ▶ Fig. 38.8.

## Pearls and Pitfalls

- The posterior fossa structures drain toward three main collecting structures, depending on the surface. The anterior (petrosal) surface drains mainly to the superior petrosal sinus. The superior (tentorial) surface drains to the vein of Galen. The posterior-inferior (suboccipital) surface drains to the torcular and the transverse sinus.
- The venous configuration explains the posterior fossa venous congestion in dural fistulas involving the transverse sinus and torcular.
- The infratentorial veins anastomose with the vein of Rosenthal via the pontomesencephalic vein and the lateral mesencephalic vein. These anastomoses explain the posterior fossa drainage of certain carotid-cavernous fistulas.
- Small bridging veins can exist between the brainstem veins and the cavernous sinus.

# Further Reading

[1] Huang YP, Wolf BS. The veins of the posterior fossa—superior or galenic draining group. Am J Roentgenol Radium Ther Nucl Med 1965; 95: 808–821

[2] Huang YP, Wolf BS, Antin SP, Okudera T. The veins of the posterior fossa—anterior or petrosal draining group. Am J Roentgenol Radium Ther Nucl Med 1968; 104: 36–56

[3] Lasjaunias P, Berenstein A, ter Brugge KG. Surgical Neuroangiography. Vol. 1. 2nd ed. Berlin: Springer; 2006

[4] Rhoton AL, Jr. The posterior fossa veins. Neurosurgery 2000; 47 Suppl: S69–S92

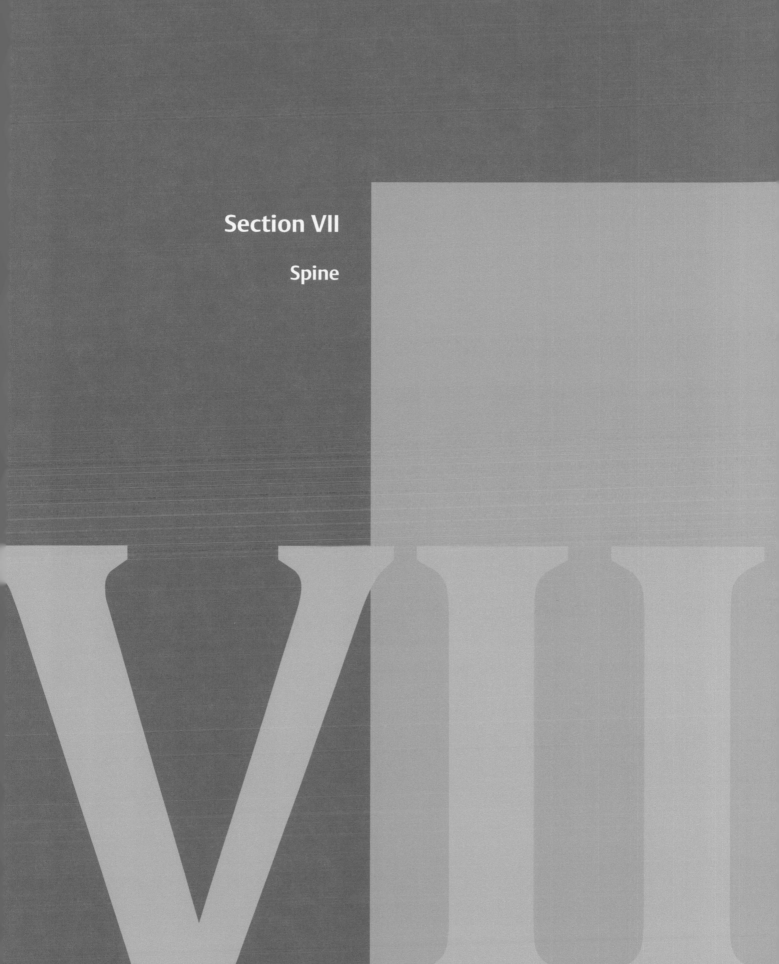

# Section VII

## Spine

# 39 The Segmental Spinal Arteries

## 39.1 Case Description

### 39.1.1 Clinical Presentation

A 24-year-old female patient complained about progressive weakness in her left leg. When she was seen, she was unable to stand on her left leg without support. Sensation, bladder, and bowel functions were not disturbed. There was evidence of hyperreflexia in her left ankle and knee with clonus and an upgoing left plantar reflex. She had a left-sided skin discoloration on her lower thoracic region that had been there since birth.

### 39.1.2 Radiologic Studies

See ▶ Fig. 39.1, ▶ Fig. 39.2.

### 39.1.3 Diagnosis

Spinal arteriovenous metameric syndrome (Cobb syndrome or juvenile spinal arteriovenous malformation) at T12.

## 39.2 Anatomy

The blood supply to a given metamere (which consists of the vertebral body, the paraspinal muscles, the dura, nerve root, and spinal cord) is derived from segmental arteries. These segmental arteries are present in the fetus for each of the 31 spinal segments. This segmental supply remains preserved in the thoracic and lumbar regions via the intercostal or lumbar arteries. In the upper thoracic region, several segmental arteries coalesce to form a common feeder, which is the supreme intercostal artery. In the cervical region, this vascular rearrangement is even more obvious: on each side, three longitudinal anastomotic arteries are established as potential sources of spinal blood supply; namely, the vertebral artery, the deep cervical artery, and the ascending cervical artery.

The vertebral artery is a chain of intersegmental anastomoses that connects the cervical segmental arteries, each of which is able to supply a cervical segment, with the most prominent being the arcade of the dens. In the upper cervical region, potential sources of metameric blood supply are via anastomoses

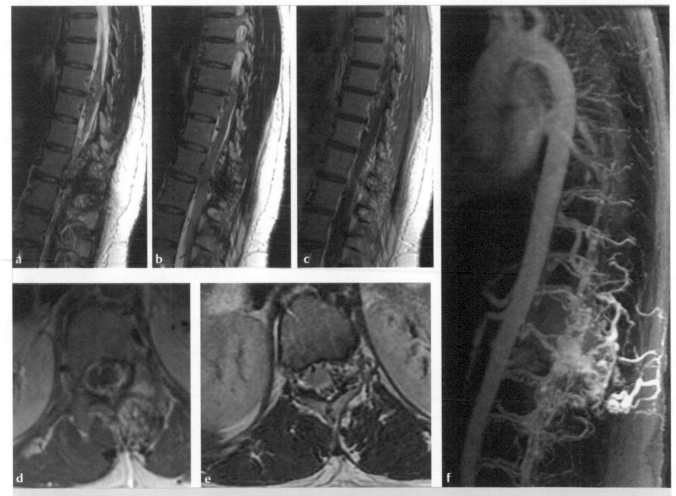

**Fig. 39.1** T2-weighted (a,b,e) and contrast-enhanced T1-weighted (c,d) sagittal (a,b,c) and axial (d,e) MRIs demonstrate an intradural intramedullary arteriovenous malformation (AVM) in addition to a paravertebral AVM with multiple dilated vessels within the left lateral pedicle of T12 and the paraspinal tissues, including the musculature at this level on the left. Magnetic resonance angiography (f) demonstrates extensive shunting in both the cord and the paraspinal soft tissues centered on the T12 level. Case continued in ▶ Fig. 39.2.

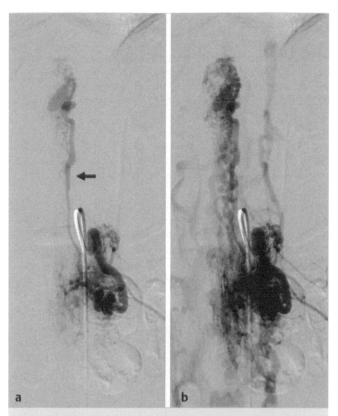

**Fig. 39.2** Spinal angiography in the anteroposterior view in early (a) and late (b) arterial phases after injection into the left T12 segmental artery reveals the paravertebral AVM with arteriovenous shunting along the segmental artery supplying the skin, paravertebral muscles, and vertebral body, as well as the origin of a dorsolateral radiculopial artery (*arrow*) that supplies a spinal cord AVM. The concurrence of arteriovenous malformations affecting multiple compartments of the same metamere gave rise to the term spinal arteriovenous metameric syndrome.

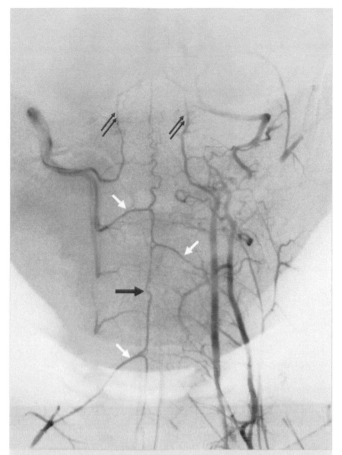

**Fig. 39.3** After injection into the left ascending cervical artery, the rich anastomotic network is well visualized. The anterior spinal artery (*black arrow*) is supplied by multiple radiculomedullary arteries (*white arrows*) that demonstrate retrograde filling to the contralateral vertebral and deep cervical arteries. The vertebral artery gives rise to the arcade of the dens (*thin double arrows*) at the C3 level.

to the external carotid artery, mainly the occipital artery (namely, the C1 and C2 anastomoses; see Case 4) and the ascending pharyngeal artery (namely, the hypoglossal artery, which anastomoses with the C3 collateral of the vertebral artery via the odontoid arterial arch that supplies the dens; see Case 30). In the sacral and lower lumbar region, sacral arteries and the iliolumbar artery (which often supply the L5 level) derived from the internal iliac arteries are the most important supply to the caudal spine.

In general, the segmental arteries supply all the tissues on one side of a given metamere, with the exception of the spinal cord. Because of its embryological origin, each metamere is centered at the level of the vertebral disk, and therefore, each vertebra is supplied by two consecutive segmental arteries on both sides that anastomose extensively both across the midline and between levels above and below. The latter is formed by an extraspinal longitudinal system that connects the neighboring segmental arteries longitudinally. The vessels course on the lateral aspect of the vertebra or transverse process. This system is highly developed in the cervical region, where the vertebral artery and the deep cervical and ascending cervical arteries form the most effective chain of longitudinal anastomoses (▶ Fig. 39.3).

In addition to this extraspinal system, an intraspinal extradural system is present that constitutes a transverse anastomosis but also has longitudinal interconnections. The retrocorporeal and prelaminar arteries are the relevant vessels for the supply of bone and dura and interconnect with neighboring and contralateral segmental arteries. These anastomoses provide an excellent collateral circulation, and it is for this reason that numerous segmental arteries can be visualized by injection of one segmental artery (▶ Fig. 39.3). The extensive network of extra- and intraspinal anastomoses protects the spinal cord against ischemia related to segmental arterial occlusion (▶ Fig. 39.4).

The segmental arteries course along the vertebral body posteriorly, supplying the periphery of the vertebral body by perforating arteries. While the muscular branch runs further posteriorly to the segmental muscles, the spinal branch of the segmental artery enters the vertebral canal through the intervertebral foramen and regularly divides into three branches: an anterior and posterior artery of the vertebral canal that supplies the bony spinal column and a radicular artery that supplies the dura and nerve root at every segmental level.

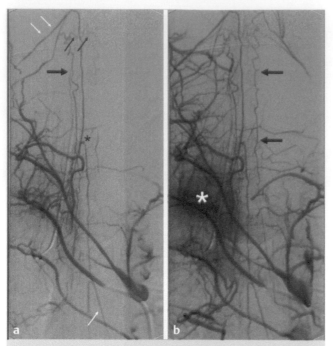

**Fig. 39.4** At various and unpredictable levels, the anterior spinal artery is reinforced by additional metameric arterial supply. In this young patient with suspected AVM, injection of the right Th4 artery in early (a) and late (b) arterial phases demonstrates the anterior spinal artery and its division into a superior and inferior branch (*small black asterisk in a*). In addition, the retrograde filling of additional feeders both superior and inferior to Th4 (*white arrows*) is visualized. Via an extensive collateral supply with longitudinal and transversel paravertebral anastomoses, and through the anastomotic network of the vasocorona (*small black arrows*), additional radiculopial arteries can be seen (*black arrows*). The level of the injected segmental artery can be deduced from the extensive vertebral blush (*white asterisk*).

## 39.3 Clinical Impact, Additional Information and Cases

Knowledge of the segmental supply of the spinal cord helps with understanding the nature of the disease encountered in the index case: a metameric disease that affects not only the spinal cord but also muscle, bone, and skin supplied by the affected vessel. Understanding the regional vascular anatomy also helps to classify different vascular shunts, depending on the feeding artery, thereby subdifferentiating spinal vascular malformations into paravertebral, radicular, dural, and pial arteriovenous malformations (▶ Fig. 39.5).

During postnatal development, a "pruning" process of the cord supply takes place that leads to regression of the number of cord-supplying arteries from the segmental arteries. This process explains why there is not necessarily cord supply from every single segmental level. Identification of cord supply is, however, of paramount importance when embarking on embolization of shunts that are fed by the radiculomeningeal arteries (such as the dural arteriovenous fistulae of the spine) or on preoperative devascularization of hypervascularized tumor metastases to the spine, because, from the segmental level that has to be embolized, vessels may arise that supply the cord (▶ Fig. 39.6; ▶ Fig. 39.7; ▶ Fig. 39.8).

The rich collateral network that is present in between the segmental arteries also explains why a proximal ligation embolization of dural arteriovenous shunts will not be successful, as other dural branches will take over the supply to the shunt with time if the liquid embolic agent does not reach the proximal "foot" of the vein (▶ Fig. 39.9).

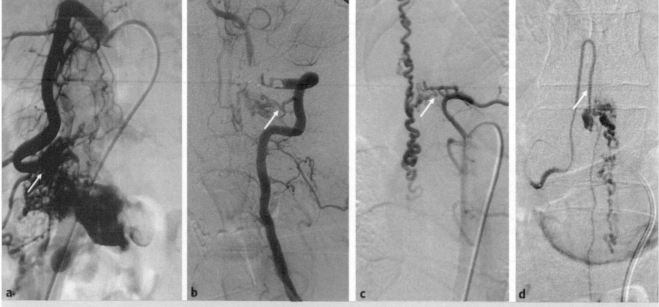

**Fig. 39.5** The type of feeding artery determines the type of arteriovenous shunt encountered (a–d). In this picture, four different arteriovenous shunts are depicted, with the arrow pointing to the feeding vessel in each case. In case (a) the shunt is derived from the segmental artery proper, thereby forming a paravertebral shunt. In case (b), the shunting artery is the radicular artery forming a radicular AVM. In case (c), the feeding vessel is a radiculomeningeal or dural branch, thereby constituting a dural arteriovenous fistula. Finally, in case (d), the feeding artery is a vessel that would normally supply the cord, thus constituting a "pial" arteriovenous malformation.

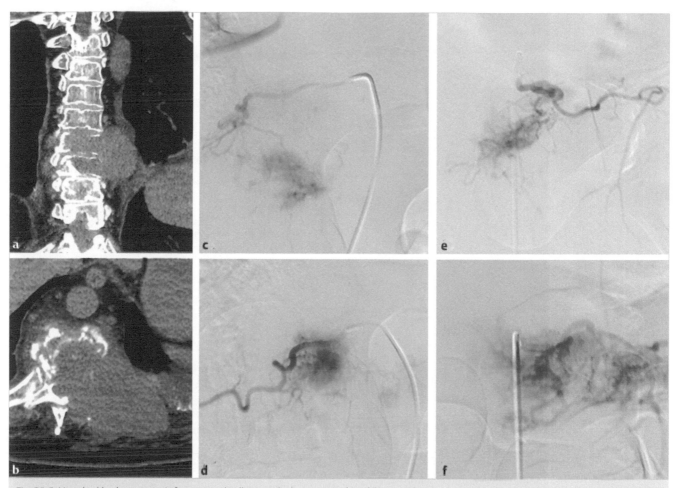

Fig. 39.6 Vertebral body metastasis from a renal cell cancer is demonstrated in plain coronal (a) and axial (b) CTs. Extensive supply from the bilateral segmental arteries is visualized on the segmental spinal angiograms (c–f). Before embolizing these lesions, it is important to make sure there is no cord supply arising from the same segmental level.

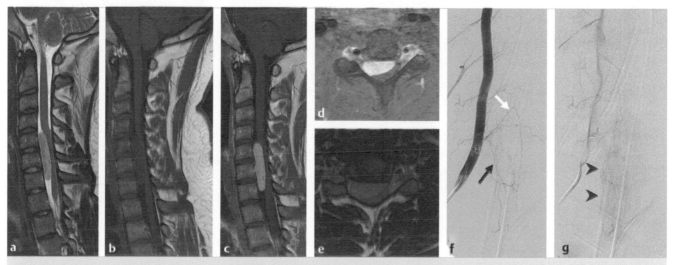

Fig. 39.7 In this patient, sagittal (a,b,c) and axial (d,e) T2-weighted (a), T1-weighted (b,e), and contrast-enhanced T1-weighted MRIs demonstrate a pathologically proven ventral schwannoma. Vertebral angiogram in arterial (f) and capillary (g) phases reveals that the supply to the schwannoma (*black arrow*) arose from the same segmental level from which the anterior spinal artery (*white arrow*) arose. Note the faint tumor blush (*arrowheads*) and the displacement of the anterior spinal artery.

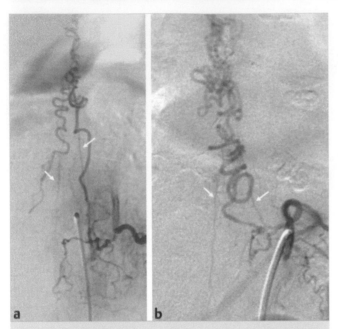

**Fig. 39.8** Spinal angiograms in two different patients (a,b) who both harbor a spinal dural arteriovenous fistula and who have additional supply to the cord (anterior spinal artery, *white arrows*) arising from the same level as the supply to the fistula. Identification of the additional cord supply is paramount to avoid inadvertent embolization into the cord supplying vessels.

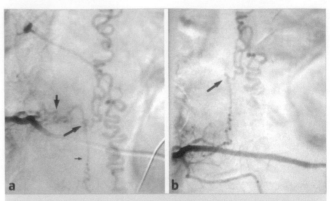

**Fig. 39.9** Injection into the right T7 segmental artery (a) revealed a dural arteriovenous shunt fed by the radiculomeningeal artery (*short arrow*), with the shunting zone (*long arrow*) underneath the pedicle of T7. On the T7 injection, a descending dural branch (*small arrow*) was noted that anastomosed to the ascending dural branch that arose from the right T8 segmental artery (b). This case demonstrates the rich collateral supply to the dura that is the cause for delayed reopening of dural arteriovenous fistulae in cases of proximal ligation of the feeding artery.

## Further Reading

[1] Geibprasert S, Pereira V, Krings T et al. Dural arteriovenous shunts: a new classification of craniospinal epidural venous anatomical bases and clinical correlations. Stroke 2008; 39: 2783–2794

[2] Krings T, Mull M, Gilsbach JM, Thron A. Spinal vascular malformations. Eur Radiol 2005; 15: 267–278

[3] Thron AK. Vascular Anatomy of the Spinal Cord: Neuroradiological Investigations and Clinical Syndromes. Vienna: Springer; 1988

### Pearls and Pitfalls

- The segmental artery gives rise at each level to vertebral, muscular, and paraspinal branches and to a radicular artery that supplies the meninges of the nerve root sleeve, as well as the nerve root itself.
- Supply to the cord may arise from this segmental artery and has to be identified before embolizing lesions like dural arteriovenous fistulas, paravertebral shunts, or hypervascularized tumors.
- The rich anastomotic network between segmental arteries may lead to inadvertent embolization of neighboring segmental arteries, especially when using liquid embolic material with high penetration capabilities.

Knowledge of the existence of these anastomoses is important when employing liquid embolic agents that slowly polymerize and that may, therefore, open anastomoses, leading to inadvertent occlusion of distant segmental arteries and their daughter vessels.

# 40 The Radiculopial and Radiculomedullary Arteries

## 40.1 Case Description

### 40.1.1 Clinical Presentation

A previously healthy 58-year-old male patient had an acute onset of quadriplegia and sensory loss in his upper and lower limbs, severe headaches, and progressive respiratory dysfunction that required intubation.

### 40.1.2 Radiologic Studies

See ▶ Fig. 40.1, ▶ Fig. 40.2, and ▶ Fig. 40.3.

### 40.1.3 Diagnosis

Spinal perimedullary arteriovenous fistula arising from an unfused segment of the anterior spinal artery.

## 40.2 Anatomy and Embryology

Although in the embryo each radicular artery gives rise to a radiculomedullary artery to supply the spinal cord, in postnatal life, the number of radicular arteries supplying the spinal cord is reduced after a transformation and fusion process. At a few unpredictable segmental levels, the radicular artery has a persistent supply to the cord that reaches either the anterior surface via the ventral nerve root or the posterolateral surface via the dorsal nerve root to form and supply the superficial spinal cord arteries. Two to 14 (on average, six) anterior radiculomedullary arteries persist as the result of this "pruning process" of the feeding vessels. The posterior radiculomedullary arteries

are reduced less drastically, mostly to between 11 and 16 vessels.

Several nomenclatures and classifications have been used to describe spinal cord arteries, which may lead to some confusion. The original classification is based on where the spinal cord arteries run (i.e., on the posterior, posterolateral, or anterior surface of the spinal cord, thereby constituting the posterior or posterolateral arteries and the anterior spinal artery). A classification proposed by Lasjaunias differentiates three types of spinal radicular arteries according to their region of supply: radicular, radiculopial, and radiculomedullary.

The spinal radicular artery is a small branch, present at every segmental level, that supplies the nerve root as well as the adjacent dura. The radiculopial arteries supply the nerve root and the dorsolateral superficial pial system (via the posterior radicular artery). The radiculomedullary arteries supply the nerve root, the superficial pial system, and the medulla (via the anterior radicular artery). This classification offers advantages for the interventional neuroradiologist when compared with the classical differentiation because it stresses the importance of the anterior supply for the gray matter of the spinal cord parenchyma. Because the anterior spinal artery has radicular, radiculopial, and medullary supply and the radiculopial posterolateral arteries may have some medullary supply (i.e., part of the posterior horns), this classification may, however, result in misunderstandings. This is why we proposed recently the following slight modification to the classification to overcome the anatomical confusions: Radicular arteries are vessels that supply the nerve root and the dura mater but do not supply the spinal cord. These arteries are present on every single segmental level, whereas the following two types may or may not be present at a given segmental level.

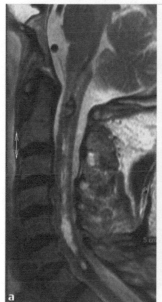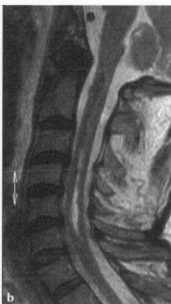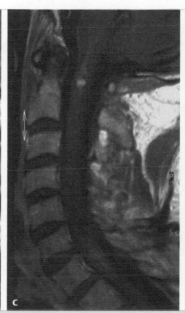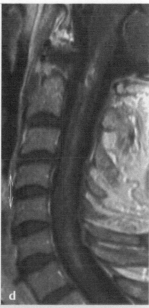

**Fig. 40.1** Sagittal T2-weighted (a,b) and T1-weighted (c,d) MRIs demonstrate hematomyelia with a localized blood clot in the center of the cord at the C2 level and no dilated perimedullary vessels. Blood was seen to extend both cranially and caudally along the central canal. The patient was first treated conservatively. After he regained consciousness, conventional angiography was performed to rule out the remote possibility of a microarteriovenous malformation. Case continued in ▶ Fig. 40.2.

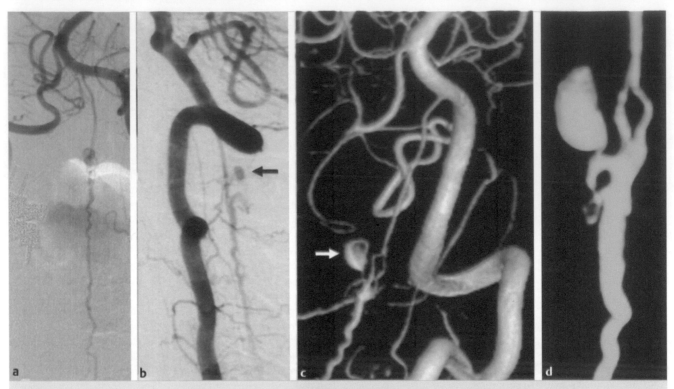

**Fig. 40.2** Left vertebral artery angiograms in anteroposterior (AP) (a) and lateral (b) views and 3D rotational reconstruction (c,d) visualized a spinal perimedullary arteriovenous fistula fed by a slightly enlarged anterior spinal artery that arose from the left vertebral artery. At the C2 level, there was a focal unfused segment of the anterior spinal artery (ASA). The fistula was selectively supplied by one of the two unfused limbs of the ASA at the level of C2 with a venous (false) aneurysm (*arrows*) as the point of rupture. Case continued in ▶ Fig. 40.3.

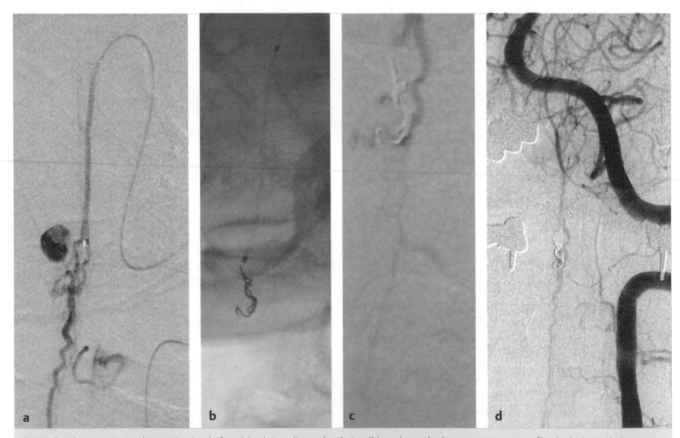

**Fig. 40.3** Selective microcatheter injection before (a), plain radiography during (b), and vertebral artery angiograms after (c,d) the embolization demonstrate deposition of two microcoils that led to occlusion of the shunt, while the ASA was preserved.

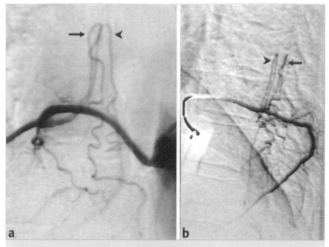

**Fig. 40.4** A segmental artery injection in AP (a) and lateral (b) views demonstrates supply from the same segmental artery to both the dorsolateral spinal artery (*arrows*) and to the anterior spinal artery (*arrowheads*). Two separate vessels arise from the radicular artery that accompany the dorsal and the ventral nerve root to reach the cord at the anterior and posterior surface. The anterior artery reaches the midline, whereas the posterior vessel forms its hairpin more laterally and more acutely.

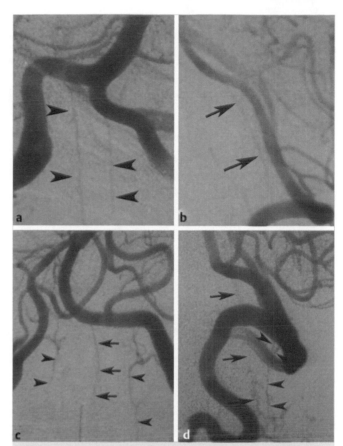

**Fig. 40.5** Vertebral artery angiograms in AP (a,c) and lateral (b,d) views in two different patients demonstrate the variable origin of the anterior spinal artery from the vertebral artery. It may arise from one or both vertebral arteries, and its junction in the midline is variable, ranging from early fusion in the anterior sulcus to a long unfused segment along the anterior surface of the cord. The upper row (a,b) demonstrates the bilateral unfused supply. The lower row (c,d) demonstrates, in addition to a unilateral supply to the anterior spinal artery (*arrows*), dorsal supply to the cord from the posterolateral spinal arteries (*arrowheads*) that may arise from the PICA (when the PICA origin is low or extradural) or the vertebral artery directly (when the PICA origin is high).

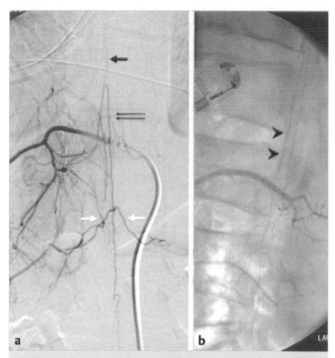

**Fig. 40.6** Right T11 segmental artery angiogram in AP (a) and lateral (b) views reveals the origin of the anterior spinal artery, with its classical hairpin curve, a small ascending branch (*arrow*), and a larger descending branch (*thin double arrows*). The white arrows denote the retrocorporeal anastomosis via which the left T12 segmental artery is supplied. On the lateral view, the anterior course of the ASA can be appreciated once it has reached the midline (*arrowheads*).

First is the anterior radiculomedullary artery, which runs with the anterior nerve root to join the longitudinal trunk on the anterior surface of the spinal cord (i.e., the anterior spinal artery). In addition to this main supply, a minor lateral contri-

bution to a superficial pial network is also derived from the anterior radiculomedullary artery.

Second is the posterior radiculomedullary artery, which accompanies the posterior nerve root and joins the longitudinal systems of posterolateral and/or posterior spinal arteries. The first one is lying laterally, the second one medial to the posterior nerve root entry zone. These arteries mainly supply the pial superficial network of vessels but may give small branches to the gray matter of the posterior horns. One has to bear in mind that these latter arteries predominantly supply the surface of the spinal cord (i.e., the white matter), whereas the anterior radiculomedullary arteries predominantly supply the gray matter of the spinal cord (▸ Fig. 40.4).

Both the anterior and posterior radiculomedullary arteries supply a system of superficial longitudinal anastomoses that are called the anterior and posterior (or posterolateral) spinal arteries. The anterior spinal artery, with a diameter of 0.2 to 1 mm, travels along the anterior sulcus and typically originates from the two vertebral arteries (▸ Fig. 40.5), whereas the typi-

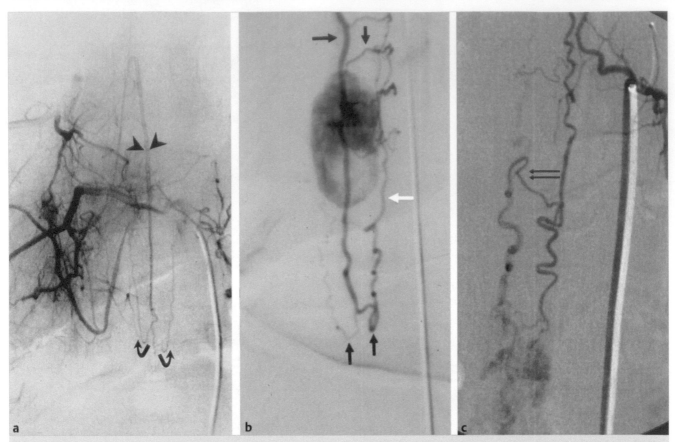

**Fig. 40.7** Three examples (a–c) of the anastomoses of the anterior and posterolateral spinal arteries. (a) The normal anatomy is visualized with a nonfused anterior spinal artery (*arrowheads*) descending to the level of the cone where the ASA connects through the arcade (*curved arrows*) to the two posterolateral arteries. (b) The arcade is dilated because of feeding of a hemangioblastoma. The anterior spinal artery (*horizontal black arrow*) is seen to anastomose not only via the arcade (*vertical upward pointing arrows*) but also via the vasocorona network (*vertical downward pointing arrow*) with the dorsolateral spinal arteries (*white arrow*). (c) Injection into one dorsolateral spinal artery opacifies the contralateral dorsolateral artery via a posterior rope ladder anastomosis (*thin double arrows*) in a patient with an arteriovenous malformation of the cone.

cally paired posterolateral spinal arteries originate from the preatlantal part of the vertebral artery or from the posteroinferior cerebellar artery (PICA) and typically have a diameter of 0.1 to 0.4 mm.

These three arteries run continuously from the cervical spine to the conus medullaris but are not capable of feeding the entire spinal cord. Instead, they are reinforced from the above-mentioned radiculomedullary arteries that derive from various (and unpredictable) segmental levels by anterior and posterolateral radiculomedullary arteries. Therefore, the blood flow in these vessels may be both caudocranial and craniocaudal. The largest of the anterior radiculomedullary arteries is the arteria radiculomedullaris magna or Adamkiewicz artery, which arises close to the thoracolumbar enlargement (between T9 and L1 [exceptionally at L2 or L3], more often on the left side; ▶ Fig. 40.6).

Additional significant ventral feeders are unusual. In the cervical region, one of the ventral radicular feeders between C5 and C8 is often distinctly larger (0.4–0.6 mm) than the others and was termed the artery of the cervical enlargement. It is more often derived from the deep and ascending cervical arteries than from the vertebral artery. The average number of anterior radicular feeders to the cervical cord is two to three. Ventral feeders to the upper cervical cord, originating from the intracranial section of the vertebral artery, may be very small,

can be uni- or bilateral, and may or may not fuse with each other. Nonfusion of the anterior spinal artery over some distance is frequent in this region. The anterior radiculomedullary arteries branch in a very typical way to reach the spinal cord. The ascending branch continues along the direction of the radicular artery in the midline of the anterior surface. The descending branch, being the larger one at thoracolumbar levels, forms a hairpin curve as soon as it reaches the midline at the entrance of the anterior fissure. Anterior radiculomedullary arteries always reach the cord at the midline, whereas the posterior arteries reach the cord slightly off-midline. The posterior radiculomedullary arteries are connected to the anterior spinal artery through two anastomotic semicircles at the level of the cone, known as the "arcade" of the cone (▶ Fig. 40.7).

Apart from these conal anastomoses, both systems anastomose via an extensive pial network to which they both contribute. This superficial pial network encircles the spinal cord and has been called the vasocorona. As stated earlier, the major contribution to this superficial pial system is from the posterior radiculomedullary arteries, whereas the supply from the anterior radiculomedullary arteries is derived just before these arteries enter the subpial space in the central sulcus. There, branches to the pial system on the anterior and lateral surface supply the ventral parts of the vasocorona.

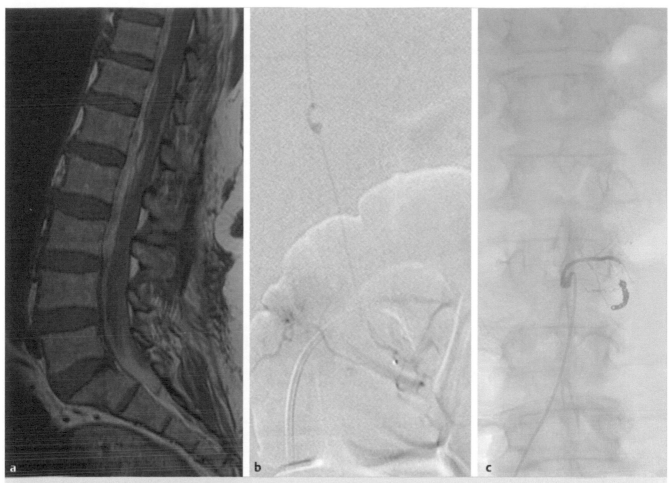

**Fig. 40.8** This patient presented hyperacutely with severe back pain and paraplegia. T1-weighted MRI (a) demonstrated massive hemorrhage in the thecal sac (hyperintense subarachnoid signal on T1-weighted scans). Spinal angiography (b) revealed a dissecting aneurysm arising from the dorsolateral spinal artery in its intradural component. The feeding radicular artery was occluded with coils (c). As this was not a shunting lesion, there was no retrograde filling to the dissecting aneurysm from other segmental arteries, and the extensive collateral network, including the basket and the rope ladder anastomoses, prevented ischemic damage to the cord.

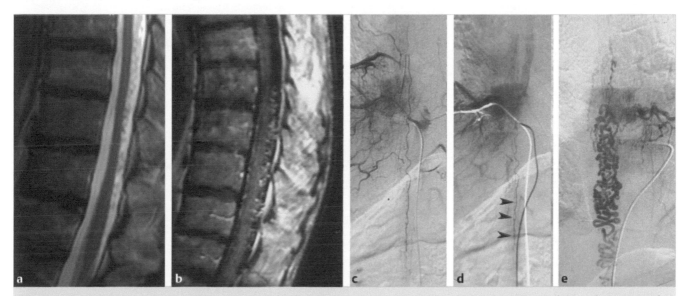

**Fig. 40.9** T2-weighted (a) and contrast-enhanced T1-weighted (b) MRIs demonstrate abnormal flow voids in this patient, indicating the presence of a dural arteriovenous shunt. Spinal angiography at the level of the artery of Adamkiewicz (c,d) reveals persistent contrast stagnation in the ASA on the delayed images in the venous phase, indicating the presence of a shunt elsewhere (*arrowheads*). In this patient, a dural arteriovenous fistula was found (e) at another level.

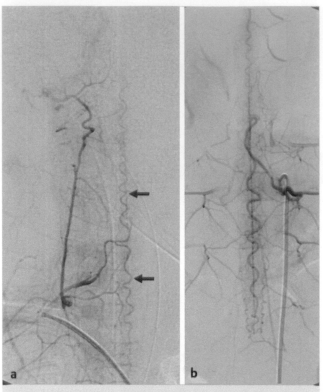

**Fig. 40.10** In this pediatric patient with diffuse cord swelling and abnormal vessels, angiography (a,b) did not reveal a shunt but, rather, cord hyperemia. The anterior spinal artery demonstrates increased tortuosity (*arrows*), a normal finding in the pediatric population that should not be mistaken for a vein.

tions in all segmental arteries that harbor cord supply are necessary. The predominant white matter supply of the dorsolateral arteries implies, in contrast to the predominant gray matter supply of the anterior spinal artery, that embolization via dorsolateral spinal arteries is considered a safer approach. In patients with isolated pathology of the dorsal spinal artery, parent vessel sacrifice may be considered, given the rich anastomotic network of the spinal cord supply (▶ Fig. 40.8). This can be important for presurgical embolization of spinal cord hemangioblastomas: As they are typically located on the dorsal surface of the cord, their usual supply is from the dorsolateral artery.

### Pearls and Pitfalls

- Arteries always run along the anterior or posterior nerve roots to reach the cord. The location of the hairpin curve at the cord surface (lateral for the posterior spinal arteries and midline for the anterior spinal arteries) can be used to identify the type of feeding vessels if you do not use a lateral view.
- Contrast stagnation in the anterior spinal artery is a seen in cases of venous congestion and indicates the presence of a shunt elsewhere that interferes with the normal arteriovenous transit (▶ Fig. 40.9).
- In pediatric patients, in patients with cord hyperemia, or in patients with distal shunting lesions, the anterior spinal artery is often rather tortuous and should not be confused with a vein (▶ Fig. 40.10). In addition, pediatric patients and patients who have harbored a shunt from early childhood will have less pruning of the cord supply (i.e., more segmental arteries will still harbor cord supply).

## 40.3 Clinical Impact, Additional Information and Cases

The rich anastomotic network implies that when embarking on embolization of spinal cord arteries, a liquid embolic material that is able to penetrate deep into this network may open collaterals via the vasocorona between the posterior and the anterior spinal arteries, which may lead to inadvertent embolization of healthy vessels. The rich network also implies that to "map" the entire supply of a spinal arteriovenous malformation, injec-

## Further Reading

[1] Krings T, Geibprasert S, Thron AK. Spinal vascular anatomy. In: Naidich TP, Castillo M, Cha S, Raybaud C, Smirniotopoulos JG, Kollias S, Kleinman GM, eds. Imaging of the Spine: Expert Radiology Series, Expert Consult. Philadelphia: Elsevier Health Sciences; 2010:185–200

[2] Lasjaunias P, Berenstein A, ter Brugge KG. Surgical Neuroangiography. Vol. 1. 2nd ed. Berlin: Springer; 2006

[3] Thron AK. Vascular Anatomy of the Spinal Cord: Neuroradiological Investigations and Clinical Syndromes. Vienna: Springer; 1988

# 41 The Intrinsic Arteries of the Cord

## 41.1 Case Description

### 41.1.1 Clinical Presentation

A 37-year-old patient presented with acute onset of stabbing back pain followed by paraplegia and complete loss of sensation below her midthoracic dermatomes.

### 41.1.2 Radiologic Studies

See ▸ Fig. 41.1, ▸ Fig. 41.2.

### 41.1.3 Diagnosis

Pial nidus-type arteriovenous malformation (AVM) with a false aneurysm arising from a sulcocommissural artery of the anterior spinal artery.

## 41.2 Anatomy

The main source of arterial supply to the cord is the anterior spinal artery (ASA) on its ventral axis. The arteries directly supplying the spinal cord that arise from the ASA are the central (sulcal and sulcocommissural) arteries that originate from the anterior spinal artery and the perforating branches arising from the superficial pial network, covering the spinal cord. Sulcal arteries are centrifugal, have a diameter between 0.1 and 0.25 mm, and supply the largest part of the gray matter. They penetrate the parenchyma to the depth of the anterior fissure, course to one side of the cord, and branch mainly within the gray matter (▸ Fig. 41.3).

These arteries can anastomose via transmedullary arteries with deep perforating arteries from the vasocorona or the posterolateral arteries. These perforating arteries arise from the superficial pial covering of the cord (vasocorona) and penetrate

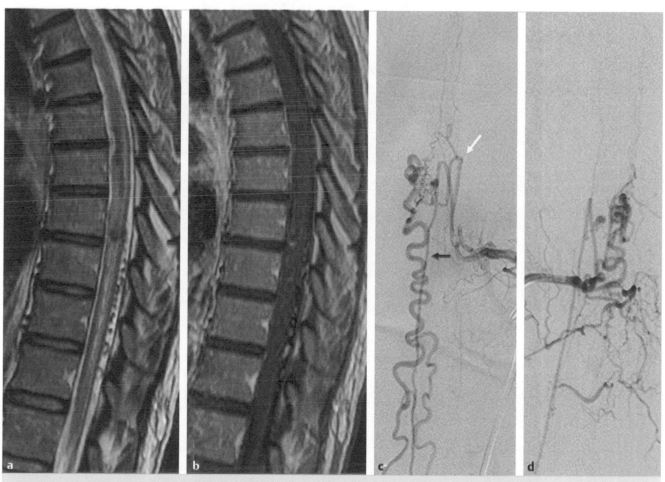

**Fig. 41.1** Sagittal T2-weighted (a) and T1-weighted (b) MRIs demonstrate hematomyelia, cord edema, and posteriorly located perimedullary flow voids that enhance after contrast administration in the mid and lower thoracic region, raising suspicion of a spinal cord AVM. Left T10 segmental artery angiograms in AP (c) and lateral (d) views reveal a shunting lesion that was fed by both the anterior (*arrow*) and the posterior (*white arrow*) spinal arteries. As an anatomical variation, the supply to both the anterior and the posterior axis arose from the same segmental artery. An aneurysm that is located in the midline and centrally within the cord is noted as the rupture point. Case continued in ▸ Fig. 41.2.

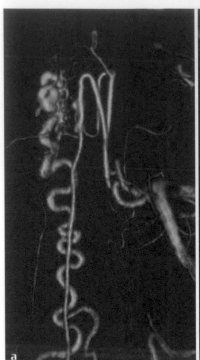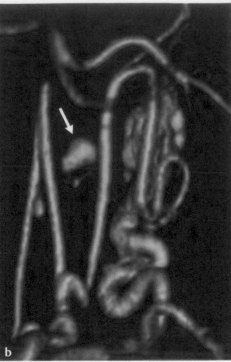

**Fig. 41.2** 3D rotational reconstruction images (a, b) demonstrate that the aneurysm (*arrow*) arose from a sulcocommissural artery that interconnects the anterior and the posterior spinal arteries.

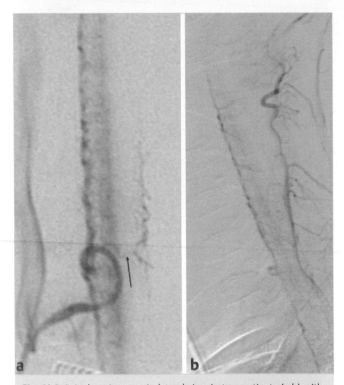

**Fig. 41.3** Spinal angiograms in lateral view in two patients (a,b) with cord hyperemia demonstrate the sulcocommissural arteries that supply the anterior aspect of the cord. The arrow points to a transmedullary anastomosis that connects the anterior axis to the posterior axis through the cord.

white matter tracts from the periphery, thus constituting a centripetal system. These vessels are numerous, with a diameter of up to 0.05 mm. The posterior and posterolateral spinal arteries distribute blood to the dorsal third of the vasocorona, and in this way, they share with central artery branches the supply of the posterior horn and marginal parts of the central grey matter. The posterior/posterolateral arteries do not have a distinct territory of supply similar to the anterior spinal artery, which means that they predominantly reinforce the rope ladder–like network of posterior pial arteries. The number of central arteries varies in the different levels: at the cervical enlargement, about five central arteries are present per (longitudinal) centimeter. They take a horizontal course. The number of central arteries is two to three per centimeter for the thoracic region, with a relatively high prevalence of steeply ascending and descending central artery branches. The densest concentration of central arteries is found in the thoracolumbar enlargement, where six to eight vessels per centimeter can be found (▶ Fig. 41.4).

## 41.3 Clinical Impact, Additional Information and Cases

The dense connections between the anterior and posterior spinal arteries have to be kept in mind when embolizing with a liquid embolic material with high penetrance, as they will be opened and may lead to inadvertent occlusion of healthy vessels. Intramedullary spinal AVMs (i.e., nidus- or glomus-type) will almost always be supplied from both the anterior and posterior spinal artery systems, given the rich transmedullary and perimedullary connections via the sulcocommissural and the vasocorona vessels, respectively (▶ Fig. 41.5).

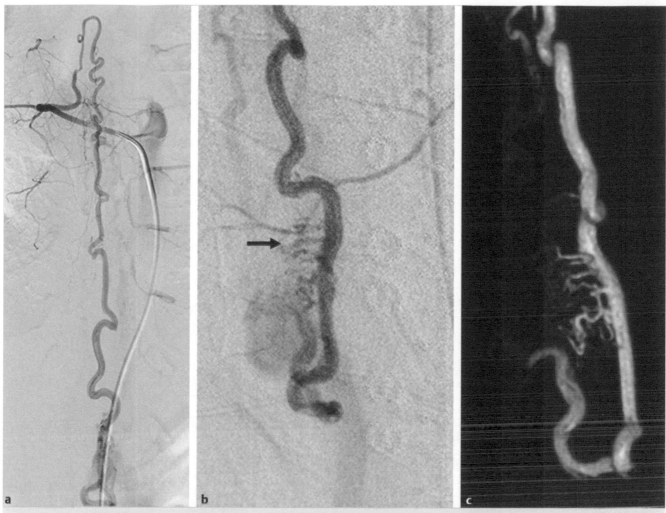

**Fig. 41.4** Spinal angiogram of the ASA in AP (a) and oblique (b) views and 3D rotational reconstruction (c) reveal a high-flow fistulous AVM supplied by the dorsolateral arteries that is indirectly filled from the anterior spinal artery via the basket anastomosis. In addition, multiple enlarged sulcocommissural arteries (*arrow*) that course through the thoracolumbar enlargement to reach the dorsal surface are seen to be sumped into the fistula.

Similar to their counterpart, the pial brain AVMs, the spinal intramedullary AVMs may be mono- or multicompartmental and can have multiple feeders or a single feeder (▶ Fig. 41.6).

Secondarily induced angiopathic changes with dilatation of normal vessels may be present and have to be differentiated from true shunting lesions. In comparison with the intramedullary AVMs, the perimedullary fistulas are supplied (again similar to their cranial counterpart, the pial cerebral AV fistulaes) by only a single feeder. Depending on the location of the transition between the artery and the vein, this may be the anterior or posterolateral spinal artery, a rope-ladder anastomosis, or the vasocorona. In the latter two cases, supply to the fistula will be seen from multiple feeders; however, it has to be kept in mind that this is related to the described anastomoses between the intrinsic cord arteries. In these cases, one can choose the most direct and/or the safest access to the fistula to treat the shunt. The large variety of potential collateral pathways and anastomoses explains the wide variety of types of cord infarctions, as depicted in ▶ Fig. 41.7.

## Pearls and Pitfalls

- The intrinsic arteries of the cord can be subdivided into those that arise from the anterior spinal artery, which supply the central cord and exhibit a centrifugal course, and those that arise from the posterior spinal artery, which supply the cord periphery (including the white matter) and have a centripetal course.
- They can anastomose via the vasocorona peripherally and via the sulcocommissural central arteries through the depth of the cord. The rich anastomoses explain the variability of cord infarctions on axial sections.
- Perimedullary fistulas have typically a single feeder, although indirect filling can be seen from various cord–supplying arteries, given their rich anastomotic network, whereas central intramedullary AVMs most commonly have multiple direct feeders.

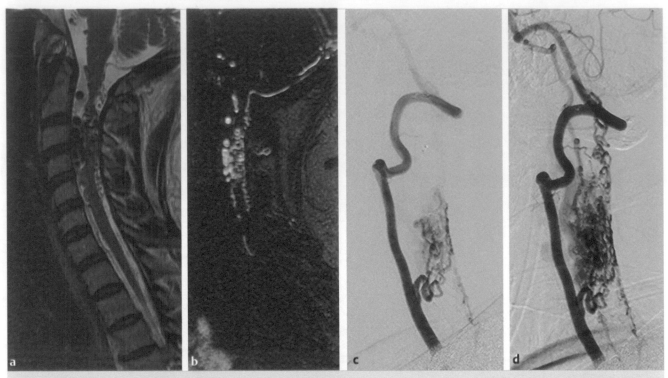

**Fig. 41.5** Sagittal T2-weighted MRI (a) and contrast-enhanced MRA (b) demonstrate an intramedullary AVM. Left VA angiogram in lateral view in early (c) and late (d) arterial phase confirms the presence of the AVM, which is seen to be primarily supplied by the ASA but transgresses the entire cord. Abnormally dilated vessels are also noted on the posterior cord surface, owing to a rich network of anastomoses between the anterior and posterior spinal arteries.

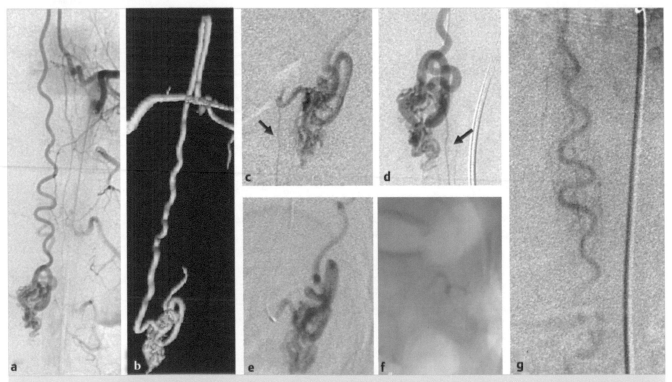

**Fig. 41.6** Injection into the segmental artery harboring supply to the anterior spinal artery (a) reveals predominant supply to a pial intramedullary AVM by the ASA. The 3D rotational reconstruction image (b) demonstrates that a single sulcocommissural artery supplied the nidus. A microcatheter injection of the ASA just proximal to the feeding sulcocommissural artery in the lateral (c) and anterior (d) planes reveals the normal-caliber ASA running further caudally (*arrows*). Distal microcatheter injection (e) demonstrates the catheter location, which allowed for glue deposition just within the sulcocommissural artery (f) that enabled complete exclusion of the AVM and preservation of the normal ASA (g).

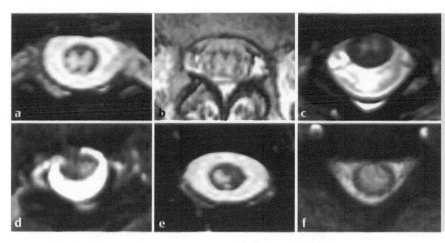

**Fig. 41.7** Six different patients with anterior spinal cord infarctions on axial T2-weighted MRIs. The upper row (a,b,c) demonstrates the typical anterior spinal artery territory with the "owl-eye" appearance of T2 hypersignal in the central gray matter of the cord, predominantly supplied by the anterior spinal artery, whereas the white matter is still preserved, as it is primarily supplied by the superficial vasocorona network that is mainly supplied by the posterolateral arteries. The potential transmedullary anastomotic pathways and further distal ischemia of only the lateralized sulcocommissural arteries can explain the different patterns of ischemia, as seen in the lower row (d,e,f).

# Further Reading

[1] Krings T. Vascular malformations of the spine and spinal cord: Anatomy, classification, treatment. Clin Neuroradiol. 2010 Mar; 20(1):5-24

[2] Krings T, Thron AK, Geibprasert S et al. Endovascular management of spinal vascular malformations. Neurosurg Rev 2010; 33: 1–9

[3] Thron AK. Vascular Anatomy of the Spinal Cord: Neuroradiological Investigations and Clinical Syndromes. Vienna: Springer; 1988

# 42 The Artery of the Filum Terminale

## 42.1 Case Description

### 42.1.1 Clinical Presentation

A 62-year-old man presented with a 6-month history of progressive bilateral lower extremity paresthesias and weakness. Three months before admission, bladder incontinence developed, and 1 month later, the patient became impotent.

### 42.1.2 Radiological Studies

See ▶ Fig. 42.1, ▶ Fig. 42.2.

### 42.1.3 Diagnosis

Spinal arteriovenous fistula of the filum terminale.

## 42.2 Embryology and Anatomy

The primordia of the filum terminale forms during secondary neurulation. This process occurs after closure of the caudal neuropore. Degeneration, regression, and retrogressive differentiations of the secondary neural tube then lead to the development of the filum terminale, which remains as a fibrous structure connecting the conus medullaris to the coccyx. The filum terminale has two components. The filum interna is an extension of the primary pia mater that connects the conus medullaris to the dura mater of the terminal thecal sac. The filum externa extends from the termination of the thecal sac to the coccyx.

Classically, the arterial supply to the filum terminale was described as singular, fed by the artery of the filum terminale. This artery is the caudal extension of the anterior spinal artery, which arises at the conus medullaris. Most commonly, the anterior spinal artery bifurcates at the conus medullaris and forms the anastomotic arcade, and the artery of the filum arises from one of the branches of the bifurcation. Anatomic variants have been described, including a trifurcation of the anterior spinal artery, with one of the branches continuing caudally as the artery of the filum.

The argument for singular arterial supply to the filum terminale is supported by the fact that no nerve roots originate caudal to the conus medullaris, and thus all radiculomedullary arterial supply must be carried caudally from the conus to the filum via the artery of the filum terminale. However, this singular supply theory has come into question after a number of

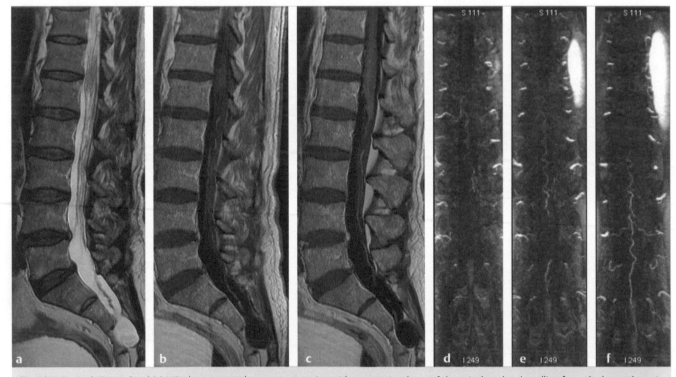

**Fig. 42.1** Sagittal T2-weighted (a) MRI demonstrated venous congestion with vasogenic edema of the spinal cord and swelling from the lower thoracic levels to the conus medullaris, along with flow voids suggestive of enlarged perimedullary veins. Contrast-enhanced T1-weighted (b,c) sequences revealed a moderate degree of diffuse enhancement of the lower thoracic spinal cord, indicative of chronic venous ischemia. Contrast-enhanced MRA (d,e,f) of the spine showed a dilated midline vessel, likely the ASA, down to the filum terminale. The patient underwent conventional angiography for further evaluation. Case continued in ▶ Fig. 42.2.

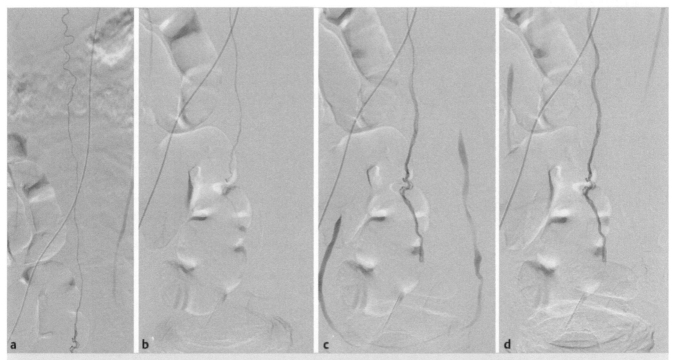

**Fig. 42.2** Right T8 segmental artery angiogram (a–d) demonstrates an abnormally enlarged and tortuous anterior spinal artery leading to an arteriovenous fistula that is located well below the cone at the level of the filum terminale at S2–S3. The single fistulous communication was noted to occur between the artery and the vein of the filum terminale with venous outflow in a cranial direction along the filum terminale, draining cranially into the perimedullary veins.

published reports have described fistulae of the filum terminale supplied by both the artery of the filum terminale and branches from the infra-aortic spinal arteries, such as the middle and lateral sacral arteries. It appears that the arterial supply to the filum terminale is instead derived concurrently from the artery of the filum terminale and branches of the infra-aortic spinal arteries carried via the lumbar and sacral nerve roots.

The venous drainage of the filum terminale is singular, carried by the vein of the filum. The vein runs dorsal to the artery of the filum and is uniform in caliber along the extent of the filum terminale. It traverses the dura at the caudal extent of the filum terminale interna and is continuous with the anterior spinal vein at the cranial extent of the filum. The venous flow can either be cephalad or caudad.

## 42.3 Clinical Impact

Arteriovenous fistulae of the filum terminale result in increased spinal venous pressure and decreased drainage from the normal spinal veins. This leads to venous congestion and ischemia of the spinal cord. Patients with these vascular lesions typically present with progressive myelopathic symptoms that necessitate intervention in nearly all cases. The goal of definitive management is to obliterate the point of fistulization. To this end, direct surgical disconnection of the arteriovenous communication is the method of choice. Endovascular embolization is an option; however, it is associated with substantial risk for ischemic injury to the spinal cord because of the need for catheterization of the anterior spinal artery, often over multiple segments. In addition, the narrow caliber of the artery of the filum terminale often precludes the possibility of endovascular access.

These fistulaes have an intradural location on the pia mater of the filum interna and receive radiculomedullary arterial supply via the anterior spinal artery to the artery of the filum terminale. This has led to their generally accepted classification as perimedullary arteriovenous fistulae. However, filum terminale arteriovenous fistulas (AVFs) are notably different than their perimedullary counterparts found in the more rostral segments of the conus medullaris and spinal cord, which have an exclusive radiculomedullary supply. Filum terminale AVFs appear to behave as transitionary shunts that may derive arterial flow from branches of the infra-aortic spinal arteries that supply the dura mater of the lumbar and sacral nerve roots in addition to the radiculomedullary flow carried to the fistula by the artery of the filum.

This makes selective spinal catheter angiography of all thoracic and lumbar segmental arteries, as well as both internal iliac arteries, essential for the diagnostic workup of a suspected arteriovenous fistula of the filum terminale. A potential pitfall in the management of these lesions is the failure to identify all arterial feeders to the fistulous communication. An incompletely defined lesion of the filum terminale may lead to complications at the time of surgical intervention or persistence of symptoms despite apparent curative intervention.

## 42.4 Additional Information and Cases

Arteriovenous fistulaes of the filum terminale need to be distinguished from perimedullary AVF of the caudal spinal cord and conus medullaris. At this location, the arterial supply to these perimedullary AVFs is often solely by the anterior spinal artery, and the venous drainage pattern and clinical presentation of these lesions are so similar to AVFs of the filum terminale that they have been previously classified together. However, accurate localization of the fistula is critically important for proper treatment planning. Access for microsurgical obliteration of a fistulous communication on the filum terminale is quite feasible in most circumstances. The paucity of functional neural elements within the filum allows for surgical sectioning of the filum at the fistulous communication. The surgical management of perimedullary AVFs of the conus or caudal spinal cord is much less straightforward, particularly if the fistula is located on the anterior aspect of the spinal cord. In these cases, the role of endovascular intervention certainly warrants stronger consideration, and in some particularly challenging cases, conservative management might be considered.

Another important consideration in the differential diagnosis of AVFs of the filum terminale is the much more common spinal dural arteriovenous fistulas in the lumbosacral region. These fistulas are located within the dural sleeve of a nerve root or the adjacent dura. Their arterial supply is derived from a radiculomeningeal artery and drainage into the spinal perimedullary veins via a radicular vein. The venous drainage pattern and clinical presentation of these dural AVFs is similar to AVFs of the filum terminale; however, their treatment warrants different considerations. Dural AVFs are classically located directly under the pedicle of a vertebral body but can be located anywhere along the adjacent dura, and surgical exposure differs from that for AVFs of the filum terminale. In addition, the endovascular approach to these lesions is often considered safer and, in many cases, is given primary consideration, with surgical intervention reserved as a secondary option. For these reasons, clear differentiation of an AVF of the filum terminale from other fistulous communications of the lumbosacral region is highly important before considering and carrying out treatment (▶ Fig. 42.3; ▶ Fig. 42.4).

> **Pearls and Pitfalls**
>
> - Filum terminale AVFs present with symptoms similar to those of dural AVF; however, recognizing them as entities separate from a dural AVF is of utmost importance when contemplating embolization of these lesions.
> - Filum terminale AVFs can recruit supply from both the artery of the filum terminale and the dural branches.

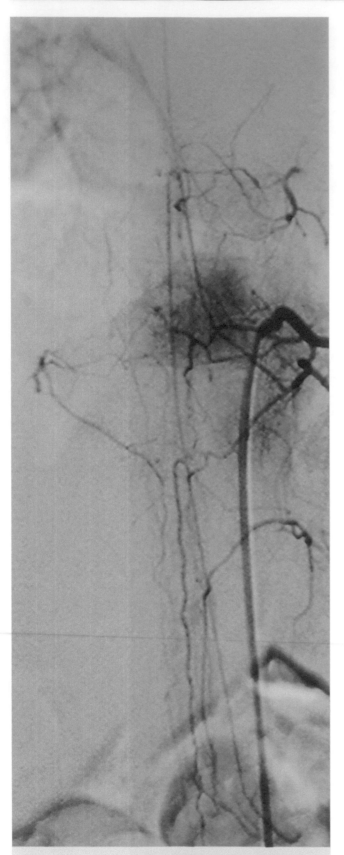

**Fig. 42.3** Spinal angiogram of the Adamkiewicz artery demonstrates continuation of the ASA below the cone as the artery of the filum terminale, which does not give any supply to the spinal cord.

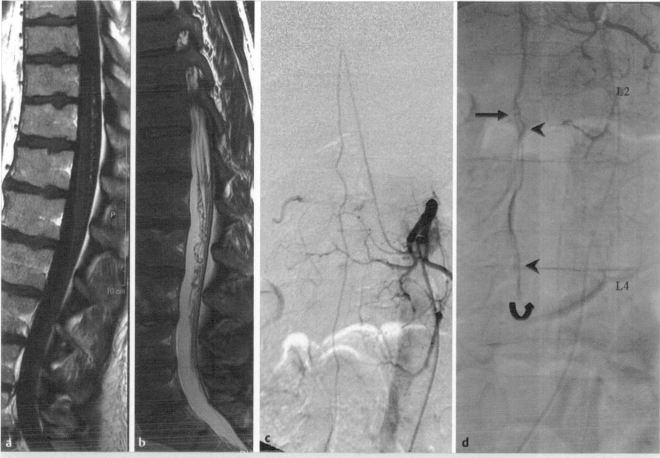

**Fig. 42.4** Contrast-enhanced T1-weighted (a) and T2-weighted (b) MRIs reveal abnormal dilated perimedullary vessels at the lumbar and lower thoracic regions. Spinal angiogram (c,d) of the Adamkiewicz artery shows an arteriovenous fistula at the L4 level (*curved arrow*), supplied by the artery of the filum terminale (*arrow*), draining cranially into the filum terminale vein (*arrowheads*) and perimedullary veins, respectively.

## Further Reading

[1] Djindjian M, Ribeiro A, Ortega E, Gaston A, Poirier J. The normal vascularization of the intradural filum terminale in man. Surg Radiol Anat 1988; 10: 201–209

[2] Fischer S, Aguilar Perez M, Bassiouni H, Hopf N, Bäzner H, Henkes H. Arteriovenous fistula of the filum terminale: diagnosis, treatment, and literature review. Clin Neuroradiol 2013; 23: 309–314

[3] Jin YJ, Kim KJ, Kwon OK, Chung SK. Perimedullary arteriovenous fistula of the filum terminale: case report. Neurosurgery 2010; 66: E219–E220, discussion E220

[4] Lim SM, Choi IS, David CA. Spinal arteriovenous fistulas of the filum terminale. AJNR Am J Neuroradiol 2011; 32: 1846–1850

[5] Lasjaunias P, Berenstein A, ter Brugge KG. Surgical Neuroangiography. Vol. 1. 2nd ed. Berlin: Springer; 2006

# 43 The Spinal Cord Veins

## 43.1 Case Description

### 43.1.1 Clinical Presentation

A 6-year-old child was investigated for an objective thrill at the back of her neck and mild headaches. Because abnormal flow voids were described at the craniocervical junction, she was transferred to our institution, where a spinal MRI was performed, followed by a conventional angiography.

### 43.1.2 Radiologic Studies

See ▶ Fig. 43.1, ▶ Fig. 43.2, and ▶ Fig. 43.3.

### 43.1.3 Diagnosis

Congenital absence of the jugular foramen bilaterally with brain drainage via the perimedullary spinal veins.

## 43.2 Anatomy

The pattern of spinal venous drainage deviates substantially from that of the arteries, the most important difference being that the spinal arteries always follow the nerves, whereas the veins do not necessarily do so. Their arrangement is described according to the direction of venous drainage from the spinal cord parenchyma out to the epidural plexus.

The blood of the spinal cord parenchyma is drained by intrinsic veins in a radial pattern in an axial plane until the radial veins reach the surface of the spinal cord. They show a horizontal, radial, and symmetrical course in most parts of the spinal cord. Only in the lower thoracic cord, from the lower lumbar enlargement to the cone, are the sulcal veins (0.1–0.25 mm) larger than the numerous radial veins. At the level of the spinal pia mater, blood is accumulated in essentially two longitudinal collectors: the anterior and posterior median spinal vein. The anterior midline vein is located underneath the anterior spinal artery in the subpial space. It has its largest diameter lumbosacrally. In about 80% of cases, it courses together with the filum terminale as a sometimes very large terminal vein to the end of the dural sac. The venous longitudinal system on the anterior and posterior surface of the cord is more variable in course, size, and localization than the arterial system. The longitudinal midline veins are not always continuous and may be replaced by secondary systems of a smaller caliber.

The posterior median spinal vein takes a course independent from the posterolaterally located arteries and is especially large cranial to the thoracolumbar enlargement. Varicose convolutions are frequent. The posterior veins of the thoracolumbar enlargement are located in the perimedullary subarachnoid space. Having the largest diameter of all perimedullary vessels (including the arteries), at up to 1.5 mm, they are the vessels most likely to be seen on normal MRI scans. The vessels are part of a pial vascular network that has been called the venous or coronal plexus of the pia mater.

Intraparenchymal transmedullary venous anastomoses can be present. These midline anastomoses, 0.3–0.7 mm in diameter, connect the anterior and posterior median veins while

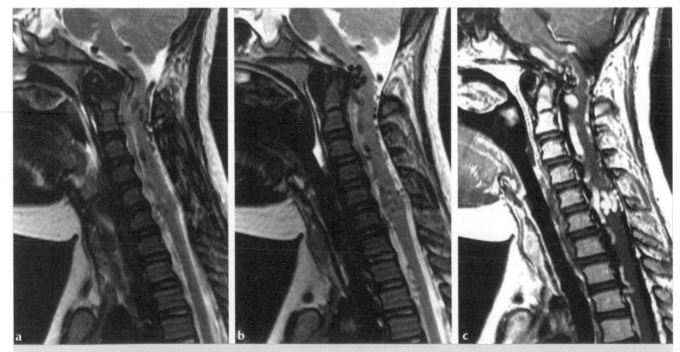

**Fig. 43.1** Sagittal T2-weighted (a,b) and contrast-enhanced T1-weighted (c) MRIs demonstrate abnormal vessels surrounding the craniocervical junction and in the perimedullary region. At the C5/6 level, there appears to be a conglomerate of abnormal vessels in the cord. There is no cord edema. Case continued in ▶ Fig. 43.2.

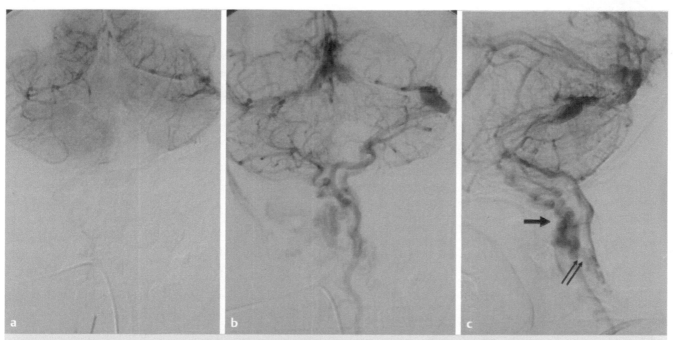

**Fig. 43.2** Vertebral artery angiogram in capillary (a) and venous phase (b,c) in anteroposterior (AP) (a,b) and lateral (c) views fails to demonstrate an arteriovenous shunting lesion. Both transverse sinuses, the sigmoid sinuses, and the jugular bulbs and internal jugular veins are missing. The brain drainage is solely via the anterior perimedullary veins, and further downward, via a transmedullary anastomoses at C5/6 to the posterior medullary venous system of the cord. Further caudad, the drainage was via the normal radicular veins into the epidural venous plexus. Case continued in ▶ Fig. 43.3.

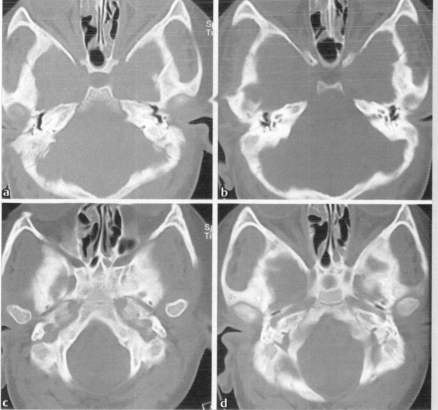

**Fig. 43.3** The cause for this peculiar drainage pattern was thought to be a benign variant of brain drainage with congenital absence of the jugular foramen, as verified on computed tomography in the bone window (a–d). This case highlights the potential role for the cord to drain the brain, via the perimedullary veins, their intramedullary connections, and their outflow routes to the epidural vertebrovenous plexus.

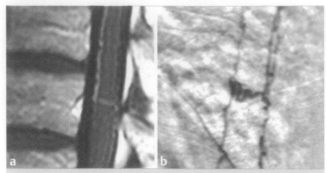

**Fig. 43.4** MRI sagittal contrast-enhanced T1-weighted image (a) and corresponding spinal angiogram in venous phase on lateral view (b). Transmedullary venous anastomoses can connect the anterior and the posterior perimedullary venous systems. They sometimes can be visualized on contrast-enhanced MR and are normal variants of the cord drainage. These normal transmedullary veins explain why there are no developmental venous anomalies in the cord: transmedullary anastomoses between the different venous systems are the norm and are not a variation of drainage (which is the case for developmental venous anomalies in the brain where the transcerebral veins typically regress and the deep and superficial venous systems become separated).

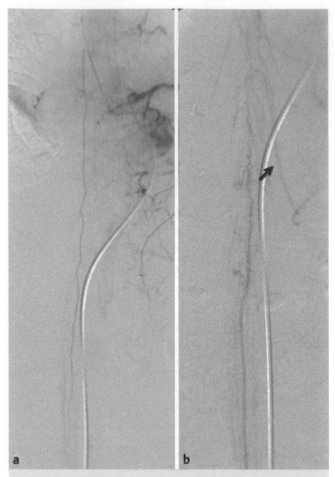

**Fig. 43.5** Selective injection into the segmental artery from which the anterior spinal artery originates in arterial (a) and venous (b) phase demonstrates the classical hairpin curve of the anterior spinal artery in the arterial phase. However, it becomes apparent in the venous phase that the venous drainage via the radicular veins can have a similar hairpin course (*arrow*). As the veins are typically larger in diameter than the arteries, depiction of a "hairpin" vessel on static MR angiogram or CTA could therefore be related both to a slightly enlarged anterior spinal artery (because of increased flow) or a normal-sized venous vessel.

receiving no tributaries from the intrinsic spinal cord veins (▶ Fig. 43.4). Because of their size, they may be seen on contrast-enhanced MRI.

Through these large anastomoses, blood can easily be directed from one side of the cord to the other. They are most often found in the thoracic region. At the cervical level, the anterior and posterior median veins connect to the brainstem veins and basal sinuses around the foramen magnum.

The superficial venous blood collectors drain into the epidural venous plexus through radicular veins. The transition of the midline vessel to the radicular vein forms a hairpin course similar to the arterial configuration (▶ Fig. 43.5).

Therefore, on angiographic images, the vein might be mistaken for an artery, particularly when an arteriovenous shunt with early venous filling is present. For the same reason, it may be impossible to distinguish the anterior spinal artery from a radicular spinal vein on non–time-resolved MR or CTA. The number of venous outlets is large. An average number of 25 radicular veins can be identified on the anterior and posterior surfaces of the cord. If smaller veins (< 0.25 mm in diameter) are excluded, the number of radiculomedullary veins draining the spinal cord is 6 to 11 for the anterior and 5 to 10 for the posterior systems. With age, it is likely that the number of radicular veins decreases, as they may fibrose and obliterate.

Drainage of blood from the spine and spinal cord is directed to the epidural plexus from multiple radicular veins, whereas retrograde flow from the epidural venous plexus to spinal cord veins (e.g., during spinal epidural phlebography) is usually not encountered and has only rarely been described in the literature. Moreover, in anatomical cadaver studies, it is nearly impossible to inject spinal cord veins from the periphery (i.e., the intercostal veins). The nature of this reflux-impeding mechanism has been a matter of dispute. The presence of venous valves was excluded in anatomical studies. Instead, an antireflux system was present within the transdural course of the radicular veins resulting from narrowing and zig-zagging of the vein while crossing the dura.

Microangiography and histology confirmed these findings and were able to demonstrate two structural features capable of acting as an antireflux structure: a substantial narrowing and a bending of the vessel at its transdural course. This bending resulted either from close vicinity of a nerve root or from the presence of a bulge of dural collagenous fibers with a glomus-like appearance. Therefore, differentiation into a slit- or bulge-type valve can be made. Because during spinal angiography, epidural shunts without reflux to the perimedullary veins are rarely found, this mechanism functions normally even in the presence of an arterialized epidural plexus.

The epidural venous plexus extends as a continuous system from the sacrum to the base of the skull and is located within the fatty and fibrous tissue of the epidural space (▶ Fig. 43.6).

This valveless system consists of thin elastic walls and is connected with the azygos and hemiazygos venous systems by

## 43.3 Clinical Impact, Additional Information and Cases

As the anterior venous system is subpial in location, arteriovenous shunts (especially if they have a low shunt volume) that drain into the anterior system only may present with cord edema because of venous congestion even before abnormal flow voids are visualized. This constitutes a diagnostic challenge, as the differential diagnoses for cord hyperintensity on T2-weighted scans are manifold and may delay diagnosis and treatment (▶ Fig. 43.7; ▶ Fig. 43.8).

Venous congestion occurs if the arterial overload into the venous system can no longer be compensated for by the venous radicular outlets. This may be a result of high-flow shunts, even in the presence of sufficient radicular venous outlets, or more commonly, as a result of progressive occlusion of venous outlets. We have encountered cases of "asymptomatic" spinal dural arteriovenous fistulas with the classical imaging pattern of an abnormal communication between a radiculomeningeal artery and a perimedullary vein, with retrograde drainage toward the cord; however, without cord edema. In all of these patients, there was evidence for persistent venous radicular outflow at levels close to the fistula site into the epidural venous plexus, indicating that the arterialized pressure in the perimedullary veins was immediately "released" into the epidural venous system, and therefore away from the cord, thereby protecting the cord from congestion. All the patients in whom we encountered this imaging pattern were younger than the typical demographics in symptomatic spinal dural arteriovenous fistulas. One can therefore hypothesize that as aging occurs, progressive fibrosis and occlusion of the radicular venous outlets will decrease the outflow options for the arterialized perimedullary veins, thereby increasing the likelihood of venous congestion (▶ Fig. 43.8; ▶ Fig. 43.9).

Shunts into the paravertebral venous plexus (so-called vertebra-venous fistulas) rarely present with cord congestion because of the reflux-preventing mechanism from the epidural venous plexus to the radicular veins described earlier. Instead, they may become symptomatic because of compression of neural elements resulting from massively dilated venous pouches or vertebrobasilar insufficiency, given the large shunt volume. These shunts, if not traumatic or iatrogenic, may point toward an inborn vasculopathy, such as Marfan syndrome or neurofibromatosis (▶ Fig. 43.10; ▶ Fig. 43.11).

The reflux mechanism described for the transition of the radicular veins into the epidural veins may, in rare cases, fail to work. As a consequence, shunts into the epidural venous plexus (which are not uncommon) can, in the rare circumstance of a failed antireflux mechanism, lead to perimedullary reflux and may mimic a dural arteriovenous fistula. Recognizing this peculiar type of arteriovenous shunt is important for choosing treatment. In these cases, the goal has to be to prevent reflux into the perimedullary veins, and a surgical disconnection of the radicular vein form the epidural plexus is therefore recommended. Because shunts into the epidural venous plexus are not uncommon, and as the epidural venous plexus communicates from the base of the skull to the sacrum, a shunt at a different level may lead to reconstitution of the fistula if the refluxing vein is not disconnected. Therefore, it will be difficult to

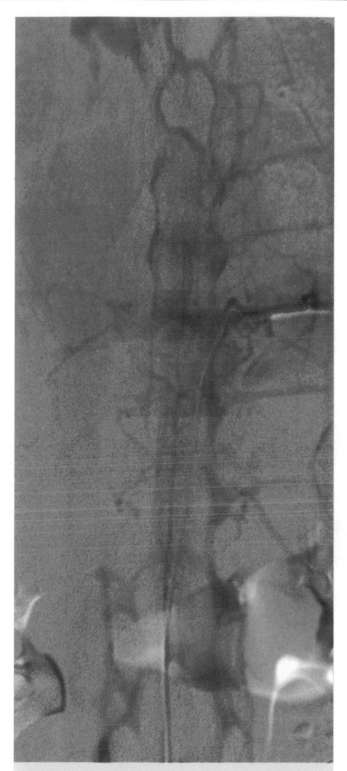

**Fig. 43.6** Spinal angiogram in AP view in late venous phase demonstrates the epidural venous system. The epidural venous plexus extends from the base of the skull to the sacrum and drains into the azygos and hemiazygos system.

intercostal or segmental veins and in the cervical region with the vertebral and deep cervical veins. The segmental veins in the lumbar region are connected by the ascending lumbar vein, joining the azygos (right side) and hemiazygos vein (left side).

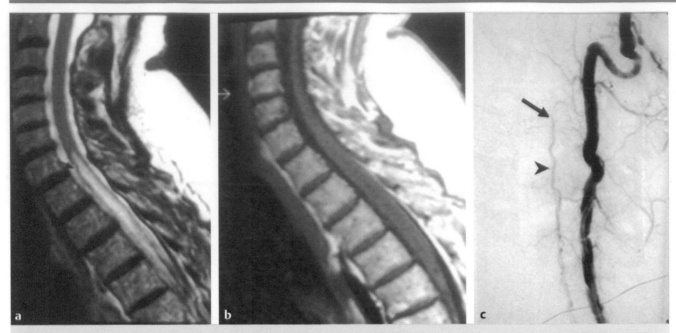

**Fig. 43.7** Sagittal T2-weighted (a) and T1-weighted (b) MRIs demonstrate extensive cord edema with enlargement of the cord without abnormal flow voids in the region. As symptoms were progressive, a catheter angiography (c) was performed that demonstrated a perimedullary low-flow shunt arising from the anterior spinal artery (*arrow*) and draining into the anterior spinal vein (*arrowhead*) that, given its subpial location and small size, was not visualized on the conventional MRI sequences.

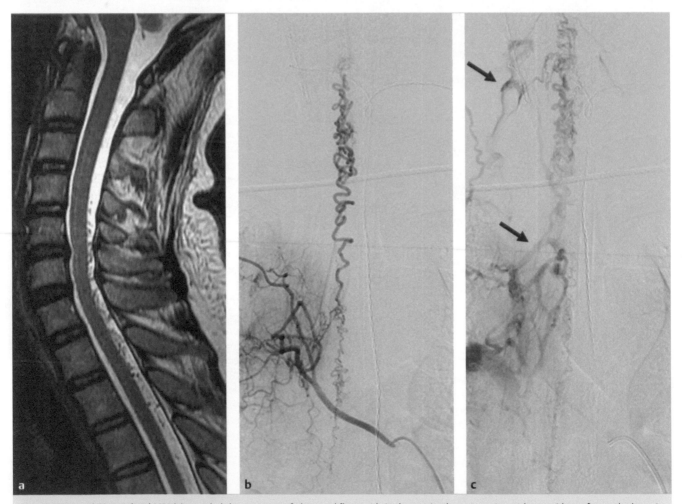

**Fig. 43.8** Sagittal T2-weighted MRI (a) revealed the presence of abnormal flow voids in the cervicothoracic region without evidence for cord edema in this asymptomatic patient. Spinal angiogram in arterial (b) and late venous (c) phase revealed a spinal dural arteriovenous fistula that drained retrogradely toward the perimedullary veins but in which the shunt was released via adjacent radicular veins into the epidural venous plexus (*arrow* in c), therefore protecting the cord from venous congestion.

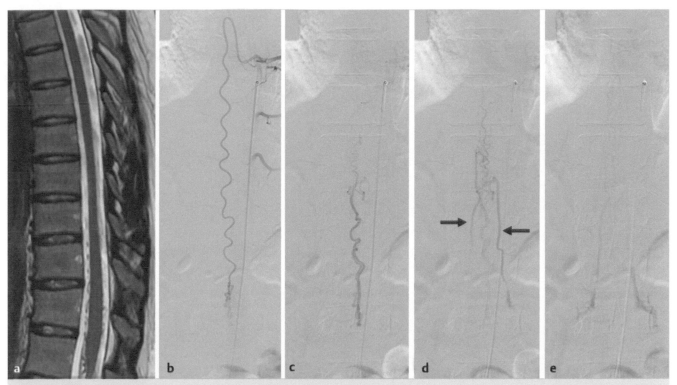

**Fig. 43.9** As a companion case to the patient in ▶ Fig. 43.8, this young patient had abnormal flow voids on T2-weighted scans without cord edema and no symptoms. On angiography, a fistula of the filum terminale was seen that drained retrogradely toward the perimedullary veins and that opened at multiple levels into radicular veins, thereby preventing cord congestion. Note that the anterior spinal artery empties rapidly, whereas in patients with cord congestion, there is stasis of contrast in the anterior spinal artery.

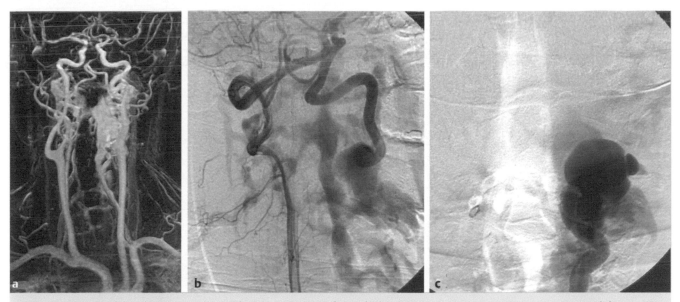

**Fig. 43.10** Contrast-enhanced MRA (a), right vertebral artery (b), and left vertebral artery (c) angiograms in AP view in a patient with known NF1 demonstrate extensive shunting from his left vertebral artery into the paravertebral and epidural venous plexus with massively dilated venous pouches. Despite the high shunt volume, no reflux to the perimedullary veins is present.

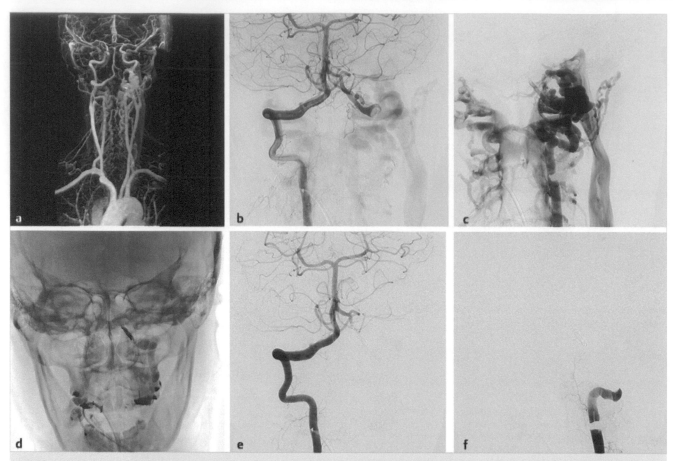

**Fig. 43.11** Similar to the patient depicted in ▶ Fig. 43.10, contrast-enhanced MRA (a), right vertebral artery (b), and left vertebral artery (c) angiograms in AP view in another patient also reveal a vertebrovenous arteriovenous fistula with high-flow shunting into the epidural veins. As these lesions will sump away blood flow, the treatment rationale is to trap the diseased segment, first distally and then proximally, with parent vessel occlusion employing coils, balloons, or a combination thereof, as seen in the plain radiography (d). Right vertebral artery (e) and left vertebral artery (f) angiograms in AP view posttreatment demonstrate complete closure of the fistula.

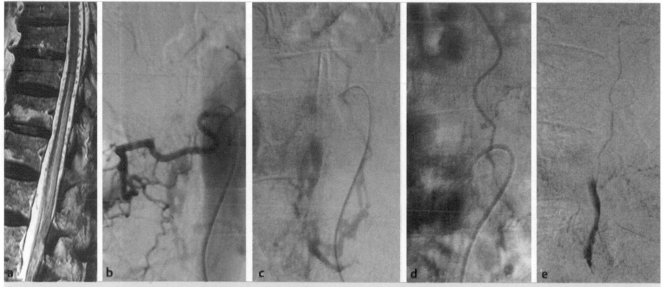

**Fig. 43.12** This patient presented with MR imaging and clinical findings that were suggestive of a spinal dural arteriovenous fistula. Sagittal T2-weighted MRI (a) demonstrates findings of cord edema with dilated perimedullary veins. Spinal angiograms (b–e) reveal an epidural shunt that drained first caudally and then crossed over to the site, where it later connected to a perimedullary vein that ascended cranially to reach the cord, leading to venous congestion of the cord.

**Pearls and Pitfalls**

- Transmedullary veins may be visible on enhanced T1-weighted scans and are normal routes of drainage to connect the anterior and posterior spinal perimedullary venous systems.
- As the anterior spinal veins are subpial, they will only be visible when grossly dilated, whereas the posteriorly located veins are subarachnoid in location and, therefore, more readily visible on routine MR sequences, even if they are only mildly dilated. This peculiar arrangement can explain why some arteriovenous shunts (that drain into the anterior system) may pose a diagnostic challenge, as they may only present with edema but no apparent abnormal venous flow voids.
- A hairpin course can be present both for the anterior or posterior spinal arteries and the radicular vein. As the veins are larger, static computed tomographic angiography or MR angiography will not be able to differentiate whether a "hairpin" vessel is arterial or venous in origin.
- In rare instances, the epidural venous plexus can interconnect with the perimedullary veins if the reflux mechanism of the epidural venous plexus is insufficient.

achieve a cure by a transarterial endovascular route, as the refluxing vein may be some distance away from the epidural shunt location (► Fig. 43.12).

## Further Reading

[1] Krings T, Mull M, Bostroem A, Otto J, Hans FJ, Thron A. Spinal epidural arteriovenous fistula with perimedullary drainage. Case report and pathomechanical considerations. J Neurosurg Spine 2006; 5: 353–358

[2] Sato K, ter Brugge KG, Krings T. Asymptomatic spinal dural arteriovenous fistulas: pathomechanical considerations. J Neurosurg Spine 2012; 16: 441–446

[3] Thron AK. Vascular Anatomy of the Spinal Cord: Neuroradiological Investigations and Clinical Syndromes. Vienna: Springer; 1988

# Index